D1621700

NURSING

242/243

Human Sexuality

McGRAW-HILL SERIES IN POPULATION BIOLOGY

consulting editors
PAUL R. EHRLICH, Stanford University
RICHARD W. HOLM, Stanford University

BRIGGS: Marine Zoogeography
EDMUNDS and LETEY: Environmental Administration
EHRLICH, HOLM, and PARNELL: The Process of Evolution
GEORGE and McKINLEY: Urban Ecology
GOLDSTEIN: Human Sexuality
HAMILTON: Life's Color Code
POOLE: An Introduction to Quantitative Ecology
STAHL: Vertebrate History: Problems in Evolution
TRESHOW: The Human Environment
WATT: Ecology and Resource Management
WATT: Principles of Environmental Science
WELLER: The Course of Evolution

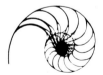

Human Sexuality

Bernard Goldstein

Department of Physiology and
Behavioral Biology
San Francisco State University

McGRAW-HILL BOOK COMPANY
New York   St. Louis   San Francisco   Auckland
Düsseldorf   Johannesburg   Kuala Lumpur   London
Mexico   Montreal   New Delhi   Panama   Paris
São Paulo   Singapore   Sydney   Tokyo   Toronto

HQ
35.2
.G64
C.1

HUMAN SEXUALITY

Copyright © 1976 by McGraw-Hill, Inc. All rights reserved.
Printed in the United States of America. No part of this publication
may be reproduced, stored in a retrieval system, or transmitted, in any
form or by any means, electronic, mechanical, photocopying, recording, or
otherwise, without the prior written permission of the publisher.

1234567890DODO798765

This book was set in Times Roman by Black Dot, Inc.
The editors were William J. Willey, Janet Wagner, and Douglas J. Marshall;
the cover was designed by Jo Jones;
cover illustration by Dan Long;
the production supervisor was Charles Hess.
The drawings were done by Eric G. Hieber Associates Inc.,
and drawings of human figures were done by Graphic Arts International.
R. R. Donnelley & Sons Company was printer and binder.

Library of Congress Cataloging in Publication Data

Goldstein, Bernard,   date
    Human Sexuality.

    (McGraw-Hill series in population biology)
    Includes index.
    1. Sex instruction for youth. I. Title.
[DNLM: 1. Sex behavior. 2. Sex Manuals. HQ21 G621h]
HQ35.2.G64   612.6'007   75-25803
ISBN 0-07-023691-7
ISBN 0-07-023690-9 pbk.

Contents

ACA 3197

627607

Preface

Another sex book? Readers have been inundated with a variety of books on sex, some highly technical, others highly sensuous, and still others a bit limited in scope. When I started teaching a human sexuality course at San Francisco State University some six years ago, I wanted to present the subject primarily in the context of the general population. At that time (and to a large extent currently) most textbooks did not clearly distinguish between evidence based on statistical analysis of the general population and evidence based on observations of psychiatric patients. Clinical impressions often do not reflect the situation found in a random sample of people. One of my reasons for writing a new textbook on human sexuality was to produce classroom material that clearly shows this difference. My second reason was to provide the student with easy-to-understand summaries and critiques of the findings of recent research. The rapid changes occurring in all areas of human sexuality require that new books be published fairly frequently; texts become anachronistic in a short time unless revised.

The objective of this book is to provide the reader with up-to-date, accurate, and in-depth information on human sexuality. A sound biological foundation is provided, and this is rounded out by including basic psychological, social, and legal aspects of the subject. Each major topic is discussed as fully as possible from several points of view and often includes references to the scholarly literature. The text is designed for the general human sexuality course and can be used no matter what the approach. No previous knowledge of biology or of the social sciences is required. An extensive bibliography appears at the end of each chapter so that the student may follow a subject through for a term paper and the instructor can investigate supporting research data. A glossary and an appendix are also included. The Appendix contains illustrations of the specific neural pathways involved in erection and ejaculation; it also contains a graph and an explanation of vaginal changes during the menstrual cycle—topics that are presented in less technical detail within the chapters. After reading the book, the student should have the satisfaction of understanding the basics of human sexuality, and he will have the tools for distinguishing between good, scholarly research and mere opinion or myth.

Although I am fully responsible for the contents of this text, I wish to acknowledge Janet Wagner, editor for McGraw-Hill. She has provided firm but enlightened advice throughout all phases of this project, and her thoughtful suggestions have contributed to a better book and a happier author. I also wish to express thanks to the following people who have reviewed the manuscript in various stages of its development: Paul R. Ehrlich, Robert G. Fossland, Richard W. Holm, Joseph LoPiccolo, Thomas R. Manley, Maxine Peterson, Eldra Solomon, Bruce Voeller, K. E. F. Watt, P. B. Weisz, and E. W. Wickersham.

I am especially indebted to my wife, Estelle, who typed the original manuscript and whose patience and understanding through the long struggle has facilitated the laborious and eased the difficult. And to my son, David, thanks for simply being David.

BERNARD GOLDSTEIN

Human Sexuality

Chapter 1

Introduction

The study of *human sexuality* deals with the following types of questions: What, in the physical sense, constitutes a male and a female? What events take place in our bodies as we become sexually aroused and reach orgasm? What social relationships must we participate in because we are born male or female? These questions relate to our physical form and function, which are the inevitable results of our inheritance. Since our sexuality is inevitable and natural, we should be able to communicate our answers to the proposed questions easily and without embarrassment.

This text will deal with many aspects of human sexuality, but it is not a "how to" or a "what to do" book. If you wish to increase your knowledge of sexual techniques, you will find many books on the market that discuss such methods. The question of "what to do" requires answers that should be dealt with only on an individual basis. The study of human sexuality and behavior is still in a state of infancy, and a great many theories and opinions are reported by the press. When you have finished the last chapter in this book, you will have some tools with which to evaluate research and to separate probable fact from opinion. You will also know enough about human sexuality to make personal decisions based upon biological fact and upon your own moral concerns and emotional needs rather than on myths. I shall report the news and you can interpret, assimilate, or reject information as you wish.

INHERITED VERSUS LEARNED BEHAVIOR

Researchers and writers sometimes try to separate human sexuality and behavior into two components: that which is inherited and that which is learned through interaction with the social environment. This is an artificial separation that is impossible to accomplish, since each aspect of our sex lives contains both inherited and learned components. A male inherits the structural and functional equipment for impregnating a female. Whether he does so depends on many variables: his attitudes about parenthood and about having sexual intercourse with a woman, learned and inherited factors that may affect the male's self-identity as a mate, and psychological factors and biological disorders that can affect his potency. Whether heredity or learning contributes more to our sexuality is not as important as discovering how these factors interact to produce a given type of sexual activity.

PROBLEMS WITH EXPERIMENTATION

Much of the information on which we base theories of human sexuality actually comes from experiments on and observations of nonhuman species. Obviously, scientists cannot perform experiments directly on humans; for instance, male sex hormones cannot be injected into a human female fetus in order to see if sex is reversible. Also, because of the tremendous variety of sexual behavior exhibited by humans, adequate controls, where all factors except the one under consideration are maintained constant, cannot easily be achieved. For example, courtship behavior in nonhuman species often involves predictable patterns of ritualized activity which are obviously influenced by heredity. Human courtship is so various that even within one culture so many specific differences exist that generalizations are difficult to make. Data derived from nonhuman animals provide a valuable basis for discussing human sexuality, but differences between species can be very great. Therefore, one cannot just assume that human sexuality is the same as rat or monkey sexuality. Of course, the closer the species is to the human, in terms of evolution, the more applicable the data. Observation of nonhuman primates (monkeys, great apes) has provided much valuable information about our own species, and this is better than no data at all.

When you evaluate the conclusions of an experiment, you should also be aware of what is called sampling error. Suppose you wish to find the average height of the United States citizen. You pick as your samples 15 people from your classroom or neighborhood and calculate the group average. You then look up the figure for the national average and discover that your results are in error. Since you have rechecked your mathematics and can find no mistakes there, you rightly conclude that the small sampling of people you chose does not accurately reflect the rest of the United States. You will obtain much better results if you subsequently measure 1,000 people from different geographic locations, with different diets, and with different ethnic backgrounds.

SEXUAL DIMORPHISM

Dimorphism is a concept that underlies many discussions of human sexuality. To say that a species is sexually dimorphic means that there are average differences between the males and females. Some species show great dimorphism in size, shape, color, and behavior. Humans are sexually dimorphic but not to as obvious a degree as many other species. For instance, the differences in size, weight, and strength between a human male and female are not as great as those between a male and a female gorilla. Actually there is a great deal of overlap in dimorphic characteristics among humans. Some women are taller than the average male and some men are shorter than the average female. Humans tend to rely very much on dress and hair styles to signal their maleness or femaleness to the stranger. Witness the complaints of parents that, since unisex styles have become popular, they cannot tell the men from the women.

But what about the more "obvious" physical differences? On one occasion in class, students were interpreting the meaning of femininity, masculinity, femaleness, and maleness. After considerable debate and agitation, one male student irritatingly said, "Why don't we simply call a spade a spade? Men have a penis, and women have a vagina." This provoked a young female student to remark, "No, you don't! Women have a penis and a vagina, and men have no vagina." The young man, thinking he had been very liberal in his original statement and remembering that a clitoris was something like a penis, could utter not much more than "Wow, I dig it, I dig it." I informed the group that as a starting point both were as good as most definitions, but biologically and culturally they had a number of weaknesses. Granted, a large number of sex-related anatomical characteristics possessed by one sex are also present in the other sex in modified form. Such organs, which develop from the same embryological tissue, are said to be *homologous.* Thus the penis is homologous to the clitoris.

Yet some distinct differences do exist. Biologically speaking, we are reduced to the inescapable fact that women can become pregnant, have menstrual cycles, and nurse; men cannot. Culturally, we are affected by the fact that others consider us to be a male or female and expect us to act in ways that our society considers masculine or feminine. However, since concepts of so-called masculinity and femininity vary so much from culture to culture and from time to time even within one culture, we shall not attempt to deal with strict cultural definitions in this book.

SOME BASIC FACTS

In the next four chapters we shall describe the anatomy and physiology of the adult male and female sex-related organs, show how they arise during fetal life, and discuss some of the biological changes that take place during puberty. But before we embark on these topics, you need to learn a few general terms. One of these terms is *anatomy,* which refers to the structure of a unit of living material. This unit may be as small as a cell or as large as the human body. *Physiology* describes the ways in which a unit of living material functions.

This text pays particular attention to the anatomy and physiology of a pair of organs called the *gonads*. These are the ovaries, which produce eggs and sex hormones, and the testes, which produce sperm and sex hormones. Conception, which is technically called *fertilization,* occurs when a sperm unites with an egg; thus the gonads have a primary responsibility for fertility. In addition, the sex hormones secreted by the gonads are responsible for the development and maintenance of the internal and external genitalia. The *internal genitalia* are all the internal structures involved in reproduction except the gonads (e.g., the female womb and birth canal and the male sperm ducts). The *external genitalia* are the reproductive organs that are externally visible, e.g., the male penis and female clitoris. Structures such as breasts, beards, and underarm hair, which are not directly involved in the conception and development of the fetus, are called *secondary sex characteristics* rather than genitalia.

Male Sexual Architecture and Function

The male genitalia produce sex hormones and sperm and provide a system for conveying the sperm from the male gonads to the vagina of the female. These organs consist of the following (see Fig. 2-1): the two male gonads, or testes, which are housed in the scrotum; a series of ducts that drain the sperm from the testes to the exterior of the body; a number of glands that discharge beneficial substances into the sperm-containing fluid; and the penis.

SCROTUM

Since the testes lie outside of the body cavity, they need some protection from mechanical injury. They also need to be kept at a stable temperature in order to function well. The organ that provides most of this protection is the *scrotum*, the sac that hangs down behind the penis and contains the testes. In man, the scrotal sacs consist of an outpouching of abdominal wall located in the groin. If one could travel through the scrotum from the outside via a tiny tunnel, the following primary layers would be encountered successively: the skin; the tunica dartos, which is composed of muscle plus a strong, tough tissue called connective tissue; the cremaster, which consists of muscle surrounded by connective tissue; and finally the capsule of the testis itself. The highly

5

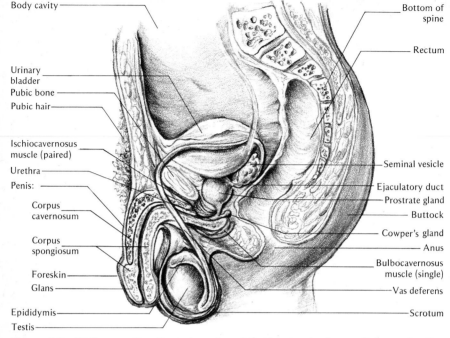

Body cavity

Bottom of spine

Rectum

Urinary bladder
Pubic bone
Pubic hair

Ischiocavernosus muscle (paired)
Urethra
Penis:

Corpus cavernosum

Corpus spongiosum

Foreskin
Glans

Epididymis
Testis

Seminal vesicle
Ejaculatory duct
Prostrate gland
Buttock
Cowper's gland
Anus
Bulbocavernosus muscle (single)
Vas deferens
Scrotum

Figure 2-1 Midline section through male pelvis showing testis, genitalia, and adjacent structures.

wrinkled, relatively hairless skin actually forms a single outer covering; whereas the tissue underneath is fashioned into a pair of sacs, each surrounding a testicle. One testis, usually the left, hangs lower down in its pouch than the other.

The testes of the early-stage male fetus lie inside the abdominal cavity. But before pregnancy becomes very far advanced, the fetal testes start to produce chemicals called male sex hormones. Under the influence of the male sex hormones, each fetal testis descends through an *inguinal canal* located in the groin and down into the scrotal sacs. By the time the fetus is born, the testes are usually in place, and the inguinal canals close off. The process of descent is not clearly understood but appears to include two components: an "apparent" motion where growth and enlargement of adjacent organs appear to displace the testes, as well as an "actual" movement through the inguinal canals.

Failure of the testes to descend into the scrotal sacs is termed *cryptorchidism* and occurs at birth in 1 to 7 percent of males. In about 70 percent of all cases of cryptorchidism, both testes have failed to descend; this is called bilateral cryptorchidism (Campbell). Descent may occur spontaneously, usually during the first year of life, but if it is not completed by puberty, surgery or hormonal therapy will be necessary. Hormonal treatment consists of giving doses of male sex hormones in the hope that they will stimulate the testes to descend on their own. Despite the availability of treatment, physical examinations of eighteen-year-olds performed at Army induction centers still reveal the incidence of cryptorchidism to be about 0.23 percent. Occasionally, testes become migratory, traveling up and down through inguinal canals that have failed to close off at birth. Sometimes part of the intestinal tract may protrude into the scrotal sacs through the open canals (Fig. 2-2). Whenever a part of the intestine bulges into an area where it does not belong, the individual has a *hernia,* and in this case an inguinal hernia. Hernias can be treated with surgical techniques (Campbell).

People with bilateral cryptorchidism produce normal amounts of male sex hormone, but they are usually infertile if the condition goes untreated. Testes remaining in the abdomen function poorly because the central body temperature is too high for normal sperm production. Tessler and Krahn showed that the average temperature of the scrotum in seven males with normally descended testes was 3.1°C (5.6°F) lower than the body temperature of 37°C (98.6°F).[1] In a wide variety of other mammals, the temperature inside the scrotum is regulated at 2 to 5°C below that of the core body temperature. This suggests that a cooler environment is necessary for adequate sperm production and for the maintenance of low mutation rates. A *mutation* is a change in a gene. Since genes are actually segments of the large and very complex chemicals called chromosomes, a mutation is really a change in the chemical structure of a

[1]°C stands for degrees Celsius, which is the metric system's unit of heat. As the United States switches over to metric measurements, you will come across the term more and more often. At present, though, our thermometers are calibrated in degrees Fahrenheit, which is written as °F. Normal body temperature is around 98.6°F, which equals 37°C.

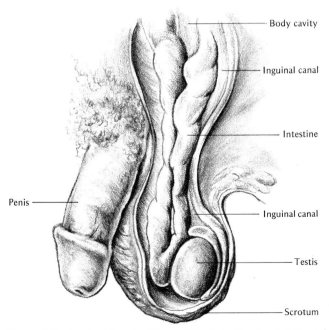

Figure 2-2 Inguinal hernia. A loop of the intestine has left the body cavity and is protruding into the scrotal sac.

segment of a chromosome. Mutations occur spontaneously in all animals, but
the number of mutations can often be increased by factors such as radiation,
chemicals, and temperature extremes. Usually when a mutation occurs in a
sperm or egg cell, the cell dies or is too abnormal to participate in conception.
Occasionally conception does occur, and in this case the mutant gene is passed
on to the offspring. If the mutation brings about a severe abnormality in the
offspring, usually the fetus does not live until birth, and a miscarriage results.
Some mutations, however, cause often undetectable "abnormalities" that may
actually be beneficial. For example, the development of the human brain
occurred through a series of mutations. Thus mutations are the raw materials
on which the process of evolution goes to work.

By comparing naked and clothed men standing at room temperature, L.
Ehrenberg et al. showed that the simple act of wearing light clothing raised the
temperature of the scrotum an average of 3°C (5.4°F) above optimum. These
workers suggested that even this slight increase could raise the mutation rate in
the genetic material of sperm by about 85 percent, accounting for half the
spontaneous mutations occurring in the human species. Garments that tend to
squeeze the scrotum up against the body are particularly hazardous for sperm
production. Robinson and Rock found that the use of a special jock strap raised
the temperature of the scrotum by almost 1°C (1.7°F). Wearing the device every
day for 7 weeks was associated with about a 25 percent drop in the number of
sperm. Waites and Setchell (1964) state that, at higher temperatures, sperm-
producing cells use much more oxygen, but the rate of blood flow bringing
oxygen to them is not increased. Depletion of oxygen from the blood then
becomes too rapid to sustain sperm production. These effects were only
temporary, and a return to normal was seen following the end of experimentation. Perhaps a drastic change in the design of men's athletic garments and
other types of clothing is needed to reduce the problems of high mutation rate
and temporary sterility.

Effects similar to those with jock straps can be produced in several other
ways: taking a steam bath in a sauna; submerging the scrotum in a 43 to 47°C
(109.4 to 116.6°F) water bath for 30 min[2] daily; holding a 150-watt light bulb
close to the sacs for 30 min every day for 14 days (Watanabe, Procope,
Robinson et al.).

In light of these facts, Cowles has suggested that evolution of the scrotal
sacs in mammals (animals that nurse their young) occurred simultaneously with
the physiological ability to maintain high constant body temperature. Actually,
many reptiles attain high body temperatures by sunning themselves, but their
testes are less vulnerable to heat. The reptile group from which mammals
evolved probably maintained a lower body temperature—they were nocturnal
animals that slept away the hot hours of the day in cool caves or burrows. Quite
possibly the testes of these animals lost their tolerance for heat, and some
cooling device had to evolve as the warm-blooded mammal body developed.

[2]Abbreviations of units of time used in this book are second (s), minute (min), and hour (h).

Thus, over a period of millions of years, the location of the testes shifted to pouches actually outside and away from the central abdominal cavity and core temperature. However, Portmann believes that the scrotum evolved not as a thermoregulatory device but as a sexual adornment like the colorful posteriors of baboons, which serve to attract females and to keep unwanted males out of their territory.

How then does the scrotum keep its cool? Certainly scrotal architecture with its thin, often naked skin and little or no fat to act as insulation plays a significant role in temperature control. Many small blood vessels also permeate the surface, where increased flow causes heat loss directly to the environment. Sweat glands abound and can enhance cooling by evaporation of sweat, which causes a loss of about 0.6 cal of heat for every g of water vaporized. Receptors that detect when the air around the scrotum gets too warm or too cool are abundant. This sensing of changes in air temperature influences the degree of contraction of the tunica dartos muscle directly under the skin. The tunica dartos is classified as a *smooth muscle.* Smooth muscle contracts and relaxes without our conscious, voluntary control and is found in many of the body's organs. For example, it is responsible for stomach movements that churn food and for intestinal movements that propel food products from the stomach to the anus. Being smooth muscle, the dartos continuously adjusts its contraction in response to surrounding temperatures without the man's conscious control. When cooled, the dartos contracts, wrinkling the skin and pushing the testes up toward the groin. When the scrotum is heated, the muscles are relaxed, the skin is smooth, and the testes hang down in a fully extended position. The other major scrotal muscle, the cremaster, is a *striated muscle.* Striated muscles can generally be contracted at will, but they can sometimes contract involuntarily as well. Most of the striated muscle in the body is found alongside bones, where it is responsible for the movements of our head, neck, back, arms, and legs. Contrary to some textbook accounts, the cremaster is incapable of sustained contractions and does not play a major role in temperature regulation. However, sexual excitement, fear, and anxiety may cause powerful contractions of the cremaster, which in turn increase the flow of blood from the testes back into the body. Stroking the inner surface of the thighs can lead to this contraction and hence is called the *cremasteric reflex.*

One final adaptation is worth mentioning. It is a heat-exchange mechanism of a countercurrent variety which helps maintain the cooler scrotal temperatures. Arteries supplying the testes and the veins that drain them run so closely parallel to each other that they are separated by less than a few micrometers, a term that is now used instead of the older term "microns." (One micrometer, symbolized as μm, equals only $^1/_{25,000}$ in!)[3] The blood flowing in opposite

[3]Metric units of length that you will come across in this text are the following:
meter (m) = 39.37 in
centimeter (cm) = 0.01 m = 0.3937 in
millimeter (mm) = 0.001 m = 0.03937 in
micrometer (μm) = 0.0000001 m = 0.00003037 in

directions allows for heat exchange from the warmer blood in arteries to cooler blood in veins, hence the term *countercurrent exchange* (see Fig. 2-3). Blood in arteries entering the scrotum will thus be cooled by about 3 to 4°C to what the temperature should be for healthy sperm production.

THE TESTES

The two male gonads, or *testes*, are oval-shaped organs about 1 in wide and 1.5 in long (Figs. 2-1 and 2-4*a*). Each contains some cells that multiply at astonishing rates and become the sperm, and still other cells that secrete sex hormones. The outer layer of each testis is a sac called the *capsule.* Recently it has been shown that the capsule contains smooth muscle whose contractions aid the process of sperm transport out of the testes and into the next major duct (Davis et al.).

The interior of the testis is divided into about 250 chambers in each of which exist one or more highly coiled *seminiferous tubules* (Fig. 2-4*b*). These are the tubules, collectively measuring almost a mile in length, that manufacture sperm throughout the life of an individual. The seminiferous tubules and the cells that lie around them are rather delicate structures. We have already described how the scrotum and the countercurrent exchange system provide a great deal of protection. In addition, the extreme coiling of the arteries carrying blood to the testes weakens the pulse and blood pressure, which would otherwise damage the testicular machinery. The seminiferous tubules them-

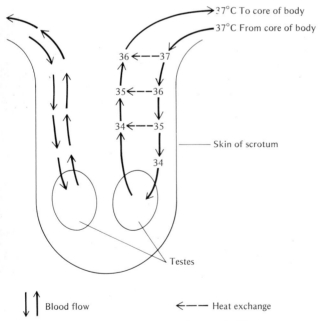

Figure 2-3 Countercurrent heat exchanges in the scrotum.

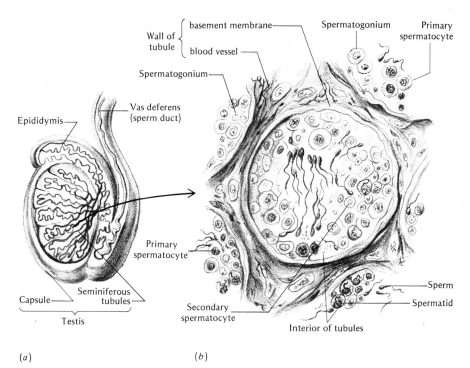

Figure 2-4 Sections through a human testis. (*a*) A testis and the ducts through which sperm leave the testis (epididymis and vas deferens). (*b*) Seminiferous tubules magnified 100x; note that the germ cells are in various stages of spermatogenesis.

selves are composed of an outer basement membrane so protective of the cells inside that some scientists have called it the blood-testes barrier (Waites and Setchell, 1969). Only oxygen, carbon dioxide, water, and glucose can readily travel across the basement membrane; and so only these materials move easily between the blood and the cells inside the tubules. Hormones and other substances can get across, but only slowly. This fact makes the fluid inside the tubules quite different from other fluids in the body and at the same time very stable.

Sperm Production

Certain cells inside the seminiferous tubules go through a series of changes that ultimately produce sperm. To understand how this occurs, you need first a quick briefing on chromosomes and cell division.

Chromosomes and Cell Division   A sperm is a very special type of cell, as is an egg. As you probably know, cells are the microscopic units of living material that make up the body, somewhat as bricks make a wall. All cells contain, or originally contained, minute structures called *chromosomes*. Chromosomes are essentially protein-wrapped packages containing the genes, which are responsible for a person's inherited characteristics. All human cells, except the sperm and mature eggs, contain 23 *pairs* of chromosomes. Regulation of chromosome number is vital to the body, and it is guided by two processes: mitosis, which occurs in all cells, and meiosis, which takes place only in the cells that are becoming sperm or mature eggs.

Mitosis   In order to grow or to replace injured or worn-out cells, the body must produce new ones. Cells multiply by dividing in half—a process called cell division—to form two daughter cells which, in turn, increase in size and then divide, and so on. However, most of the cells in the body contain 23 pairs of chromosomes, which is called the *diploid number.* Obviously then, the chromosomes in a cell must be duplicated if both daughter cells are to have the full 23 pairs. *Mitosis* is the term that describes the duplication of the chromosomes and the subsequent distribution of the original 23 pairs to one daughter cell and the 23 duplicates to the other daughter cell. The details of mitosis are somewhat complicated, but the overall process is quite simple and is illustrated in Fig. 2-5a.

Meiosis   Now consider what would happen if a sperm having 23 pairs of chromosomes fertilized an egg that also contained 23 pairs. The new child would have 92 chromosomes, which is twice the normal number. And if this process continued, the chromosome number would double with each generation. It should not surprise you, then, to learn that eggs and sperm have only 23 *single* chromosomes—one chromosome from each of the original pairs. When a cell has lost half the original chromosomes, it is said to contain the *haploid number.* Sperm and egg cells become haploid through two special cell divisions called *meiosis,* which are illustrated in Fig. 2-5b.

Meiosis starts off with replication of all of the genes inside the chromosomes, but the chromosomes themselves do not increase in number. Thus, when the cell divides, the two daughter cells will be haploid. That is, each daughter cell will obtain only one chromosome from each of the original pairs. However, a second cell division must take place in order to get rid of the duplicated genes. During this second meiotic division, the duplicate genes separate from the parent chromosome and form new chromosomes of their own. As the cell divides, the newly formed chromosomes are distributed to each of the haploid daughter cells.

Later on, when the sperm unites with the egg, the resulting single cell will have the full 23 pairs of chromosomes—23 single chromosomes from the mother and the 23 missing mates from the father.

Spermatogenesis   Two kinds of cells are present in the seminiferous tubules (Fig. 2-6). One type is the germ cells, which are in various stages of becoming sperm—a process called *spermatogenesis.* The other kind are the Sertoli cells. Most substances reaching the interior of the tubules are first processed within the Sertoli cells before they are fed to the germ cells; the Sertoli cells also coordinate spermatogenesis. The germ cells closest to the basement membrane are the *spermatogonia,* or sperm stem cells. These continually divide by mitosis, forming a pool of new stem cells that act as a

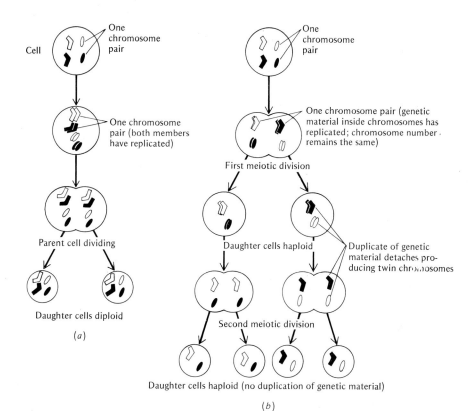

Figure 2-5 Division of a cell whose diploid number = 4. (*a*) Mitosis produces two diploid daughter cells. (*b*) Meiosis requires two cell divisions and results in four haploid daughter cells (haploid number = 2).

reserve contributing sperm throughout the life of the person. Periodically, groups of stem cells enlarge into cells called *primary spermatocytes*. Each primary spermatocyte then undergoes the first meiotic division, thereby producing two haploid daughter cells called *secondary spermatocytes*. Whereas the primary spermatocyte has 23 chromosome pairs, the secondary spermatocytes receive only 23 single chromosomes. Each secondary spermatocyte then goes through the second meiotic division to produce two *spermatids*. Each spermatid develops a head and a tail, at which point it is called a *sperm* and is released from the testis. Thus a spermatogonium gives rise to four sperm, the whole process taking 74 days.

A mature human sperm averages about 60μ m in length and consists of a head, neck, midpiece, and tail (see Fig. 2-7). The head contains the chromosomes plus an acrosome. The acrosome secretes an enzyme type of chemical called hyaluronidase that dissolves away the protective coating of cells that usually surround an egg. This allows the sperm to penetrate to the egg and thereby facilitates the process of fertilization. The midpiece of the sperm

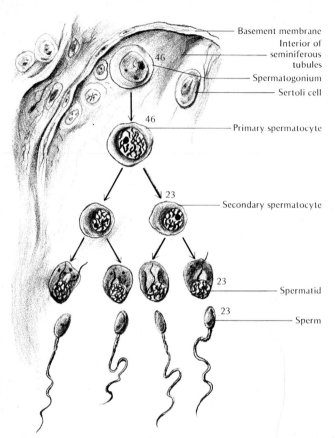

Figure 2-6 Human germ cell undergoing spermatogenesis. Diploid number = 46; haploid = 23.

contains very small particles called mitochondria. Mitochondria essentially break down sugars and fats and trap the energy released from these compounds into smaller, more useful packets of chemical energy. This energy is used when a sperm swims by lashing its tail back and forth.

   Two Kinds of Sperm?   In a developing human, two of the chromosomes, called the *sex chromosome* pair, determine whether the individual's gonads will become testes or ovaries. In the female, the two sex chromosomes are identical and are given the designation XX, whereas in the male, the sex chromosome pair consists of one X, like the female's, and a shorter chromosome called a Y.

   But during meiosis, the original chromosome pair separates so that a mature egg contains only one X chromosome and a sperm contains either an X or a Y. An X-bearing sperm is called a *gynosperm,* and a Y-bearing sperm an *androsperm.* Whether a new individual will become a male or a female depends on whether a gynosperm fertilizes the egg, in which case the offspring will be

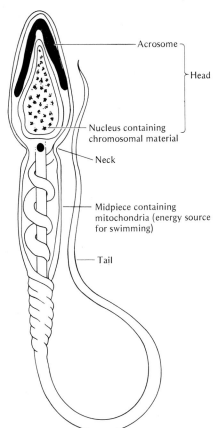

Figure 2-7 Human sperm. Length = 55-65 μm (0.00217 to 0.00256 in).

female (XX), or whether an androsperm does the fertilizing, in which case the offspring will be male (XY).

Many authors have tried to identify measurable differences between androsperm and gynosperm, and this has led to considerable controversy. Shettles not only claims to have done so, but based upon his evidence, has developed a scheme for predicting the sex of future children by timing intercourse with the particular days of the month when the woman is fertile. He identified the following characteristics of androsperm: They have less specific gravity (weight in proportion to size), longer tails, smaller, rounder heads, greater velocity when swimming, and more susceptibility to environmental changes. Shettles concludes that, in order to conceive a boy, intercourse must take place as close to the time of the woman's fertility as possible. During this time the woman's vaginal fluids become less acid and thus less hostile to all sperm. Since the androsperm will survive in the less acid environment and since they are faster swimmers, they will swim quickly to the egg, leaving the gynosperm behind. The egg would thus meet a plethora of Y-bearing sperm and fertilization would produce a genetic male. On the other hand, if intercourse occurred a few days before an egg was ready to be fertilized the chances are the offspring will be a female. This is primarily because the vaginal fluids would initially be relatively acid and thus more hostile to the less hardy androsperm. Gynosperm would survive, and even though they are sluggish swimmers, they would reach the egg by the time it is ready to be fertilized. A number of workers have severely criticized Shettles' observations. These criticisms have been summarized by R. A. Beatty. Shettles based his evidence primarily on observations made with special microscope techniques. However, differences between sperm as seen under the microscope could be due to many reasons other than the possession of X or Y chromosomes. Sperm that are alive or dead, from the left or right testis, with or without certain parts of sperm anatomy, mature or immature, could all appear different. In addition, recent attempts to separate sperm based on differences in specific gravity have proved to be contradictory. When sperm are placed in a fluid container, heavier ones drop to the bottom and accumulate faster than ones with less specific gravity. Artificial insemination using sperm found on the bottom theoretically should produce female offspring since these should be the heavier gynosperm. This has not been shown to be true in humans although it works experimentally with rabbits and bulls. More sophisticated techniques will be needed before the problem is finally resolved.

Sex Hormones

The second important function of the testes is to produce sex hormones. *Hormones* are chemicals that are produced by the body and that stimulate specific activities within the body. For example, some hormones stimulate bones to grow; some control the amount of sugar in the blood; still others, called sex hormones, confer "maleness" or "femaleness." The male sex hormones are a group of chemicals that are collectively called *androgens.* Every person produces both male and female sex hormones, but males produce far more androgens, and females produce more female sex hormones.

Testosterone   The chief androgen is *testosterone.* Testosterone stimulates the development and growth of the genital organs and contributes to the growth of bones and muscles. It is also responsible for the longer bones, greater musculature, deeper voice, and the type of hair distribution over the chest, legs, and face that tend to characterize the human male.

Many textbooks on sexuality state that the testes secrete testosterone, and that the cells of Leydig, located in groups between the seminiferous tubules, are the actual source. This raises the obvious question as to whether anyone has actually seen a Leydig cell secrete any hormone? The answer must be an unqualified no. Many bits of experimental information (Hall, Lipsett) give us indirect evidence that testosterone is produced within the testes and that the cells of Leydig are probably the producers. However, we are not absolutely sure that this is true. It is startling that our knowledge of so basic a function is still tenuous.

How Testosterone Turns on Genes   How does testosterone cause the body to develop in a way that is considered male? The answer is that testosterone indirectly affects the types of proteins that the body manufactures. Proteins are a group of chemical compounds that come in an almost infinitely varied array of shapes and sizes. Many proteins are the building blocks of body tissues. Others, called enzymes, construct, demolish, and remodel tissues and smaller materials within the body. However, enzymes are specialists. That is, only certain kinds of enzymes can digest the proteins in the food you eat. A whole other group of enzymes is responsible for the reassembly of digested proteins into a particular body structure. The manufacturing of all proteins, including enzymes, is directed by the genes. In fact, a gene is really a small segment of a chromosome that is the blueprint, or mold, for a particular type of protein. If you have brown eyes instead of blue, it is because your body manufactures the enzymes that promote the manufacture and deposit of certain types of pigment in the eye.

Recent evidence suggests that the androgens as well as a group of female sex hormones called estrogens may cause protein synthesis by "turning up" the operation of genes turned off by other genes (Villee). To illustrate: A particular type of protein is molded by a single gene, which we shall call a *worker gene.* Several worker genes are, in turn, controlled by another type of gene, which will be called a *trigger gene.* The trigger plus all the worker genes under its control are called an *operon.* When a trigger is turned on, the workers will mold their respective proteins. When the trigger is turned off, these proteins will not be manufactured. Whether the trigger is on or off depends on still another gene, the "boss." Each operon has its own "boss," which produces a chemical that can keep the trigger gene turned off. Some researchers hypothesize that when testosterone enters the system, it blocks the action of the boss gene, allowing the trigger to fire and proteins to be synthesized (see Fig. 2-8). Increased protein synthesis is the basis of growth and development in the male, as well as in the female. Exactly what bodily structures develop depends on which operons are turned on. Estrogen probably turns on different operons than testosterone does.

Other Testicular Hormones   Estrogen and androgens other than testosterone are also secretory products of the testes. However, the specific source and function of estrogen remains controversial. Estrogen may also be derived from the adrenals, two glands that are located above the kidneys, and from conversion of androgens in the blood. Estrogen appears to play a role in controlling spermatogenesis.

EPIDIDYMIS AND VAS DEFERENS

The seminiferous tubules drain via small channels directly into the highly coiled *epididymis,* a duct that lies just outside the testis (see Fig. 2-4a). Although some disagreement exists, it has been proposed that sperm are transported to the epididymis by smooth muscle contractions of the testicular

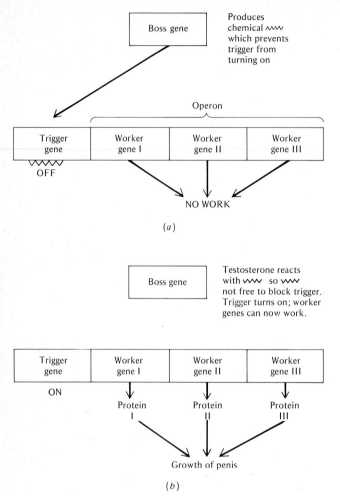

Figure 2-8 Operon concept of how testosterone turns on genes leading to protein synthesis. The diagrams show a portion of a chromosome in a penis cell. In (*a*) no testosterone is present; in (*b*) testosterone is present.

capsule and possibly by contractions of the seminiferous tubules. In addition, the tubules are lined with cilia, tiny hairlike structures that can whip like the tail of a sperm. The cilia are supposed to beat continuously, forcing fluid containing sperm to the epididymis from the tubules.

Sperm that are surgically removed from the seminiferous tubules are not able to swim and have a low capacity for artificial insemination. It has been suggested that a period of maturation, or ripening, is necessary for the sperm and that this occurs in the epididymis. Transport through the epididymis requires from 2 to 4 weeks, but the exact time is dependent upon the number of ejaculations per week. Freund has estimated that depletion of the entire reserve of sperm in the epididymis and vas deferens would take place if an adult male had an average of 2.4 ejaculations per day for a period of 10 days.

In every "normal" sample of ejaculate, there are always some sperm that are abnormal in shape, size, and motility (movement). In guinea pigs, abnormal sperm are selectively removed from the epididymis by certain amoeboid cells that wander around the body, engulfing foreign material such as bacteria and other single-celled organisms. Thus the epididymis in man is theorized to be not only a ripening but also a chamber where abnormal sperm are removed. However, in man sperm can also appear in the urine; so "leakage" could be an additional mechanism for transporting aged, unused, or unhealthy sperm.

The epididymis drains into the *vas deferens,* a long tube that runs up and out of the scrotum, curves around the urinary bladder, and then turns downward, where it opens into a short ejaculatory duct (see Fig. 2-1). The two ejaculatory ducts (one from each testis) connect with the single urethra. The *urethra* isthe tube that runs the length of the penis and drains sperm and urine from the body. Between ejaculations, the vas deferens serve as holding tanks for mature sperm; during ejaculation, the vas deferens, ejaculatory ducts, and urethra serve as conduits through which the sperm are propelled to the exterior of the body.

SEMEN

Human *semen* consists of sperm in a suspension of seminal plasma (Mann). Released primarily from the seminal vesicles, prostate, and Cowper's glands (Fig. 2-1) at the time of ejaculation, the composition of the seminal plasma is highly suited to its function. It consists of the following groups of substances:

1 water—vehicle for transport of sperm
2 mucus—lubrication of male ducts and tubes
3 bases—neutralize the acidity of the male urethra and female vagina, making these environments more hospitable to the sperm
4 fructose sugar—energy source for sperm
5 salts and minerals—equal in concentration to that found inside sperm
6 coagulators—temporary (20 min) clotting of semen in vagina to help prevent leakage of sperm back out of woman's body
7 prostaglandins—chemicals that cause contractions of uterus (womb) and fallopian tubes (ducts through which the egg moves from the female's gonads to her uterus). It is suspected that these contractions aid the movement of the sperm to the egg.
8 many other materials—functions unknown

For a specific description of components see Table 2-1. Actually nothing in seminal plasma is absolutely necessary to enhance the ability of sperm to fertilize an egg. It is essentially a transporting and energizing medium. Mature sperm that have never been exposed to the plasma are perfectly capable of fertilizing eggs. However, exposure to fluids within the female tract for at least 1 to 2 hours is necessary before fertilization can take place, and this is called

Table 2-1   Characteristics of Human Semen

General properties

Creamy texture; gray to yellow color
Isotonic to blood serum; i.e., has same concentration of salts as blood does
Specific gravity: 1.028 (slightly heavier than water, which is 1.000)
Average volume: 2.5–3.5 ml after 3 days of abstinence (range = 2–6 ml)
Fertility index (minimum qualifications for male fertility):
  At least 20 million sperm/ml seminal plasma (average being 120 million/ml seminal plasma)
  At least 40% sperm must show vigorous progression
  At least 60% sperm must be normal in shape and size
pH (acidity-alkalinity): 7.35–7.50 (slightly alkaline; 7.00 is neutral)

Major components		
Seminal vesicles (46–80% of total)	**Prostate (13–33% of total)**	**Cowper's gland**
Water	Water	Water
Fructose sugar	Bicarbonate buffers (neutralize acidity)	Phosphate and bicarbonate buffers
Fibrinogen (coagulator)	Fibrinogenase (participates in coagulation); fibrinolysis (returns coagulated semen to its liquid state)	Mucus
Ascorbic acid	Hyaluronidase (enzymes)	
Citric acid	Prostaglandins (cause contraction of sperm ducts and uterus, possibly enhancing sperm transport)	

Source: Mann, 1970.

capacitation. Some unknown substances in the vagina and uterus apparently stimulate the final maturation of sperm so that fertilization can take place.

Sperm may be said to be concentrated in the first one-third of a given semen sample at ejaculation. People who use withdrawal as a contraceptive technique should be aware that, if any portion of the semen is released into the vagina before withdrawal of the penis, pregnancy is quite possible. Also during coitus, but before ejaculation, the clear droplet that forms at the opening of the urethra is Cowper's gland secretion and may contain numerous sperm which can be passed to the vagina without ejaculation. Thus, a woman can become pregnant even if the man did not ejaculate.

PENIS

The *penis* is an erectile organ, covered with skin that is smooth and glistening in some and dry and leathery in others. The penis is divided into two general areas: the long *shaft* and an enlarged tip called the *glans* (see Fig. 2-9). The glans, supposedly resembling an acorn, actually has a variety of shapes—some

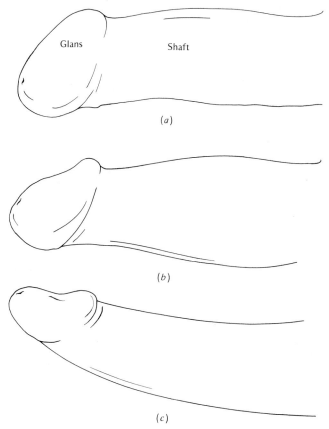

Figure 2-9 Penile shapes: (a) blunt, (b) bottle, (c) prow.

bottlelike, some flat-topped, and still others that look like the prow of a ship (Fig. 2-9). The area where the glans arises abruptly from the shaft is called the *corona*, meaning "crown" (Fig. 2-10). The glans, particularly the corona, is the most sensitive part of the penis.

If the male is uncircumcised, the skin of the shaft continues forward and forms a loose-fitting hood, or cuff, over the glans. The hood is called the *foreskin*, or *prepuce* (see Fig. 2-10). On the under surface, the glans is attached to the prepuce by a thin fold of skin called the *frenulum*. In the cavity of the foreskin and along the corona of the glans are located oil glands whose secretions when mixed with dead cells form an odoriferous, cheesy material called *smegma*.

Circumcision

Although commonly performed in hospitals throughout the country, the necessity and desirability for removal of the foreskin, an operation called *circumcision*, is currently being debated. No definitive statement one way or

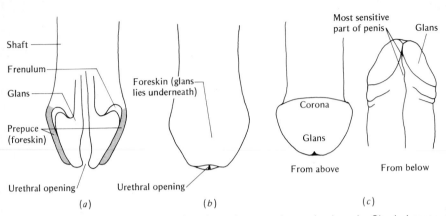

Figure 2-10 (a) Longitudinal section through an uncircumsized penis. Shaded areas are removed during circumcision. (b) Uncircumcized penis seen from above. (c) circumsized penis.

the other has ever been published by either the American Pediatric Society or the American College of Surgeons.

A circumcised penis is a symbol in many religions and the mark of a Jew or a Moslem. In many societies, circumcision is performed as part of a puberty rite and is a sign of manhood.

There are several medical arguments for circumcision. If the prepuce is tight, urine, smegma, and dirt may accumulate under it and irritate the glans penis and lead to infection. A higher rate of penile cancer is observed among uncircumcised males (Hand). There are additional claims that Jewish women show a lower incidence of cervical cancer, and this is correlated with the fact that their husbands are circumcised (Weiner et al.). However, studies of Jewish women married to uncircumcised husbands or non-Jewish women married to circumcised men would have to be done to corroborate this evidence. Apparently cervical cancer may be the result of a multiplicity of factors; which factors are most important remain controversial (Rotkin). Circumcision is the treatment of choice for problem foreskins such as seen in *phimosis*. Here the prepuce is extremely long, tight, and unretractable, often connected to the glans with strands of fibrous tissue.

Arguments against circumcision include the possibility that the foreskin may have some unknown but important function. One recalls that only a few years ago the tonsils, adenoids, and appendix were organs excised for the slightest reason. Today it is recognized that the lymphoidal tissue present in these structures contributes to an individual's ability to fight disease. Also, circumcision performed on a newborn can produce unnecessary surgical trauma with its possible ramifications. Finally, many people believe that a free glans penis unencumbered by a hood is much more sensitive to tactile stimulation and could lead to premature ejaculation on the part of the male. However, Masters and Johnson (1966) have found that no difference exists between a circumcised or uncircumcised penis in terms of sensitivity. Except for the condition of phimosis, the foreskin, when present, is generally pulled back during coitus and the glans is stimulated directly, which is the case among circumcised males as well.

Many physicians perform a circumcision immediately after birth. Others maintain that the newborn's capacity for blood clotting is not well developed during the first week of life, and to prevent excessive bleeding, they often wait until after the eighth day to perform the operation.

Size

Flaccid penises range in length from 2.3 to 4.5 in, with one authenticated record of 7.9 in measured after death in a twenty-year-old affected by tuberculosis (Dickenson). Erect penises range in length from 4.7 in to 9.2 in, with an unofficial world's record of 14 in. These statistics are based on published reports, and many exceptions probably exist. Note that the greater range in length observed among erect penises seemingly contradicts the recent statement of Masters and Johnson (1966) that erection tends to neutralize the differences in flaccid length. Supposedly penises that are shorter when flaccid gain more, whereas longer ones gain less at the time of erection and thus all would be similar in length (Masters and Johnson). Circumference does not vary much from individual to individual; it averages 3 $^3/_8$ in in the flaccid state and 4 $^3/_8$ in when erect. No known relationship exists between length and circumference of the penis and body build or height.

A boy or a sexually inexperienced man often shows a great deal of concern about the size of his penis—especially if he thinks his penis is smaller than those of his friends. Even an experienced man sometimes wonders if a longer penis would make him a better lover. These fears are needless. As you will learn in the chapter on coitus, the female receives sexual stimulation chiefly through the friction of the penis against the walls of the *exterior* opening of the vagina. The vagina itself has few nerve endings and is not a particularly sensitive structure. Fears about penis width are also unnecessary. The vaginal opening is surrounded by striated muscles, which the woman can contract at will—thus narrowing the opening. On the other hand, the vaginal opening has a good deal of stretchability and can also accommodate wider-than-average penises.

Erection

Transmission of semen from male to female requires a system of conveyance. The system includes the placement of an erect penis in the vagina followed by the propulsion, or ejaculation, of semen out of the penis.

An *erection* is defined as a penis that widens, lengthens, and hardens as it becomes congested with blood. An erection functions as a symbol of power and protection in man and as part of an aggressive display toward other males in many nonhuman primates (MacLean and Ploog). A male squirrel monkey, for example, waves his erect penis around in an attempt to establish a position of dominance within a hierarchy of other males.

In order to find out how an erection occurs, let us take a look at the inside of the penis. The interior of the penis contains three columns of spongy tissue that run through the shaft and are parallel to it (see Figs. 2-1 and 2-11). The two upper columns, or *corpora cavernosa,* are attached to the pubic part of the hipbone by a tough, tendonlike tissue. Partially surrounding each base of the corpora cavernosa are the two erector penis muscles called the *ischio-cavernosus.* The lower column of spongy tissue, called the *corpus spongiosum,* surrounds the urethra and expands at the tip of the penis to form the bulk of the glans. The somewhat enlarged area of the corpus spongiosum that lies up over the scrotum is called the *penile bulb.* The bulb is surrounded by the *bulbo-cavernosus* muscle, which is also involved in the ejaculatory process.

An erection is initiated by the stimulation of the *erection center*, which is located in the lower part of the spinal cord (at sacral segments 1 to 4, for those who are familiar with human anatomy). Look at Fig. 2-12 and notice that the erection center receives inputs from two areas: the brain and the penis. If a man thinks sexually exciting thoughts, his excitement can be transmitted from the brain to the spinal cord, where the message is passed on to nerves that run from the erection center to the penis. An erection is then initiated. Alternatively, or simultaneously, if the penis is manipulated, nerves that lie in the penis and that are sensitive to touch transmit signals up to the erection center, and the stimulated center relays its excitement to the nerves that lead back to the penis. Erection can also be brought on by another, rather unusual, type of stimulation. History recounts that when men have been decapitated, or hanged by the neck until dead, an erection and often an ejaculation occur simultaneously. Apparently the brain-to-erection center nerve fibers become momentarily activated if they are injured or severed.

Because erection is basically a spinal reflex, it can occur when the man is not psychologically aroused. However, it can be initiated as well as inhibited by psychological states within the brain. Students who wish to know the names of the nerves that are involved in erection should turn to Fig. A-1 in the Appendix.

Actual erection of the penis starts when the penile nerves bring about the relaxation of the walls of the arteries that feed the spongy columns. As the walls relax, the diameters of the arteries increase and more blood surges into the columns. However, blood draining out of the columns through the veins is relatively slow at all times. For one thing, it must move uphill against gravity. For another, it is farther away from the heart than is the blood in the arteries

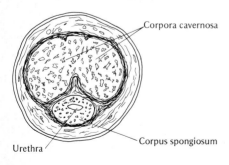

Urethra

Corpora cavernosa

Corpus spongiosum

Figure 2-11   Cross section through shaft of a penis.

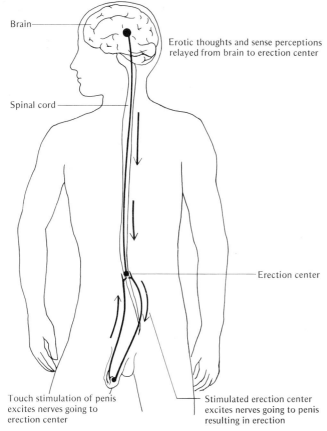

Brain

Erotic thoughts and sense perceptions
relayed from brain to erection center

Spinal cord

Erection center

Touch stimulation of penis
excites nerves going to
erection center

Stimulated erection center
excites nerves going to penis
resulting in erection

Figure 2-12   Initiation of erection.

and therefore less affected by the pumping action of the heart. In the flaccid
penis, venous outflow just barely keeps up with arterial inflow. In the erect
penis, outflow cannot keep up with inflow, and blood accumulates in the
columns. In addition, the ischiocavernosus muscles and possibly others
contract and compress the spongy columns; this further retards drainage of
blood. As the columns fill up, they become extended and rigid, resulting in the
erect penis.

The chronic inability of heavy drinkers to get an erection is apparently due
to alcoholic damage occurring somewhere in the mechanism controlling
erection. The problem becomes acute because, despite inability to perform in
coitus, many chronic drinkers maintain strong sexual desires.

Theoretically, erections occur primarily in response to sexual stimuli.
However, occasionally and sometimes embarrassingly an erection can occur
without apparent sexual input. The young teenager whose nervous system still
requires time to mature can experience an erection when he least expects

it—during a history exam or when taking a shower after a football game. Also, most men and boys never cease to wonder at the morning erection they become aware of when waking after a night's sleep. The mechanism of morning erection has never been fully explained, but it is possible that partial responsibility can be attributed to the pressure of a full urinary bladder. After all, urination involves many of the same nerves and muscles that control the mechanism of erection. In addition, friction against underpants, sheets and blankets, and erotic dreams can contribute to the phenomenon. Urination is not fully compatible with erection, and voiding the bladder usually ends in a return to the flaccid state.

Based upon studies of electrical changes in the brain, two states of sleep have been identified: slow-wave sleep interrupted every 30 to 60 min by shorter periods (10 to 15 min) of paradoxical sleep. During paradoxical sleep almost all muscles relax, and signs of body activity are limited to rapid eye movements, irregular breathing and pulse rate, and penile erections. Karacan believes that morning erections occur when a person wakes up during or at the end of a period of paradoxical sleep. Lack of erections during paradoxical sleep implies a rare, organically caused form of impotence.

Ejaculation

Mechanism of Ejaculation *Ejaculation* is the transport of semen out of the body. Like erection, it is a spinal reflex. When the erect penis becomes intensely stimulated, either by manual or oral manipulation or by intercourse, nerves in the penis relay messages to the *ejaculation center* in the spinal cord. The center lies in the midback area (in thoracic 12 to lumbar 3 segments) and relays "ejaculate" messages back to the penis.

Ejaculation itself consists of two phases. The first, or *emission,* phase occurs when sperm and seminal plasma are transported to the urethra by contractions of smooth muscles that lie in the walls of the genital ducts and glands. These muscles contract in waves, propelling the semen ahead of the areas of contraction. Meanwhile, a sphincter muscle located between the urinary bladder and urethra contracts, thereby closing off the upper end of the urethra. The closed sphincter also prevents the escape of urine into the urethra while ejaculation is occurring. During the second, or *expulsion,* phase of ejaculation, semen is exploded out of the urethra by strong contractions of the bulbocavernosus muscle of the penis. It should be mentioned that during urination, it is presumed that the sphincter is open but the ejaculatory and prostatic ducts are closed, preventing urine from entering these structures. Figure 2-13 summarizes the ejaculatory process; note that it involves the erection center as well. Figure A-2 in the Appendix illustrates the neural pathways.

Semen leaving the penis may spurt out a great distance or simply ooze out over the glans. Force of ejaculation is influenced by factors such as age, length of time elapsed between ejaculations, and degree of sexual arousal.

Ejaculation should not be construed as equivalent to orgasm, but it is

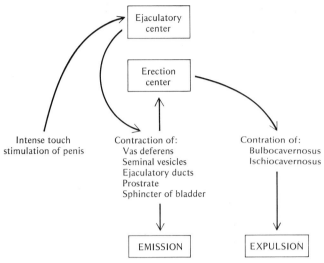

Figure 2-13 Initiation of ejaculation.

considered a part of it. Orgasm is a total body response including the person's subjective interpretation of the resulting bodily changes. Orgasm will be further discussed in the chapter on coitus.

Ejaculatory Force and Evolution The size of the penile bulb varies among males, whereas the shaft length of the penis is rather uniform. Sherfey implies that strong natural selection is not operating on the shaft, which simply functions for proper deposit of semen. On the other hand, the penile bulb is subjected to strong selective pressure which leads ultimately to wide variation in size. The largest penile bulb has the greatest capacity for "sexual tension" because it has more spongy tissue and greater "ejaculatory force" due to a correspondingly larger bulbocavernosus muscle. Some men are then more forceful ejaculators than others. However, Sherfey's conclusions are highly questionable. Indeed, a case could be made for just the opposite position on all counts. Great variation in the length or size of a particular structure among individuals of a population or between species implies a *lack* of strong selective pressures for any particular dimension (Goldstein, Badar). In other words, within reason one size is as good as any other in terms of functional capacity. Also, all things being equal, small muscles are more powerful relative to their size than larger muscles. This is why an ant can lift far more weight for its body size than a man. Thus it would appear that ejaculations are not more forceful in men with the largest penile bulbs.

Detumescence

Following ejaculation the penile arteries constrict, reducing blood flow into the penis. This allows for the emptying of the spongy columns by the normal venous outflow, and the penis returns to its flaccid state. *Detumescence* is the return of the erect penis to the flaccid state, whether or not ejaculation has occurred.

Evolution of Mammalian Penis

In an evolutionary sense, the first penis consisting of erectile tissue similar to that of mammals is found in crocodiles and turtles. Certainly copulatory organs exist in other animals, but these are in the form of modified fins, as in sharks and some bony fish, or pockets that become erect by filling with lymphatic fluid, as in the hemipenes of lizards and snakes. The presence of actual blood-containing spongy tissue interposed between arteries and veins is the characteristic that identifies a mammalian penis. Variations on the central theme include two-headed penises in marsupials and the presence of a bone (os penis) located between the cavernosus bodies. The os penis is found in rodents, bats, carnivores, whales, and certain monkeys and apes. The exact function of this bone is not clear in every species. However, in a walrus and some whales where the os may be 6 ft long, the extra support seems necessary to maintain the position of the penis during copulation in water. Otherwise the penis would oscillate like a pendulum to and fro with the wave action and thus never reach the mark. Male cats appear poorly structured for intercourse—their front legs are shorter than the rear ones; and in order to position himself, the male cat must grasp the female by the ruff of the neck. Again it would appear that the penis would suffer constant slippage if it were not for some spines located on the skin and for the os penis, which provides the additional rigidity necessary to keep it in the vagina. The os is considered one of the hardest and densest of all the hard parts in the body with the exception of tooth enamel. Why it is present in apes and monkeys but absent in humans is not known. A small bone called an os clitoris is present in the clitoris of females belonging to those species where the male has an os penis.

MALE CYCLES AND REGULATION OF SEXUAL FUNCTIONS

The ultimate control over male hormonal function and spermatogenesis rests with the brain. The *hypothalamus*, which is a rather small portion of the brain, secretes hormones called releasing factors. The releasing factors travel by a network of blood vessels to the *pituitary gland*, which lies just under the hypothalamus. The pituitary is often called the master gland of the body because it secretes hormones that control many other glands as well as the growth of bones. When stimulated by the proper releasing factors, the pituitary secretes *follicle-stimulating hormone* (FSH) and *luteinizing hormone* (LH). These two hormones travel in the blood to the testes, where FSH stimulates spermatogenesis and LH stimulates secretion.

When the amount of testosterone in the blood reaches a certain level, it reacts with the hypothalamus in such a way as to decrease the secretion of LH releasing factor. Lacking releasing factor stimulation, the pituitary then slows

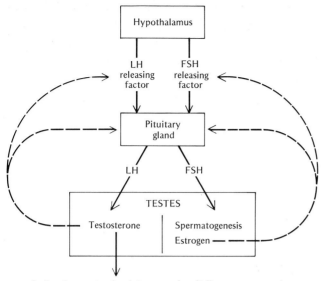

Figure 2-14 Regulation of testosterone production and spermatogenesis via negative feedback systems. Note that the system is relatively acyclic.

down secretion of LH, and consequently the testes temporarily slow down testosterone production. Then, as the level of testosterone in the blood falls below a certain amount, the hypothalamus becomes free to increase its secretion of LH releasing factor.

To summarize, rising levels of testosterone inhibit secretion of releasing factor, and falling levels of testosterone increase secretion of releasing factor (see Fig. 2-14). Thus the amount of the hormone circulating in the body is kept fairly constant. This phenomenon is an example of a *negative feedback system.* It can be compared with a thermostat located in a house. When the temperature of the house drops, the thermostat turns on the heater. As the temperature reaches a certain prescribed point, the thermostat turns off. All this stabilizes the system at a particular level.

FSH secretion in the male is also apparently controlled by a negative feedback system, but not much is known about the mechanism. Some scientists have suggested that spermatogenesis triggers release of a substance that inhibits FSH releasing factor. Although controversy still surrounds the nature of this substance, some authors have recently implicated testicular estrogen as the inhibitor (Johnson).

Sperm production and testosterone secretion have been labeled continuous, or *acyclic.* However, male functions should not be considered totally devoid of rhythms. Nieschlag and Ismail reported a daily change in blood testosterone levels, although the pattern was not the same from day to day in the same individual. Highest levels were generally at 8:00 A.M., and lowest levels around 8:00 P.M. Spermatogenesis also shows cycling. Groups of germ cells in any one area of the seminiferous tubules pass through six successive stages before the cycle of spermatogenesis begins again in that area. The cycle lasts 16 days. No correlations have as yet been shown between these cycles and male sexual behavior; however, little research has been done.

BIBLIOGRAPHY

Badar, R. S. 1955. Variable and evolutionary rate in the Oredonts, *Evolution,* **9:**119–140.

Beatty, R. A. 1970. The genetics of the mammalian gamete, *Biol. Rev.,* **45:**73–119.

Campbell, M. F. 1970. Anomalies of the genital tract, in M. C. Campbell and J. H. Harrison (eds.), *Urology,* vol. 2, chap. 39, pp. 1573–1670. Saunders, Philadelphia.

Cowles, R. B. 1965. Hyperthermia, aspermia, mutation rates and evolution, *Q. Rev. Biol.,* **40:**341–367.

Davis, J. R., et al. 1970. The testicular capsule, in A. D. Johnson et al. (eds.), *The Testis,* vol. I, pp. 281–337. Academic, New York.

Dickinson, R. L. 1949. *Atlas of Human Sex Anatomy,* 2d ed. Williams & Wilkins, Baltimore.

Ehrenberg, L., et al. 1957. Gonadal temperature and spontaneous mutation rates in man, *Nature,* **180:**1433.

Freund, M. 1963. Effect of frequency of emission on semen output and an estimate of daily sperm production in man, *J. Reprod. Fertil.,* **6:**269.

Goldstein, B. 1972. Allometric analysis of relative humerus width and olecranon length in some unspecialized burrowing mammals, *J. Mammal,* **53** (1):148–156.

Hall, P. F. 1970. Endocrinology of the testis, in A. D. Johnson et al. (eds.), *The Testis,* vol. II, pp. 1–71. Academic, New York.

Hand, J. R. 1970. Surgery of the penis and urethra, in M. F. Campbell and J. H. Harrison (eds.), *Urology,* vol. 3, chap. 65. Saunders, Philadelphia.

Hotchkiss, R. S. 1957. The nervous system as related to fertility and sterility, *J. Urol.,* **78:**173.

Hotchkiss, R. S. 1970. Physiology of the male genital system as related to reproduction, in M. F. Campbell and J. H. Harrison (eds.), *Urology,* vol. I, chap. 6, Saunders, Philadelphia.

Johnson, S. G. 1970. Investigations into the feed-back mechanism between spermatogenesis and gonadotropin level in man, in E. Rosenberg et al. (eds.), *The Testis.* pp. 231–244. Plenum, New York.

Karacan, I. 1970. Clinical value of nocturnal erection in the prognosis and diagnosis of impotence, *Med. Aspects Hum. Sex,* **4**(4):27–34.

Lipsett, M. B. 1970. Steroid secretion by the human testis, in E. Rosenberg et al. (eds.), *The Human Testis,* pp. 407–418. Plenum Press, New York.

MacLean, P. D., and D. W. Ploog. 1962. Cerebral representation of penile erection, *J. Neurophysiol.,* **25:**29–55.

MacLeod, J. 1951. Effect of chicken pox and of pneumonia on semen quality, *Fertility Sterility,* **2:**523.

Mann, T. 1970. The biochemical characteristics of spermatozoa and seminal plasma, in

E. Rosenberg et al. (eds.), *The Human Testis.* pp. 469–478. Plenum Press, New York.

Masters, H. W., and V. E. Johnson. 1966. *Human Sexual Response.* Little, Brown, Boston.

Nieschlag, E., and A. A. A. Ismail. 1970. Diurnal variation of plasma testosterone in normal and pathological conditions as measured by the technique of competitive protein binding, *J. Endocr.,* 46.

Portmann, P. A. 1952. *Animal Forms and Patterns.* Faber and Faber, London.

Procope, B. J. 1965. Effect of repeated increase of body temperature on human sperm cells, *Int. J. Fert.,* **10:**333–339.

Robinson, D., and J. Rock. 1967. Intrascrotal hyperthermia induced by scrotal insulation: effect on spermatogenesis, *Obstet. Gynecol.,* **29:**217.

Robinson, D., et al. 1968. Control of human spermatogenesis by induced changes of intrascrotal temperature, *J. Am. Med. Assoc.,* **204:**290.

Rock, J., and D. Robinson. 1965. Effect of induced intrascrotal hyperthermia on reticular functions in man, *Am. J. Obstet. Gynecol.,* **93:**793.

Rotkin, I. D. 1967. Epidemiology of cancer of the cervix. Sexual characteristics of a cervical cancer population, *Amer. J. Public Health,* **57:**815.

Sherfey, M. J. 1966. The nature and evolution of female sexuality in relation to psychoanalytic theory, *J. Amer. Psychoanalytic Assoc.,* **14** (1):28–128.

Shettles, L. B. 1961. Differences in human spermatozoa, *Fert. Steril.,* **12:**20–24.

Tessler, A. N., and H. P. Krahn. 1966. Varicocele and testicular temperature, *Fert. Steril.,* **17:**201–203.

Villee, C. A. 1967. Hormonal expression through genetic mechanisms, *Amer. Zool.,* **7:**109–113.

Waites, G. M. H. 1970. Temperature regulation and the testes, in A. D. Johnson et al. (eds.), *The Testis,* pp. 241–279. Academic Press, New York.

Waites, G. M. H., and B. P. Setchell. 1964. Effect of local heating on blood flow and metabolism in the testis of the conscious ram, *J. Reprod. Fert.,* **8:**339–349.

Waites, G. M. H., and B. P. Setchell. 1969. Physiology of the testis, epididymis and scrotum, in A. Mc Laren (ed.), *Advances in Reproductive Physiology,* vol. 4, pp. 1–63. Academic Press, New York.

Watanabe, A. 1959. The effect of heat on the human spermatogenesis, *Kyushu J. Med. Sci.,* **10:**101.

Weiner, L., et al. 1951. Carcinoma of the cervix in Jewish women, *Am. J. Obst. & Gynec.,* **61:**418.

Chapter 3

Female Sexual Architecture and Function

The female genitalia (Fig. 3-1) include the vulva, a collective term for the external genitalia; the vagina, or birth canal; the uterus, or womb; two ovaries, whose functions are analogous to those of the testes; the two fallopian tubes, which are ducts leading from the ovaries to the uterus; and a number of glands.

VULVA

The external female genitalia, collectively called the *vulva*, have probably been the least studied area of the human body. Volumes have been written about the ovary, and treatises have described the vagina. Only the healthy vulva, like love, remains obscure and up until Masters and Johnson (1966) almost totally neglected as a subject of research. The reluctance of inquiry parallels the social control placed upon "the provocative gesture of exposing the female genitals" (Ford and Beach). The one universal sign of sexual readiness, more than the naked breasts, is the exposed vulva. Even in cultures where clothes are not worn at all men are required by custom or law to avoid staring directly at the external genitalia of a nonchalantly passing woman. Indeed, among many nonhuman primates the color, odor, and enlargement of the vulva become a supreme flag of sexual enticement. (Primates are the group of mammals to

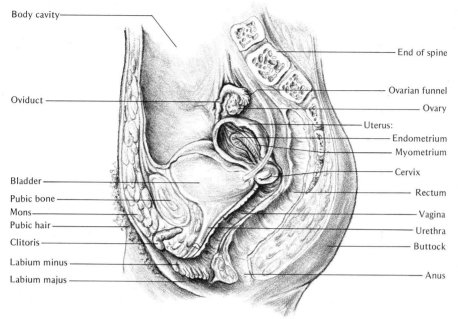

Figure 3-1 Midline section through female pelvis showing ovary, genitalia, and adjacent structures.

which shrews, lemurs, monkeys, apes, and humans belong.) Little wonder then that there is a scarcity of scientific investigation into vulval structure and function. So many fear that cold scientific inquiry would erase the "ah, sweet mystery of life," replacing it with facts.

The vulva should be studied simply because it exists, or for the sake of curiosity about a multifaceted human characteristic (Fig. 3-2). After all, the vulva possesses the mons veneris, a fatty prominence covered with pubic hair; the clitoris, an organ whose *sole* function is to receive and transmit sexual information; the hymen, a part devoid of biological function but abundant with cultural concern; and the labia majora and labia minora, the lips that protect the delicate port of entry into the vagina.

The *mons veneris,* a pillow of fat underlying the pubic hair, is a highly sensitive organ possessing far more receptors to touch (although fewer pressure receptors) than the clitoris (Krantz). A receptor is a nerve ending that is sensitive to stimuli such as touch, pressure, and temperature. Indeed, during masturbation, many women stimulate the mons area rather than the clitoris, which is a highly sensitive erectile tissue. Further proof of mons sensitivity comes from the fact that women who have had their clitoris surgically removed (clitoridectomy) can still reach orgasm during masturbation and intercourse by stimulating the mons area (Masters and Johnson).

The color, thickness, and distribution of pubic hair varies among women but generally forms an inverted triangle confined to the mons. In some 25 percent of women, the pubic hair forms a line reaching to the umbilicus (naval).

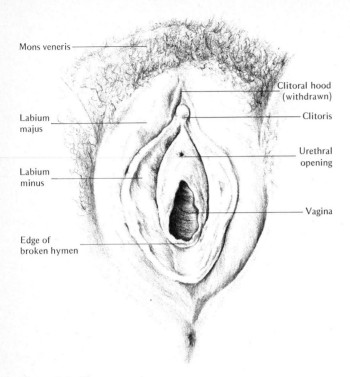

Mons veneris

Clitoral hood
(withdrawn)

Clitoris

Labium
majus

Urethral
opening

Labium
minus

Vagina

Edge of
broken hymen

Figure 3-2   The open vulva.

     The two *labia majora*, meaning "large lips," form the outer boundaries of
the vulva and protect the vaginal opening, labia minora, and urinary opening.
The labia majora are homologous to the scrotum, which means that these
organs arise from the same tissue in the embryo. When not sexually excited,
and if not altered by pregnancy, the major lips fold over the internal structures,
meet, and form a deep cleft in front. Pubic hair extends downward and covers
the outside of the labia majora, and sweat glands are abundant along the inside.
The major lips possess an array of receptors to touch, pressure, pain, and
temperature that are much more extensive than in the labia minora but less than
in the mons. Thinning of the skin due to low estrogen may leave the nerve
endings more exposed to the environment and, consequently, more susceptible
to stimulation by very mild friction; this situation may result in severe itching.
During sexual excitement, the major lips separate and flatten against the inner
surface of the thighs, exposing the minor lips and vaginal opening. Multiple
pregnancies can modify this reaction especially if blood vessels and channels
have accumulated in the majora. In these instances, the lips become distended
with blood and do not separate completely. Nevertheless, ensuing intercourse
is rarely hampered (Masters and Johnson).
     The two *labia minora* lie just inside the labia majora. They are two folds of
smooth, pigmented skin, which extend upward to form the foreskin or prepuce

of the clitoris and downward to guard the vaginal opening. Lacking hair and fat cells but possessing many blood vessels and sweat- and oil-producing glands, the minor lips show great variation in the quantity of sensory receptors. Some women have few receptors, others have them evenly distributed throughout the tissue, and still others have receptors concentrated at specific locations. It would appear, based on numbers of receptors, that the labia minora would rank somewhat lower as an erogenous zone than both the clitoris and mons. The minor lips undergo vivid color changes due to the influx of blood that occurs with mounting sexual tension and are thus called the "sex skin." The intensity of color change is directly proportional to the level of sexual arousal. Women who have never been pregnant possess pink or colorless labia that become bright red with an increase in sexual excitement. The labia of women who have been pregnant usually contain an extra number of blood vessels, particularly veins, that give off a red hue even during rest. As sexual tension increases, these veins turn deep wine in color—the darker the color, the more the pooling of blood and the greater the level of arousal. The changes in color are a definitive sign of approaching orgasm (Masters and Johnson). All of these changes tend to remove the curtain of protection over the vaginal opening in readiness for intercourse.

Lying beneath the minor lips are the two *Bartholin's glands*, each communicating with the outside by a 5-mm-long duct, opening directly on each side of the hymen. The Bartholin's glands are homologous to the male Cowper's glands, and they were thought at one time to make an important contribution to vaginal lubrication and alkalinity. However, the Bartholin's glands have recently been relegated to the category of "function unknown" (Masters and Johnson). Secretions are mucuslike, clear, stringy, and alkaline. One or two drops are formed during sexual arousal, but this occurs long after fluid from other sources has lubricated the internal surface of the vagina. Indeed, women with artificial vaginas lack Bartholin's glands, yet adequate lubrication similar to that in the natural vagina is still maintained (Fink). Also, the minute amount of secretion produced by the Bartholin's glands could not possibly contribute to the change in the vaginal fluid toward alkalinity that occurs during sexual arousal. Women after the age of thirty generally show wasting of the Bartholin's glands, and secretion gradually decreases. One must then wonder as to the significance of such structures. Masters and Johnson report that with prolonged sexual intercourse, Bartholin's glands may contribute a large quantity of secretion which would then act to lubricate the opening of the vagina. How prolonged intercourse must be for this to occur seems not to have been mentioned.

Rarely in the annals of medical science has one organ of the human body been so often discussed yet so widely misunderstood as the *clitoris*. For years the function and structure of the clitoris was a center of scientific controversy, and even conclusions from current research contradict each other. No two references are in complete agreement about the structure and function of the clitoris—let alone about the subjective perceptions of clitoral changes. Some researchers have called the clitoris "minute," "miniscule," or "a penile remnant." If this type of thinking is expanded, the penis could be described as a gargantuan clitoris that somehow got stuck to the urinary bladder. Although their embryological origins are similar, the penis and clitoris are distinct organs, and one should never be viewed as an offshoot of the other—shades of Adam's rib? The following description has been derived from dissections of cadavers as well as from interpretations of the literature.

The clitoris (Fig. 3-3) includes the body or *shaft*, composed of fused corpora cavernosa which, like those of the penis, split into two legs or *crura* (singular, *crus*). The corpora are made of blood sinus tissue and are attached to the hip bone. (Readers who have studied human anatomy may be interested in knowing that the place of attachment is the ischium.) The shaft protrudes forward but is bent on itself and points down toward the vaginal opening. Capping the end of the shaft is the *glans,* which is about $^1/_5$ in in diameter. Much controversy about the structure and embryological history of the glans still exists. Krantz claims "cavernous tissue homologous to the corpus spongiosum of the male is not found in the clitoris." Recall that the male glans is made up of this material. However, Reid claims that the clitoris is formed from two sources of erectile tissue. The shaft is composed of fused corpora cavernosa, but the glans is formed from corpus spongiosum which also makes up the *vestibular* bulbs in the female (Fig.3-3). The largest portion of each bulb is located not in the clitoris but beneath the labia minora on each side of the vaginal opening. Only a small piece of each bulb fuses in front to form the

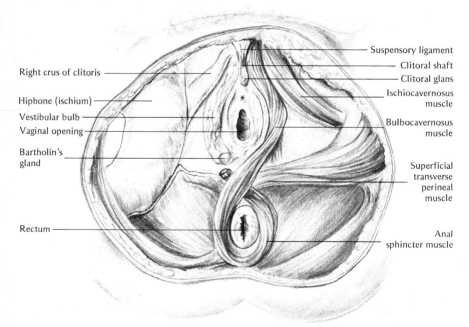

Figure 3-3 Front view of clitoris (hood removed), vestibular bulbs, and clitoral muscles. The ischiocavernosus and bulbocavernosus muscles have been removed from one side so that the underlying crus and vestibular bulb can be seen.

glans. Dissections on cadavers appear to support Reid's contention. Veins leaving the glans and larger parts of each vestibular bulb appear to interconnect. This implies a common embryonic origin for both vestibular bulbs and glans clitoris.

Most of the clitoris, except the glans, is hidden from view by the hood or prepuce, which is formed from the upper portion of the labia minora. Further, during intense sexual excitement the clitoris elevates upward and disappears beneath its hood, often to the surprise of someone concentrating on its stimulation. A clitoris rarely becomes "erect" in the same sense as the penis does. It may become tumescent, or swollen, and muscles may elevate it, but it rarely extends outward from the body.

The clitoris functions principally as a receptor and transformer of erotic stimuli (Masters and Johnson). It is particularly well endowed with pressure receptors. Surprisingly, relatively few touch receptors are present in the clitoris compared to the mons veneris; however, a larger number of temperature receptors are present, especially in the glans (Krantz). All of these receptors ultimately hook up to the dorsal nerve of the clitoris, which joins a nerve from nearby areas (the pudendal nerve) just before entering the lower part of the spinal cord at sacral vertebrae 2, 3 and 4.

The following is based on Masters' and Johnson's observations of clitoral changes during sexual excitement (see Fig. 3-4): During early arousal, called the excitement stage, the clitoral glans always develops a microscopic increase in size which can be detected only by using special magnifying equipment. Less than one half of the women in the study developed an additional increase in glans size that could be seen without the aid of a microscope. The clitoral shaft usually increases in diameter but in only 10 percent of cases does it increase in length. In the advanced stage of sexual arousal that occurs just prior to orgasm, the clitoral muscles, suspensory ligaments and crura retract the clitoris beneath its hood (Fig. 3-4c).

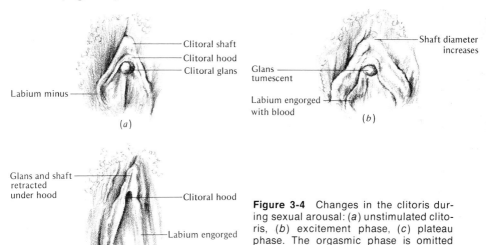

(a) Clitoral shaft / Clitoral hood / Clitoral glans / Labium minus

(b) Shaft diameter increases / Glans tumescent / Labium engorged with blood

(c) Glans and shaft retracted under hood / Clitoral hood / Labium engorged

Figure 3-4 Changes in the clitoris during sexual arousal: (a) unstimulated clitoris, (b) excitement phase, (c) plateau phase. The orgasmic phase is omitted because of lack of information. (*Adapted from Masters and Johnson, 1966.*)

The most common type of *hymen* is called *annular* and consists of a thin ring of tissue partially enclosing the vaginal opening (see Fig. 3-5). Other forms, which are relatively uncommon, more totally block the vaginal opening and therefore require surgical removal before intercourse. Particularly rare is the *imperforate* hymen which consists of a thick piece of tissue closing the vaginal opening completely. Sometimes going unnoticed during the childhood years, this problem must be diagnosed before the girl's first menstrual period.

Incorrectly called the maidenhead, the presence of a hymen does not indicate virginity. In some women, a hymen may be present even after extensive coital experience or absent with no such activity. No biological function has as yet been attributed to the hymen.

VAGINA

Connecting the vulva with the uterus is a thin-walled muscular tube called the *vagina* (Latin meaning "sheath") which encircles the penis during intercourse and serves as a passageway for the birth of a baby. The vagina is about 5 to 6 in long. As it ascends into the pelvis, it changes direction at least three times and thus resembles the italic letter *f*. The wall of the vagina consists of a thin outer serosa, which is part of the membrane that lines the body cavity and covers its organs; a middle layer of smooth (involuntary) muscle, which is continuous with that of the uterus; and an inner layer of moist mucous membrane called the *mucosa.*

Most of the time the walls of the vagina are thrown into numerous inwardly directed folds, or *rugae,* that meet each other in the center of the passageway. Under pressure of an inserted penis or a baby's head, the rugae unfold, allowing the diameter of the vagina to become quite large. The diameter of the vaginal canal and its opening may be controlled by voluntary contractions of the striated muscles of the pelvic floor: the bulbocavernosus, ischiocavernosus, superficial and deep perineal muscles, pubococcygeus, sphincter

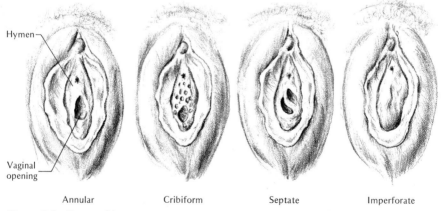

Annular   Cribiform   Septate   Imperforate

Figure 3-5 Types of hymens.

of urethra, and external anal sphincter (see Fig. 3-3). Many of these muscles also control the urinary process and are often cited as the ones to exercise for maximum manipulation of the penis during intercourse. The inner lining, or mucosa, has few touch and pressure receptors, but it does contain scattered free nerve endings. Numerous small blood vessels weave through the vaginal walls, and during sexual excitement these vessels become markedly engorged with blood. This massive congestion of blood occurs within 10 to 30 s after the start of sexual stimulation and is the source of lubrication (Masters and Johnson). Under the pressure of the dammed-up blood, small droplets of fluid are squeezed through the vessel walls and the mucosa and appear as "beads of sweat" on the inner surface of the vagina. As sexual tension mounts, the beads coalesce to eventually form a layer of shiny lubricant covering most of the inner mucosa (Masters and Johnson).

The vaginal mucosa changes in response to the fluctuations of estrogen during the menstrual cycle. Cells of this layer continually slough off and are replaced by younger ones. The cells that are ready to come off can easily be picked up on a swab and then transferred to a glass slide; the material on the slide is called a smear. The smear can then be examined under a microscope. The characteristics of the cells in any given smear will vary with the stage of the menstrual cycle and thus with estrogen level. High estrogen levels occur at the time of ovulation (the time when an egg is released from an ovary) which causes a degree of cornification, or hardening, of sloughed off vaginal cells. These cells manufacture a tough protein called keratin which causes the partial cornification. A similar process of hardening is found in the skin. Observation of these cornified vaginal cells serves to identify when and if ovulation is taking place. Examination of vaginal smears can be useful in diagnosing infertility problems. Students who have had these smears taken or are planning careers in medicine will find Fig. A-3 in the Appendix interesting. However, Fig. A-3 will be more helpful if you first read the remainder of this chapter.

At the time of ovulation, mucosal cells also tend to accumulate considerable amounts of a carbohydrate called glycogen. It has been suggested that the glycogen is a nutrient for sperm. Glycogen can also be fermented to lactic acid by the Döderlein's bacilli (bacteria) which normally inhabit the vagina. The fermentation process maintains a vaginal environment that is relatively acid and thus hostile to many disease-causing bacteria and yeasts. Antibiotics can destroy the Döderlein's bacilli population, and it is not uncommon for a vaginal infection to make its appearance when a woman is undergoing antibiotic treatment for some other infection.

UTERUS

Lying between the urinary bladder and rectum is the hollow, thick-walled *uterus,* which is suspended in place by a series of ligaments. One of the most changeable organs in the body, the uterus constantly shifts its position relative to the degree of fill in the rectum and bladder (see Fig. 3-6). During pregnancy it

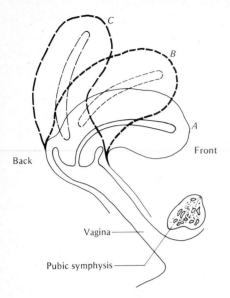

Back

Front

Vagina

Pubic symphysis

Figure 3-6 Approximate positions of uterus in standing woman. (*a*), bladder and rectum empty; (*b*), bladder and rectum full; (*c*), full bladder and empty rectum.

changes size as well as position. In addition, tissue modifications can be observed during the menstrual cycle and pregnancy.

The uterus is composed of a thin outer connective tissue called the serosa or *perimetrium,* a thick middle layer of smooth muscle, the *myometrium,* and the inner mucus membrane, the *endometrium.* The myometrium consists of muscle fibers running in several directions: an outer and inner layer that run from the top to the bottom of the uterus and a thick middle layer that encircles the organ in figure eight patterns. The arrangements of these muscle fibers are responsible for the complex contractions of the uterus that occur during increases in sexual tension, orgasm, childbirth, and nursing. In its nonpregnant state, the uterus is about the size and shape of an inverted pear. During pregnancy it enlarges and the muscle fibers increase in length from 50 to 500 μm. In addition, new fibers are formed by cell division of preexisting ones and by development of embryonic connective tissue and lymphocytes (a kind of white blood cell).

The endometrial lining is the site where a fertilized egg implants and begins its development into a new individual. Once every 28 days or so, a portion of endometrial lining grows and secretes fluids and nutrients in readiness for a fertilized egg. These changes occur in response to cyclic fluctuations in sex hormones and will be described in a later section.

Hanging down into the vagina is the *cervix,* which is the neck of the uterus. The inner lining of the cervix differs from true endometrium in that it contains special glands which secrete varying amounts of mucus that plugs the opening into the uterus. Certain changes in the cervical mucus indicate that the woman is ovulating, and therefore studies of the mucus plug are useful in determining causes of infertility. The mucus is most copious, less thick, and more readily penetrable by sperm at the time of ovulation. At this time it is also at its maximum weight, is very stringy, shows high elasticity, lacks stickiness, forms crystalline patterns resembling fern leaves when dry, and contains a high salt (NaCl) level. All of these characteristics are associated with the high estrogen levels found in the blood at the time of ovulation. A series of examinations of the mucous plug can tell the physician when and how often the woman ovulates. In other words, it indicates when and how often the ovaries release an egg that can be fertilized by a sperm. A consistent absence of these mucous plug characteristics means that the woman probably is not ovulating. Of interest, during pregnancy these characteristics are lacking, and the mucus is usually quite sticky (Loraine and Bell).

THE OVARY

The female gonads are the *ovaries*. Homologous to the testes, the ovaries produce eggs and secrete female hormones as well as small amounts of androgen.

The human female has two ovaries, one located on each side of the pelvic region of the abdominal cavity. Each ovary is attached to the uterus and pelvic wall by large ligaments. An adult ovary ranges from $4/5$ to 1 in in length, is flattened like a large bean, and consists of two relatively indistinct regions—the central *medulla* and outer *cortex* (Fig. 3-7).

The medulla consists essentially of the large, tortuous ovarian blood vessels exiting and entering through a matrix of connective tissue. The arteries entering the ovary form spirals which provide the organ "with a uniform blood supply under somewhat reduced pressure" (Franchi). At times, hormones stimulate an uncoiling of the arteries which allows the blood to be distributed unevenly. This means that more blood can go to regions where eggs are maturing and in need of increased oxygen. Scattered throughout the matrix are hilus cells, which are remnants of embryonic testicular tissue. Very rarely, hilus cells increase their rate of cell division and form a kind of tumor that secretes an excess amount of male hormone.

The cortex, or outer zone, contains the eggs, which are called *oocytes.* Each egg is surrounded by a variable number of cells called *granulosa.*

Oogenesis

The development of an oocyte starts about the fifth or sixth week of fetal life, when germ cells emigrate from the yolk sac and arrive at the gonads. (The yolk sac is a structure that arises from the embryonic gut but lies outside the embryo's body.) The germ cells proliferate, and, by the fifth month of fetal life, give rise to approximately 7 million future eggs cells called *oogonia.*

The development of an oogonium into a mature egg is called *oogenesis* (see Fig. 3-8). Oogenesis begins during the last half of fetal life and ends when an oocyte of the sexually mature woman is fertilized by a sperm. The following describes the process: Before the female child is born, certain oogonia

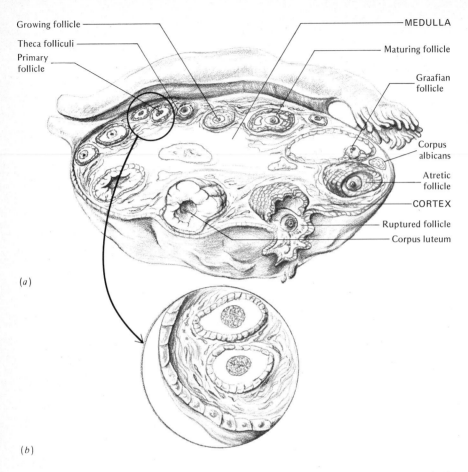

Growing follicle

Theca folliculi

Primary follicle

MEDULLA

Maturing follicle

Graafian follicle

Corpus albicans

Atretic follicle

CORTEX

Ruptured follicle

Corpus luteum

(a)

(b)

Figure 3-7 (a) Diagram of a composite mammalian ovary. (b) Close-up of a primary follicle.

duplicate their genes and enlarge into cells called *primary oocytes.* A primary oocyte plus a single surrounding layer of granulosa cells is called a primary *follicle* (see Fig. 3-7). At birth, each ovary contains about 1 million primary follicles—all that will be formed in the woman's lifetime. This contrasts sharply with the human male, in whom primary spermatocyte formation occurs throughout most of his life.

The first meiotic division does not occur until the female reaches sexual maturity. During the girl's first menstrual cycle and about every 28 days thereafter, a primary oocyte undergoes the first meiotic division. As in spermatogenesis, both daughter cells receive a member of each pair of chromosomes, and are therefore haploid. Unlike spermatogenesis, one of the cells, called the *secondary oocyte,* also receives most of the cytoplasm (semifluid contents of the cell), nutrients, and enzymes that will be necessary for survival of a fertilized egg. The other daughter cell is called a *polar body.* It

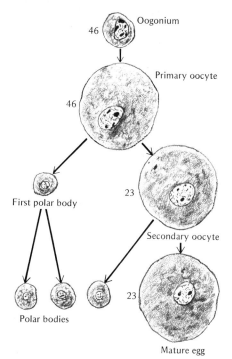

Oogonium

46

Primary oocyte

46

First polar body

23

Secondary oocyte

Polar bodies

23

Mature egg   **Figure 3-8** Oogenesis.

will either disintegrate or divide again and form two new polar bodies, which eventually die.

A secondary oocyte, along with several granulosa cells, leaves the ovary at each ovulation, but the oocyte undergoes the second meiotic division only if it is fertilized by a sperm. Again, as in spermatogenesis, the second division gets rid of the duplication of genes. One of the daughter cells is called a polar body; it receives very little of the nutrients and cytoplasm and disintegrates. The other daughter cell is the fertilized egg, which is now called a *zygote.* Some confusion exists about the terms ovum and zygote (Franchi). Theoretically an ovum is the mature unfertilized germ cell that results from a completion of meiosis and is equivalent to a mature sperm. But since the second meiotic division does not occur until after fertilization, the existence of an ovum in humans is impossible and the term should be discontinued. Fertilization restores the full number of chromosomes in the zygote and initiates the series of mitotic cell divisions which ultimately give rise to a new individual.

Why So Many Oocytes and Sperm?

From the time of birth until the change of life, which is called menopause, a large number of primary oocytes undergo a process of degeneration called *atresia.* Atresia has not yet been fully explained, but it is known that the 2 million primary oocytes present at birth are reduced to twenty to sixty thousand at puberty and to only a few hundred by menopause. A woman who experiences her first menstrual period at twelve and menopause at forty-eight will release only about 400 secondary oocytes. Herein lies one of the most difficult problems to explain. Why so many eggs, when only a few will ever contribute to the future population? Is nature wasteful?

During cell division, chromosomes may trade off genes with each other, or a segment of a chromosome may attach to another chromosome, making one shorter and the other longer. Cohen has suggested that, because of these trade-offs and acquisitions and because of spontaneous mutations, each oocyte in an ovary may have a slightly different arrangement and/or assortment of genes. The same is true of sperm. Thus, the offspring does not receive a perfect copy of half of each parent's chromosomes. This phenomenon allows the species to experiment with a wide variety of genetic combinations. Combinations that produce harmful effects may cause miscarriage; whereas highly beneficial combinations may lead to healthier offspring who will be able to leave behind many descendants.

Because sperm do the traveling, an additional explanation for their huge numbers has been proposed. The human female reproductive tract can be viewed as a tortuous series of traps and dead ends that include blind alleys in the vagina, small and therefore hard-to-find openings into the uterus and into the fallopian tubes, attacking white blood cells, cervical mucus, and an acid environment. These traps help prevent disease-causing bacteria from reaching the oocytes, but they are also hostile to sperm. The prodigious number of sperm ensures that a few will pass these barriers.

Ovarian Hormones

The ovaries produce two types of female sex hormones, estrogens and progesterone, plus male androgens.

The *estrogens* are a group of closely related hormones that produce a wide variety of effects. They control the first half of the menstrual cycle, prime the oocyte for ovulation, and are responsible for the neutralization of the vagina during ovulation, for female fat distribution, and for breast development. Recent evidence indicates that, like testosterone, estrogens probably enter cells and turn on particular genes. *Progesterone* controls the second half of the menstrual cycle, influences breast development, and retards smooth muscle contraction of the uterus during pregnancy. Androgens appear to increase sexual motivation.

Estrogens, progesterone, and androgens are collectively included in a chemical category called steroids. Of considerable interest are the chemical similarities between steroids—not only are they alike in chemical structure, but their synthesis involves many of the same steps and enzymes. The raw material for the manufacturing of steroids is cholesterol. If, say, estrogen is to be manufactured, the process starts with the secretion of FSH from the pituitary. FSH activates an enzyme, found in certain cells of the ovary, that can change the cholesterol into a substance called pregnenolone. Pregnenolone is, in turn, converted by a series of steps into progesterone-androgen and eventually into estrogen.

The similarities among steroids are clinically important. For example, contraceptive pills contain synthetic estrogen and progesterone. A few kinds of contraceptive pills contain a type of synthetic progesterone that is easily converted to estrogen once inside a woman's body. This conversion could possibly result in an excess of estrogen and thus lead to a number of adverse side effects. It should be stressed, however, that the majority of pills contain a synthetic progesterone that is termed an *antiestrogen* and does not undergo conversion.

FALLOPIAN TUBES

The fertilization of an oocyte by a sperm actually takes place in one of the two *fallopian tubes*, or oviducts, which extend between the ovaries and the uterus. The zygote then moves slowly down the tube and implants itself in the wall of the uterus several days later. The chief function of the fallopian tubes is to serve as an environmentally hospitable conduit for the transport of sperm, oocytes, and zygotes. Transport of sperm and oocytes must occur in opposite directions, and no one has yet discovered how this happens. Information we do have comes mostly from observations on rabbits (Clewe and Mastroianni, Blandau). Following ovulation in a rabbit, oocytes and their entourage of granulosa cells are brushed from the site of ovulation into the ovarian funnel of the oviduct by long, fingerlike extensions of the ovary like a carpet sweeper (see Fig. 3-1). In addition, the granulosa cells appear to be sticky—a condition that facilitates the transfer. Once the oocyte enters the tube, it is helped along its way by cilia that line the tube and beat downward. Although the opening into the oviduct lies very close to that of the ovary, the two are not attached. Nor is the ovary completely surrounded by the fingerlike mouth of the oviduct. Occasionally a tube misses an egg that has just been released and the egg ends up in the abdominal cavity, where it will usually degenerate. Even more unusual is the possibility that it could survive, be fertilized, and become implanted somewhere in the abdomen, forming a type of *ectopic pregnancy* which usually dies in a few days. An ectopic pregnancy is an implantation of a zygote anywhere outside the uterus.

The carpet-sweeper account discussed above is not totally sufficient to explain how an oocyte is picked up by a woman's fallopian tube. For example, evidence indicates that some women with one ovary and one fallopian tube located on opposite sides may still have proper pickup. Perhaps oocytes are chemically attracted to the tube or wander and find it by chance.

Sperm transport up the tubes seems to occur in two stages—a rapid phase followed by a slower, more lengthy phase (Bedford). A small quantity of sperm is first transported rapidly by muscle contractions. Sperm have been known to arrive in the upper one-third of the human oviduct 30 min after coitus has taken place. Many sperm, however, remain stuck in the cervical mucus and are liberated gradually. Once within the oviduct, some sperm, by chance, find troughs where ciliary activity is lacking and thus can swim up toward an advancing oocyte. Rapid transport of sperm can be inhibited by extreme stress, which causes the body to release epinephrine, an "alertness" and quick-energy hormone. Secretion of epinephrine by the woman can decrease the rapid phase of sperm transport by inhibiting the smooth-muscle contraction of tubes and uterus.

Fertilization usually takes place in the upper one-third of a fallopian tube. The human oocyte is capable of being fertilized for only a short time after ovulation—6 to 24 h. Beyond this time, it is called overripe and will disintegrate. If fertilization takes place, the zygote will take approximately 3 days to travel along the tube into the uterus where implantation takes place. Cilia in the tube which beat toward the uterus plus smooth muscle contractions transport the zygote. Hormones such as estrogen and progesterone will accelerate and retard transport, respectively. Indeed, the postcoital pill, which is taken after sexual intercourse, is composed of a powerful dose of synthetic estrogen. It prevents implantation in two ways: (1) by speeding up transport of a zygote and thereby allowing it to arrive in the uterus before it is capable of implantation, and (2) by making the endometrial lining inhospitable to reception of a zygote.

THE MENSTRUAL CYCLE

The menstrual cycle is a series of bodily changes that occur repetitively from the time of the first menstrual period until menopause. The events of the cycle include the development of a secondary oocyte, release of the oocyte from the ovary, buildup of the uterine lining in preparation for a possible pregnancy, and a sloughing off of part of the lining if a pregnancy does not occur. The ovaries, uterus, vagina, indeed the whole body, change with various portions of the cycle. All these changes are controlled by the hypothalamus, with modifications coming from even higher centers of the brain. As much a part of life as eating and breathing, menstruation, nevertheless, is viewed negatively or at the very least with mixed emotions by a majority of women (Bardwick). It would be a rare person indeed who said, "Gee, I can't wait for my menstrual flow," unless she was worried about pregnancy. Advertisements for tampons and sanitary napkins indicate that proper use would make a menstruating woman "appear normal." By implication, the menstrual flow is relegated to the "abnormal." It is difficult for a young adolescent experiencing her first period to suddenly shift her attitudes about a loss of blood from a concept of hemorrhage to one of health. Even with proper sex education, it is natural for people anticipating a novel event, such as their first menstrual period, intercourse, or pregnancy, to have feelings of fear and concern. Possible discomfort caused by the bodily changes, attitudes of the culture, and a girl's self-concept derived from years of living within a specific family milieu will affect the final degree of acceptance. Anne Frank in *Diary of a Young Girl* summarizes the complexities with the comment, "Despite all the pain, unpleasantness and nastiness . . . I have a sweet secret, and that is why although it is nothing but a nuisance to me in a way, I always long for the time that I shall feel that secret within me again" (Frank).

Phases of the Cycle

The menstrual cycle is divided into three phases, which overlap each other. These are the proliferative and secretory phases and the menses.

Proliferative Phase   The *proliferative* (or follicular or preovulatory) phase starts while the woman is still experiencing menstrual flow, lasts from 9 to 17 days with an average of 14, and ends just after ovulation. *Ovulation* is the release of the secondary oocyte from the ovary. During this phase the lining of the uterus builds up, or proliferates, and, in the ovary, a primary oocyte becomes a secondary oocyte—activities that prepare the woman's body for pregnancy. Body temperature tends to be a little below the "normal" 98.6°F (37°C) at this time.

On the first day of the woman's period, several follicles start to grow and to develop many layers of granulosa cells. A fluid-filled space forms in the center of the follicle where the primary oocyte resides (see growing follicle in Fig. 3-7). This early growth takes place spontaneously without hormonal control.

A few days later, the proliferative phase is initiated by secretion of FSH releasing factor by the hypothalamus. The releasing factor triggers release of FSH from the pituitary, and FSH travels in the blood to the ovaries. FSH stimulates one of the enlarged follicles to grow to a diameter of 8 mm, at which point it is called a *Graafian follicle* (Fig. 3-7). It is not known why, out of many follicles, generally only one develops. It has been suggested that those closest to ovarian blood vessels are likely to receive the strongest dose of FSH. Or one of the follicles may have reached a level of maturity, making it more susceptible to FSH influence.

Note in Fig. 3-7 that several layers of cells called *theca folliculi* surround the maturing follicle. FSH stimulates the thecal cells to secrete increasing amounts of estrogen. Estrogen, in turn, is responsible for the buildup of the endometrium, which lines the uterus. In addition, estrogen, along with FSH, brings on the final changes in the maturation of the Graafian follicle that occur a few hours before ovulation. These changes include the division of the primary oocyte into a secondary oocyte and a polar body. The secondary oocyte then works loose from most of the granulosa cells and floats free in the fluid-filled space with only a few cells around it.

As estrogen level rises throughout the proliferative phase, it causes FSH secretion to decrease via a negative feedback system (see Fig. 3-9). One or two days before ovulation, estrogen reaches a peak level, and the pituitary releases a sudden surge of LH, which is the hormone that brings on ovulation. Recent evidence suggests that the high level of estrogen is the trigger for LH release (Vande Wiele et al.). If so, then this is an example of one of the few *positive* feedback systems in the body. Interestingly, FSH secretion shows a moderate increase at this time, despite the fact that it has previously been inhibited by rising estrogen (Fig. 3-10). Ross et al. have suggested that this second rise in FSH may be a fail-safe mechanism or back-up helping LH to cause ovulation.

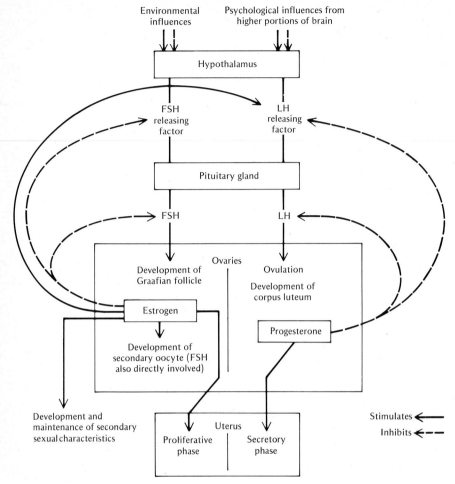

Figure 3-9 Regulation of menstrual cycle.

In any case, it appears that a precise ratio between LH and FSH is required for ovulation to take place.

Ovulation occurs approximately 36 h following the surge of LH. The effects of LH on the Graafian follicle and the changes leading ultimately to rupture are not completely understood. However, the follicle must have been previously primed by FSH and estrogen before it will respond to the sudden and sharp influence of LH.

It has been proposed that LH functions in two ways to cause ovulation (Loraine and Bell). One is to stimulate enzyme production by some granulosa cells. The enzymes produced will erode and weaken a small portion of the follicular and adjacent ovarian walls. Second, LH causes an increase in blood flow to the ovary. Blood pressure rises and tends to break up capillaries adjacent to the eroded area mentioned above. The cells of this portion of the

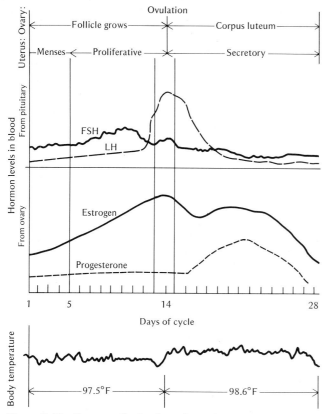

Figure 3-10 Hormone fluctuations throughout the menstrual cycle. The fluctuations control the phases of the cycle, influence body temperature, and may affect mood.

follicle do not receive oxygen and will degenerate. The area then becomes thin and translucent and forms a clear blister called the *stigma.* Eventually the stigma tears and the follicular fluid and egg trickle out.

In the human female the exact timing of ovulation is determined spontaneously by some internal biological clock. In rabbits, cats, ferrets, camels, and raccoons, it is part of a reflex mechanism triggered at the time of coitus.

Secretory Phase   The *secretory* (or luteal or postovulatory) phase of the menstrual cycle begins immediately after ovulation, averages 13 days in most women, and ends on the first day of the woman's period. Thus ovulation generally occurs 2 weeks before the first day of menstrual flow, regardless of total cycle duration. During this time the lining of the uterus secretes the carbohydrate glycogen, which would provide nourishment for a zygote—hence the name of this phase. Visible signs include a rise in body temperature to 37°C (98.6°F) and often swelling of the breasts and some weight gain because of water retention.

Following ovulation, LH stimulates changes in the granulosa cells that had just previously surrounded the secondary oocyte: the ruptured Graafian follicle, which is still in the ovary, is invaded by blood vessels and by cells of the theca folliculi. The granulosa cells then enlarge, and the former Graafian follicle becomes a yellowish body known as the *corpus luteum* (Fig. 3-7). The corpus luteum secretes progesterone and estrogens. Progesterone is responsible for the secretory function of the endometrium and for the maintenance of pregnancy, should it occur. The estrogens enhance this action of progesterone. A negative feedback system is now set up whereby progesterone inhibits LH secretion and estrogen inhibits FSH (Figs. 3-9 and 3-10).

If fertilization does not occur, the corpus luteum eventually degenerates into a whitish scarlike body called the *corpus albicans.* The exact reason for this degeneration in humans is not known. Experiments with the cow, pig, and guinea pig indicate that if implantation of a fertilized egg in the uterus does not take place, the endometrium produces a substance called luteolysin which causes degeneration of the corpus luteum. If implantation does take place, luteolysin is not produced and the corpus luteum remains functional. However, luteolysin has not been found in the human uterus. The luteal hormones, progesterone and estrogen, help maintain the pregnancy in humans for at least 3 months, until the placenta is sufficiently developed to secrete its own hormones (Caldwell).

Degeneration of the corpus luteum is coupled with a decrease in secretion of progesterone and estrogen (Fig. 3-10). Decreases in these two hormones trigger the onset of the menstrual flow. The most recent hypothesis describing the events leading to the flow comes from direct examination of the endometrial tissue at various stages of development as well as observation of pieces of living endometrium transplanted into the eyes of monkeys and rabbits (Markee, Okkels, Bartelmez). Low levels of estrogen and to a lesser extent progesterone cause a reabsorption of fluid from the endometrium into the blood stream. This shrinks the endometrium and buckles certain arteries bringing blood to the uterus. As they buckle, the arteries collapse or close off and circulation is slowed down, leading to a lack of oxygen in the endometrium. The oxygen-starved tissue begins to die and releases histamine and serotonin, substances which cause a sudden increase in the diameters of the formerly collapsed arteries and thereby cause a sudden surge of blood flow. The sudden increase in blood pressure causes the small, weak capillaries to bleed. In addition, some of the arterial blood is shunted to large venous lakes or storage depots of blood, which eventually break up. About three-quarters of the endometrium dies; the remaining will contribute to the regeneration of the endometrium for the next cycle. Much of the dead tissue is reabsorbed, and menstrual flow consists mostly of blood. Figure 3-11 shows the changes that occur in the lining of the uterus throughout the cycle.

The Menses   The menstrual flow, called the *menses*, lasts from 3 to 7 days and overlaps with the beginning of the next cycle. In fact, since the onset of the menses is the most obvious and dependable clinical sign of the cycle and since

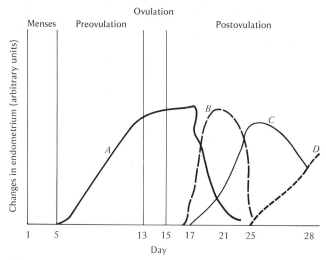

Figure 3-11 Histological changes in endometrium in a 28-day menstrual cycle. (*a*) Gland proliferation or buildup; extensive cell division. (*b*) Buildup of the carbohydrate glycogen in gland cells—a sign that ovulation has occurred. Glycogen is nutrient source for possible zygote implantation. (*c*) Visible secretion of glycogen from glands. (*d*) Visible shrinkage of endometrium due to reabsorption of fluid into blood stream; occurs just prior to menses.

proliferation of the follicles starts at this time, the first day of the menstruation is generally called day 1 of the cycle.

Approximately two-thirds of the menstrual discharge is blood, with the remaining material consisting of endometrial tissue, mucus, vaginal cells, and a variety of chemicals. The quantity of menstrual discharge varies for each cycle ranging from 1 to 6 oz (30 to 180 ml), with an average of 2.5 oz. Women with an intrauterine contraceptive device often experience a heavier-than-average menses, whereas use of the combination pill is usually associated with a reduced discharge.

Contrary to popular belief, the "clots" observed in the discharge are not blood clots but fragments of endometrium with other adherent substances. Pepper and Lindsay have found that the menstrual discharge contains few blood platelets. Platelets are cell-like bodies found in normal blood, and they are essential to blood-clot formation. Pepper and Lindsay suggest that during endometrial disintegration the blood that forms clots then becomes unclotted by an unknown chemical agent. Because of this previous clotting, blood that leaves the female tract has lost many of the platelets and will remain in the fluid state. Israel further mentions the possibility that blood in the menstrual discharge is lacking in the essential clotting chemicals of prothrombin and fibrinogen.

Before the end of menses, low levels of estrogen allow for an increase in FSH-releasing factor, the proliferative phase starts, and the menstrual cycle begins again. Table 3-1 summarizes the cycle. Arrows pointing upward indicate an increase of hormonal level; arrows pointing downward indicate a decrease of hormone level.

**Table 3-1 Summary of the Menstrual Cycle
(The events are listed in order of occurrence.)**

1 FSH ↑ = follicular growth and estrogen secretion from follicles
2 Estrogen ↑ = proliferative buildup of endometrium
                        inhibition of FSH
                        stimulation of LH "surge"
3 LH surge and smaller increase in FSH = ovulation and corpus luteum formation
4 Corpus luteum secretes estrogen and progesterone
5 Estrogen ↑ = inhibits FSH
    Progesterone ↑ = secretory phase in uterus
                        inhibits LH
6 FSH ↓ LH ↓ = corpus luteum degenerates if fertilization doesn't take place
7 Estrogen ↓ Progesterone ↓ = menstrual flow
8 Estrogen ↓ = FSH ↑ cycle begins again

Duration of Menstruation

Females in our society generally experience *menarche*, the first menstrual period, between the ages of nine and seventeen. Following menarche, many adolescent females experience wide variation in the length of the cycle and in the amount of menstrual flow (Israel). Sometimes an interval of 5, 6 or 7 months can occur between the onset of menstruation and the second cycle. A lack of ovulation or uncompleted cycles is the rule for at least a couple of years, but eventually a more consistent and stable rhythm is established. Established cycles vary from 11 to 63 days with an average of 28.86 days (Bailey and Marshall). These workers also found that cycle length declines slightly between the ages of twenty and forty-four and in some cases becomes quite irregular after the age of forty-five.

The Menstrual Cycle and Daily Activity

Many unresolved problems remain with respect to the menstrual cycle and individual concern. Should women perform strenuous exercise or even moderate activity during the menses? Should women take a bath during the menses? What are the causes of menstrual cramps? These questions would not exist were it not for the misconception that the menses is a time of withdrawal from normal behavior. Of interest is a study made on 66 women athletes competing at the Tokyo Olympics. The women were asked how the menstrual flow affected their athletic prowess. Seventy percent said there was no difference in mental or physical capacity during menses as compared with the other phases of the cycle. Fifteen percent said they perform better during the menses, and 15 percent said they performed comparatively worse.

Many physicians recommend that the temperature of bath water be nearly that of the body. If the water temperature diverges sharply from body temperature and if exposure is abrupt, this may lower the resistance against infection on the part of anyone, let alone a menstruating woman. Also the menstrual flow may increase in a hot bath but decrease when the water is cold.

A common problem that sometimes limits the activities of a woman during the first part of the menses is menstrual cramps. The cramps are caused by contractions of the muscle layer of the uterus and its cervix, and they range in intensity from a feeling of slight abdominal discomfort to severe pain. Menstrual cramps occur most often on the first day of the menses, but may last until about the third day. Some women never experience these symptoms; some suffer from severe cramping; whereas many women experience mild to moderate discomfort on occasion.

The cause of menstrual cramps has not been determined. Some physicians claim that cramps have a psychological origin, some say the cause is strictly biological, while still others compromise and claim both a psychological and a physiological basis.

Recent evidence indicates that attitudes about menstruation in conjunction with certain religious training may be correlated with menstrual cramps (Paige). Among Jewish women, for example, cramps were most severe in those who felt intercourse during menses was distasteful. Catholic women with high menstrual discomfort tended to believe in premarital chastity, and had few ambitions to pursue a career, and were strongly oriented toward home and family life. Protestant women who suffered the most were individuals predisposed to psychological stress and who tended to complain more easily about illness and bodily changes.

However, it appears that a number of physiological causes also exist. Masters and Johnson report that some women experience a decrease in cramps following orgasm. They suggest that the increased pelvic congestion at the time of menses could cause cramps and is more quickly relieved by the uterine contractions of orgasm.

It also appears that severe cramps, at least, are heavily influenced by levels or ratios of hormones circulating in the blood. Women who are taking a contraceptive pill seldom experience severe menstrual pain, despite the fact that they may have had moderate to severe cramping before they used this method of contraception and may reexperience the same amount of pain after they give up the pill. The pills contain synthetic progesterone. One of the effects of high progesterone levels during pregnancy is that they inhibit strong or sustained contractions that might expel the fetus. Some researchers suggest that the bodies of women who suffer from menstrual cramps may produce slightly less progesterone during the secretory phase than do other women.

Menstrual Cycle and Mood

Psychological mood can influence hormone levels and fluctuations, and vice versa. For instance, when a woman travels to a foreign country, starts her first semester of college, or finds herself in other new or stressful situations, her menstrual cycle may be temporarily disrupted. The visible sign of disruption is an absence of the menses for up to several months. Other evidence has shown just the reverse—that hormonal fluctuations during a normal cycle influence mood and sometimes influence behavior. J. Bardwick (1972) administered a simple projective test to 26 college women over two menstrual cycles. These tests were scored using the Gottschalk and Gleser verbal anxiety scale, which measures anxiety about divorce, death, bodily harm, and so on. The results can be summarized as follows:

1   At ovulation, when estrogen levels are the highest, women generally felt the most self-esteem, were alert and happy, self-confident, and other-directed.

2   During the secretory phase of the cycle, women felt more passive and self-involved.

3   During the premenstrual times, 4 days before menses, women felt the most anxiety, tension, depression, irritability, helplessness, and hostility.

4   At menses, irritability and tension eased, but depression continued until estrogen levels once again increased.

Mood swings can influence behavior, and it has been reported that one-half of the women in the United States who commit criminal acts or suicide do so during the premenstrual days (4 days before menses) (Dalton). This author also reports that 45 percent of women who enter hospitals for mental or physical reasons do so premenstrually. However, it must be stated that major environmental changes can retard the above hormonal influences and that anticipation of such mood swings can heighten them.

Further evidence that hormones influence mood comes from women on the pill. The pill contains artificial estrogens and progesterones taken for 20 to 21 days beginning with the fifth day of the cycle. Under the influence of these hormones, a number of women reported a more constant mood that could be classified as "a moderate amount of anxiety" (Bardwick, 1972). This correlates well with feelings reported by women during the secretory phase of a normal menstrual cycle.

High estrogen levels are correlated with reduced quantities of the enzyme monoamine oxidase (MAO) in the brain (Bardwick, 1971). This enzyme breaks down norepinephrine, a chemical that is required for the relay of messages between certain types of nerves, including some of the nerve cells of the brain. Thus, high estrogen should be correlated with high quantities of norepinephrine. During the 4 days of premenstruation, estrogen is low, MAO is high, and norepinephrine is low. It has been shown that high MAO is often associated with depressive mental states in psychiatric patients. Whether increased levels of MAO cause the light depression that is often associated with the premenstrual syndrome remains to be elucidated.

However, we should not make the mistake of assuming that most women are blissfully happy during ovulation and emotional wrecks around the time of the menses. Bardwick's results show menstrual-related *tendencies* toward particular types of mood. They do not show full-blown neurotic behavior in women of average mental health. Furthermore, many other factors affect both mood and behavior. These include relaxed and pleasant or stressful situations in the woman's life and, just as important, the woman's ability to cope with stress. Indeed, one of the hallmarks of emotional maturity is the ability to cope with unpleasant moods and situations in ways that are not destructive to oneself or to others.

It has been substantiated and should be made clear that males have a number of 24-h cycles in hormonal secretion. It is also suspected that males have rhythms which are not as obvious as the menstrual cycle. Ramey reports an intensive 16-year study in Denmark where androgen levels in the urine of men fluctuated up and down over a period of 30 days.

Breasts

Breasts, also called *mammary glands,* are a characteristic used by scientists to define a whole class of organisms—the mammals—that suckle their young. Evidence indicates that breasts have evolved from glands associated with the production of perspiration. Milk, therefore, in an evolutionary sense may be seen as a highly nutritious derivation of sweat. Among most Americans, breasts also function as erotic organs.

The number of breasts found in a species corresponds roughly to the number of young produced per birth, ranging from one pair in humans to eleven pairs in certain primitive mammals (some shrews). The location and position of breasts varies with the species and correlates with the newborn infant's ability to reach various areas of its mother's body. For instance, cats have six functional breasts, which lie in two rows that extend from the groin to the foreleg. The kittens, who are not able to stand until a couple of weeks after birth, suckle while the mother cat is lying on her side. The cow has four mammary glands, which lie in the groin, protected by the legs. The cow stands while nursing, as does the calf, which is strong enough to get on its feet within a few hours after birth. Humans have one pair of breasts, which are located on the chest. Because the mother holds her baby, she can stand, sit, or lie while nursing.

Breasts develop in the human embryo from a raised ridge of tissue called the *milk line,* which extends from the base of the arm buds to the base of the leg buds. Most of this ridge will disappear except for a pair of thickenings that develop in the chest region. Each thickening will ultimately gives rise to a breast and its associated nipple. Occasionally, more than two breasts grow, and records of humans with up to eight functional breasts have been reported in the literature. This condition can be corrected by surgery. Sometimes the extra breasts consist of nipples only, the nipples may be fully formed or they may be small pigmented spots on the chest or abdomen. This condition is called *polythelia* and is not uncommon, even in males. In addition, adult males may show *gynecomastia,* a situation where the breasts become enlarged and can even secrete milk. Gynecomastia occurs in response to injections of estrogen given to the male as therapy for other conditions. Following birth, infants of both sexes have been known to secrete small quantities of fluid, inappropriately called witches' milk, from their breasts, apparently in response to maternal hormones that may have crossed the placenta during fetal life. This latter condition quickly disappears and is nothing to worry about.

Once formed, a female breast does not develop further until the onset of puberty. Estrogen, progesterone, growth hormone from the pituitary, prolactin, also from the pituitary, and thyroxine from the thyroid gland act together during puberty to stimulate growth of the breast to the form seen in the adult. The process takes a couple to several years, but is usually completed by the late teens. During menstrual cycles and sexual excitement, the breasts undergo changes in shape, size, and color, but these are slight compared to the changes that occur during pregnancy and during nursing, or *lactation.*

The exterior parts of a breast include the nipple and the *areola,* which is the pigmented area that encircles the nipple (see Fig. 3-12). The interior of a nonlactating breast is composed mostly of fat and connective tissue surrounding a small quantity of glandular tissue. The milk-producing glands are saclike structures with branching ducts that extend to the nipple. The amount of glandular tissue is similar in each breast; the differences in breast size and shape are primarily related to the amounts of fat and connective tissue. It is therefore impossible to predict the milk-producing potential from the external observations of breasts. Large breasts do not necessarily produce more milk than small breasts and vice versa.

Breast size and shape varies widely among humans—from large, rounded

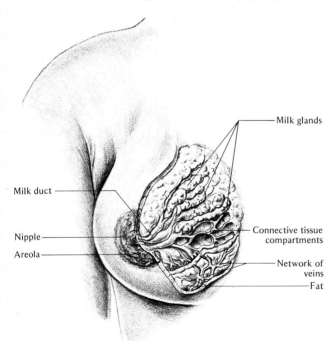

Figure 3-12 The human breast.

types to smaller and flatter ones (see Fig. 3-13). It seems that brassiere companies, with cries of "a quarter of an inch," "lifts and separates," and certain magazines and doll companies have created and help to maintain models of "perfect" breast architecture that the average woman cannot hope to achieve. This has contributed to an anxiety on the part of some women concerning their relative attractiveness and whether breast-feeding modifies or ruins this attractiveness. This concern may be correlated with the fact that only 10 percent of American women ever breast-feed. The truth is, nursing does *not* permanently alter the size, shape, or "lift" of the breasts. During pregnancy the breasts become heavier, and the ligaments that hold them in place may stretch, causing the breasts to hang a little bit lower in the future. However, nursing places no additional strain on the breasts and cannot produce further changes in their architecture.

During pregnancy the breasts grow, but milk production does not occur. However a yellowish, alkaline secretion called colostrum usually is present the last few weeks of pregnancy and for 3 to 4 days after delivery. Colostrum has a much lower fat and carbohydrate content but a higher level of protein and vitamin A than does mother's milk. According to many physiologists, milk

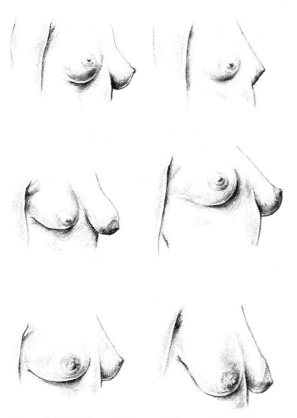

Figure 3-13 Different sizes and shapes of breasts

production during pregnancy is inhibited by high levels of progesterone secreted by the placenta. Apparently progesterone inhibits prolactin release from the anterior pituitary gland. (Prolactin is known to stimulate milk manufacture by the glands in the breast.) At the time of delivery, the expulsion of the placenta removes the inhibitory influence of progesterone. This reduced influence of progesterone coupled with uterine contractions and suckling on the nipples will cause prolactin release as well as cortisol secretion from the adrenal cortex.

Milk production refers to the manufacture of milk and does not mean the release of milk from the nipple into an infant's mouth; the latter is often called milk "letdown." Milk letdown requires a further suckling reflex. During nursing, stimulation of the nipple causes release of the hormone oxytocin from the pituitary. Oxytocin will cause contraction of the smooth muscle surrounding the milk-producing glands so that the milk is propelled into the ducts and out of the nipple (see Fig. 3-14).

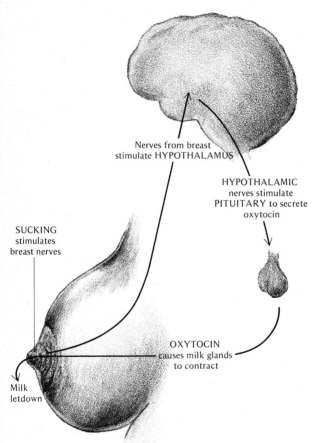

Nerves from breast
stimulate HYPOTHALAMUS

HYPOTHALAMIC
nerves stimulate
PITUITARY to secrete
oxytocin

SUCKING
stimulates
breast nerves

OXYTOCIN
causes milk glands
to contract

Milk
letdown

Figure 3-14   Sucking reflex. Sucking stimulates release of oxytocin from pituitary, and milk is let down.

Breast-feeding is a matter of individual choice. There are a number of alleged advantages and disadvantages which should be examined carefully (Silver et al.).

Advantages of Breast-Feeding:

1   Mother's milk is relatively inexpensive and more convenient.
2   Nursing causes uterine contractions which help to restore the organ to prepregnancy state.
3   Development of love and closeness between participants occurs.
4   Colostrum contains antibodies which reduce local bacterial infections and consequent digestive upsets, which include diarrhea.
5   Colostrum also contains a natural laxative that can aid the first few bowel movements.
6   Mother's milk is more nutritious and contains a better balance of constituents than cow's milk. For example, cow's milk contains more protein, which can form indigestible curds in the infant's digestive tract. These proteins, however, can be removed by boiling the milk. Cow's milk contains less sugar and vitamin C but more calcium and phosphorus salts in proportions that differ from mother's milk.
7   Nursing has been known to inhibit ovulation temporarily. But this varies and should not be used as a contraceptive technique.
8   There is a tendency to overfeed an infant with the bottle, and earlier switches to solid food often occur in such situations. Overfeeding leads to the growth and development of fat storage cells. Excessive amounts of this tissue, once formed, remain through life and are associated with obesity in adolescence (Brook).

Disadvantages of Breast-Feeding:

1   The constant high temperature of mother's milk can make weaning to cooler formulas or cow's milk difficult.
2   The amount of mother's milk obtained by an infant at any one sitting is difficult to determine.
3   Many nursing mothers develop painful cracked nipples. Cracked nipples can lead to bacterial invasion and result in inflammation of the breast, called *mastitis.*
4   Evidence from seven United States cities has shown concentrations of DDT in mother's milk that are in excess of the World Health Organization's recommended maximum concentration (Wilson et al.).

BIBLIOGRAPHY

Bailey, J., and J. Marshall. 1970. The relationship of the post-ovulatory phase of the menstrual cycle to total length, *J. Biosoc. Sci.,* **2**:123–132.
Baker, T. G. 1963. A quantitative and cytological study of germ cells in human ovaries, *Proc. Soc. London,* Ser. B., **158**:417.
Bardwick, J. 1971. *The Psychology of Women,* Harper & Row, New York.
Bardwick, J. 1972. Her body, the battleground, *Psych. Today,* Feb. Issue.

Bartelmez, G. W. 1957. The phases of the menstrual cycle and their interpretation in terms of the pregnancy cycle, *Am. J. Obstet. Gynecol.,* **74:**931.

Bedford, J. M. 1970. The saga of mammalian sperm from ejaculation to syngamy, in H. Gibian and E. J. Plotz (eds.), *Mammalian Reproduction,* pp. 124–182. Springer-Verlag, Berlin.

Blandau, R. J. 1969. Gamete transport—comparative aspects, in E. S. E. Hafex and R. J. Blandau (eds.), *The Mammalian Oviduct—Comparative Biology and Methodology,* p. 129. University of Chicago Press, Chicago.

Brook, C. G. D. 1972. Evidence for a sensitive period in adipose-cell replication in man, *Lancet,* **2:**624–627.

Caldwell, B. V. 1970. The role of the uterus in the regulation of ovarian periodicity, in H. Gibian and E. J. Plotz (eds.), *Mammalian Reproduction,* pp. 356–388. Springer-Verlag, Berlin.

Clewe, T. H., and L. Mastroianni Jr. Mechanisms of ovum pickup, I. Functional capacity of rabbit oviducts ligated near the fimbria, *Fertil. Steril.* **9:**13.

Cohen, J. 1971. The comparative physiology of gamete populations, in O. Lowenstein (ed.), *Advances in Comparative Physiology and Biochemistry,* vol. 4, pp. 268–362. Academic, New York.

Dalton, K. 1964. *The Premenstrual Syndrome.* Charles C Thomas, Springfield, Ill.

De Allende, I. L. C., and O. Orias. 1950. *Cytology of Human Vagina.* Hoeber-Harper, New York.

Fink, P. J. 1969. A review of the investigations of Masters and Johnson, in P. J. Fink and V. B. O. Hammett (eds.), *Sexual Function and Dysfunction.* Chap. 1. Davis, Philadelphia.

Ford, C. S., and F. A. Beach. 1951. *Patterns of Sexual Behavior.* Harper & Row, New York.

Franchi, L. L. 1970. The ovary, in E. E. Philipp et al. (eds.), *Scientific Foundations of Obstetrics and Gynecology,* pp. 107–134. Davis, Philadelphia.

Frank, Otto. 1952. *Ann Frank: The Diary of a Young Girl.* Doubleday, Garden City, N.Y.

Israel, S. L. 1970. Menstruation, in E. E. Philipp et al. (eds.), *Scientific Found. Obstet. & Gynec.* pp. 98–104. Davis, Philadelphia.

Krantz, K. E. 1970. The anatomy and physiology of the vulva and vagina and the anatomy of the urethra and bladder, in E. E. Philipp et al. (eds.), *Scientific Found. Obstet. & Gynec.* pp. 47–64. Davis, Philadelphia.

Loraine, J. A., and E. T. Bell. 1968. Fertility and contraception in the human female. E. & S. Livingstone, Ltd., London.

Masters, W. H., and V. E. Johnson. 1966. *Human Sexual Response.* Little, Brown, Boston.

Markee, J. E. 1950. The endocrine basis of menstruation, in J. V. Meigs and S. H. Sturgis (eds.), *Progress in Gynecology,* Grune & Stratton, New York.

Mossman, H. W. 1968. A critique of our progress toward understanding the biology of the mammalian ovary, in M. Diamond (ed.), *Perspectives in Reproduction and Sexual Behavior.* Indiana University Press, Bloomington.

Noyes, R. W. 1966. Morphological changes in the endometrium during menstrual cycle, in R. B. Greenblatt (ed.), *Ovulation,* p. 319. Lippincott, Philadelphia.

Okkels, H. 1950. *The Histophysiology of the Human Endometrium in Menstruation and Its Disorders,* E. T. Engle (ed.). Charles C Thomas, Springfield, Ill.

Paige, K. 1973. The curse of religion, *Newsweek,* **82** (19):66.

Pepper, H., and S. Lindsay. 1960. Levels of platelets, leukocytes and 17-hydroxycorticosteroids during the normal menstrual cycle, *Proc. Soc. Exp. Biol. Med.,* **104:**145.

Ramey, E. 1972. Men's cycles (They have them too, you know.), *Ms. Mag.,* Spring Issue, p. 8.

Reid, D. E. 1972. The embryology and anatomy of the female reproductive tract, in D. E. Reid et al. (eds.), *Principles and Management of Human Reproduction.* Saunders, Philadelphia.

Ross, G. T., et al. 1970. Pituitary and gonadal hormones in women during spontaneous and induced ovulatory cycles, *Recent Prog. Horm. Res.,* **26:**1348.

Silver H. K., et al. 1969. *Handbook of Pediatrics.* 8th ed., Lange Medical Publ., Los Altos, California.

Simpson, G. G. 1961. *Principles of Animal Taxonomy,* Columbia, New York.

Vande Wiele, R. L., et al. 1970. Mechanisms regulating the menstrual cycle in women, *Recent Prog. Horm. Res.,* **26:**63–95.

Vander et al. 1975. *Human Physiology,* McGraw-Hill, New York.

Wilson, D. J., et al. 1973. DDT concentrations in human milk, *Am. J. Dis. Child.,* **125:**814–817.

Young, W. C. 1961. The mammalian ovary, in W. C. Young (ed.), *Sex and Internal Secretions,* vol. I, pp. 449–496. Williams & Wilkins, Baltimore.

Zuckerman, S., et al. (eds.). 1962. *The Ovary,* vol. I. Academic, New York.

Chapter 4

The Genesis of Sexuality

There appear to be some striking differences between male and female anatomy, and yet many of these differences are really a matter of degree. As seen in Table 4-1, a large number of anatomical characters possessed by one sex are also present in the other sex but in modified form (H. W. Jones). In addition, Overzier points out that there are five basic types of urogenital systems in adult humans ranging from the "purely female" to the "purely male." The intermediates are individuals with ambiguous genitalia and are called intersexes (Polani).

But humans, by nature, tend to suffer from the "cubby-hole" syndrome—everyone must fit into a distinct classification. As Weston La Barre has said, "To be human is constantly to be burdened with self definition." One semester, "Charles" Virginia Prince, male transvestite, spoke to our class on human sexuality and gave still further evidence of the human need to classify with the statement that "she" was "feminine" but not a "female." All of this ultimately led the class into postponing the creation of precise definitions in favor of a further analysis of the factors that lead to the development and maintenance of sexuality.

What are the components that contribute to the development of sexuality?

Table 4-1 Some Homologous Portions of the Genitalia

Embryonic source	Adult male	Adult female
Indifferent gonad (medulla and cortex)	Testes from medulla	Ovary from cortex
Müllerian duct	Degenerates Remnants on appendix testis and a small bit of vaginalike tissue on the bladder	Fallopian tubes Uterus Portion of vagina
Wolffian duct	Epididymis Vas deferens Seminal vesicle	Degenerates Remnant on ovaries
Urethral primordia	Prostate Cowper's gland (bulbourethral)	Skene's glands Bartholin's glands
Genital tubercle	Glans penis	Clitoris
Genital swelling	Scrotum	Labia majora

A number of sexologists[1] have categorized several major elements, which are summarized in Table 4-2 and discussed in the following sections. Usually all ingredients correlate with one another in the production of a female or male person. Occasionally, due to unusual routes of development, one or more ingredients do not correspond with the others, and this results in one of many variations potentially possible in our species. For instance, an individual with the male chromosome pattern XY may have femalelike genitalia. Many humans often have difficulty when comparing these variations with the culturally derived but hypothetical ideal or standard, and the degree of difficulty depends on the extent of variation. Some of the variations have been called "deviates," "perverts," and just "abnormal." The remainder of this chapter will serve as an introduction to the genesis of various ingredients of sexuality.

SEX CHROMOSOMES

Sex chromosome combination is an extremely important ingredient of sexuality because it determines whether the fetal gonads will develop into testes or ovaries. In the normal genetic male, the combination is XY; and in the female, it is XX. However, a few people fall into neither of these classifications. For instance, the so-called superfemale has three X chromosomes, and the so-called supermale has one X and two Y chromosomes (see Table 4-3). Actually, "supermale" and "superfemale" are poor terms, because these people do not appear to be more male or more female than average. Furthermore, presence of an extra chromosome of any type is often likely to produce abnormalities, such as mental retardation, that have nothing to do with normal X or Y function. A few people possess a mosaic distribution of chromosomes; for example, some

---

[1]Armstrong; Hampson, 1964, 1965; Brown and Lynn; Whalen, 1966; Money; La Barre.

Table 4-2 Summary of Ingredients of Sexuality

Biological ingredients	Suggested readings
1 Sex chromosomes	Armstrong, 1964; Hamerton, 1971; White, 1954
2 Structure and function of gonads	Jones, 1968; Jost, 1970; Witschi, 1951
3 Hormones during fetal life	Jost, 1970; Mittwoch et al., 1969
4 Accessory sex organs: Internal genitalia (uterus, fallopian tubes, vas deferens, etc.) External genitalia (penis, clitoris, etc.)	Elger et al., 1970; Jones, 1968; Jost, 1970
5 Psychosexual differentiation of the brain	Phoenix et al., 1968; Beach, 1969; Money, 1969
6 Hormones during puberty	Hamburg and Lunde, 1966; Money, 1969; Phoenix et al., 1968
7 Secondary sex characteristics: Body form, composition, proportions, hair distribution, etc.	Cortes and Gatti, 1970; La Barre, 1971; Thompson, 1961
Bio-psychosocial ingredients	
1 Sex assignment (reared as male or female)	Hampson, 1964; Hampson, 1965; La Barre, 1971
2 Gender and role identity	Johnson, 1963; Kagan, 1969; Lynn, 1962
3 Gender orientation (preferred gender of sexual partner)	La Barre, 1971; Whalen, 1966
4 Sexual motivation—libido, drive, desire, etc.	Hardy, 1964; Kirkendall, 1961; Whalen, 1971

of their cells may have two X chromosomes, and other cells may have XXY. Other people may have only one sex chromosome.

People who are not biologically a "typical" male or "typical" female are called _intersex_. Accordingly, a person who has an abnormal number of sex chromosomes is considered an intersex, even though, like many XXX females and XYY males, she or he may be anatomically normal and able to have children. A frequent cause of variations in chromosome number is _nondisjunction_, which is failure of a pair of chromosomes to separate during meiosis. Thus one germ cell receives both members of the pair and the other cell receives neither. Nondisjunction of the sex chromosome pair can lead to an XX secondary oocyte or XY sperm or to an oocyte or sperm that has no sex chromosome. However, scientists are still at a loss to explain how the rare XXXX or XXXXX individual arises. We should mention here that not all intersex conditions are caused by genetic abnormalities. For instance, it is believed that an abnormal hormonal environment during certain stages of fetal development can lead to people who have both male and female genitalia; more will be said about this subject later.

Scientists can detect sex chromosome abnormalities in humans by using the following techniques:

1 _Barr Technique_ (Barr and Bertram). In the human female a tiny clump

Table 4-3 Some Human Variants and the Correlated Abnormal Sex Chromosomes

Classification	Genotype	Phenotype
"Superfemale" (poly X syndrome)	Mostly XXX; a few with XXXX or XXXXX	Body proportions normal and female. Some irregularity of menstruation but normal offspring produced. High degree of mental retardation, but most surveys done in mental institutions.
"Supermale"	XYY plus other, rarer types (e.g., XXYY)	First discovered 1960. Tall, thin with normal male genitalia; acne. All IQ levels.
Turner's syndrome (ovarian agenesis)	XO plus 20 other, rarer genotypes	A female with underdeveloped ovaries; other sexual organs also immature; short, stocky stature. Feminine psychosexual identity and not prone to mental retardation, contrary to popular belief.
Klinefelter's syndrome	XXY plus at least 11 other genotypes	Males with small testes, penis, etc. May be tall and slender but occasionally obese. IQ superior in a few, retarded in others. Sex motivation very low.
True hermaphrodites	Mostly with XX; few with mosaic (e.g., XX/XXY)	Rare—114 recorded patients beginning 1964. Ovarian and testicular tissue present. Majority reared as boys due to male-appearing genitalia but breasts may develop; female genitalia may be rudimentary. Various causes.

Source: Jones and Baramki, 1968; Money, 1969.

can be detected at the edge of the nucleus of many nondividing cells. This clump is called a *Barr* body (Fig. 4-1), and it actually represents one of the two X chromosomes. The number of Barr bodies is usually one less than the number of X chromosomes in the cell; a male, therefore, has none. Any abnormal number of X's will show up as an increase in the number of Barr bodies. This sexual difference in cells shows up as early as the sixteenth day following conception, and the technique may be used to reveal abnormalities before birth. The technique is also used prior to the Olympic games to verify whether competing female athletes are indeed female. A similar sexual difference, or dimorphism, exists between some types of white blood cells in

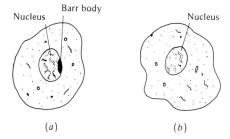

Figure 4-1 Barr Bodies. (*a*) Nucleus of normal female cell has one Barr body; (*b*) normal male has none.

males and females. The nuclei of certain white blood cells in girls and women often contain a drumstick-shaped appendage which is lacking in the male. Each "drumstick" represents one X chromosome.

   2 *Full Chromosome Counts.* During cell division the chromosomes become visually separate distinct entities. Photographs can be taken of the details seen through the microscope, and the pictures of the chromosomes can be cut out of the photograph, arranged in order of descending length, and numbered. Abnormalities in number, length, or shape will show up readily.

   3 *Fluorescence.* Laura Zech has shown that a portion of the Y chromosome will fluoresce brightly when stained with compounds formerly used to treat malaria. The presence of a Y chromosome can thus easily be shown in spermatozoa and other cells. This technique may revolutionize our ability to distinguish between X- and Y-bearing sperm and will aid in detection of chromosomal abnormalities involving the Y.

GONADAL SEX

When a human embryo is 28 days old (postconception) and less than $1/2$ in long, its gonads are in an "indifferent" stage of development and are not recognizable as either ovaries or testes. They are composed of an outer cortex, an inner medulla, and germ cells that have wandered in from the yolk sac, a region not actually part of the embryo but attached to it via the digestive system. Differentiation of the testes first becomes evident when an embryo is 7 weeks old. However, if an ovary is to develop, it will not be recognizable until much later (11 to 12 weeks). Witschi has proposed a theory that the cortex of the indifferent gonad produces a substance (which he calls corticene) and the medulla produces another chemical substance (medullarine), each of them antagonistic to the other. In a normal genetic male, medullarine predominates under the influence of the Y chromosome, causing the degeneration of the cortex and transformation of the medulla into a testis. In a genetic female, ovarian differentiation results from the converse process—corticene prevails and the cortex becomes the ovary while the medulla degenerates. A. Jost, however, has suggested that the hypothesis proposed by Witschi is unnecessarily complicated. He supports instead the alternative concept that the female sex is the neutral sex which develops in the absence of the Y chromosome. He believes that no cortical inducer such as corticene is necessary for the ovary to develop. The absence of the Y chromosome and concomitant lack of medullarine or some other chemical inducer means that a testis will not form and an ovary will. Basically, the embryo is female and will automatically continue this development unless the Y-controlled chemical inducer and male hormone reroute the direction into maleness (see Fig.4-2).

Influence of the Y Chromosome on Gonads

All evidence points to the following hypotheses concerning functions of the Y chromosome in relation to gonadal development:

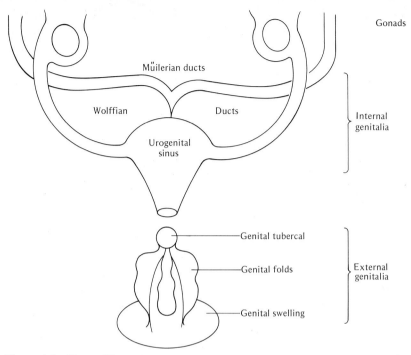

Figure 4-2 The undifferentiated genital system during the fifth to sixth week postconception (embryo is $1/5$ to $1/6$ in in length). Gonads begin differentiating at 7 weeks for male and 12 weeks for female. Internal genitalia differentiates at 10 weeks. External genitalia become distinct by the twelfth week.

    1 It stimulates testes formation, and in its absence an ovary develops (Hamerton).

    2 The Y or a portion of it may act as a control center that turns on the gene(s) responsible for actually stimulating the medulla and inhibiting the cortex (Hamerton).

    3 This gene(s) is probably located somewhere on the X chromosome (McFeely et al.).

    4 Although presently unidentified, there may be additional controlling centers that are similar to the Y in function but are located on chromosomes other than the Y or X (Hamerton).

    5 Evidence indicates that the Y chromosome in concert with the X also controls growth and the suppression of certain growth abnormalities such as early cessation of growth in the long bones (Ferguson-Smith).

    Additional Y chromosomes in the genotype such as in "supermales (XYY)" have been correlated with acne and tallness. Claims of unusual aggressiveness and mental retardation in men with XYY have also been made, but require further substantiation.

    Recent evidence regarding behavioral implications of the XYY genotype has been summarized by Ernest Hook. The XYY characteristic shows up in only 0.11 percent of the general population but has a much higher incidence (2 percent) among the males residing at mental-penal institutions. In an attempt to explain why so many men with the XYY genotype are placed in mental-penal institutions, at least three hypotheses have surfaced:

1 XYY males are more often found in environmental situations conducive to antisocial behavior than are XY males. For instance, if the parents receive poor nutrition and poor health care, they may be more likely to produce an XYY offspring. To compound matters, the frustrations of poverty may be conducive to antisocial behavior.

2 Acne and unusual tallness are physical characteristics definitely correlated with the XYY genotype, and they may well seem more threatening to juries, judges, and law-enforcement officials than the less-forbidding height and clearer complexion of the XY male. Thus, the XYY male, by virtue of his physical appearance may be more susceptible to conviction and imprisonment than the XY male.

3 Some nervous impairment or hormonal imbalance exists in the XYY individual and is responsible for his antisocial behavior.

These hypotheses are currently under investigation; the truth may involve a combination of all three or some new concept heretofore unseen.

Influence of the X Chromosome on Gonads

The X chromosome is definitely known to influence a number of characteristics not directly related to gonadal development—for example, red-green color blindness and a type of muscular dystrophy. New evidence indicates that its presence is also required for normal gonadal development and function.

1 Genes regulating testes formation are actually located on the X; however, a controlling center on the Y chromosome is necessary to activate these genes (McFeely et al.).

2 The presence of two X chromosomes is required if normal ovaries are to develop and function; however, the presence of one or more Y's is known to inhibit proper ovarian development. The presence of one X as in Turner's syndrome (XO) leads to some development of an ovary in the fetus, but this ovary will not continue to develop normally following birth if the second X is missing (Hamerton).

INFLUENCE OF FETAL HORMONES ON INTERNAL AND EXTERNAL GENITALIA

During the fifth to sixth week of gestation, organs that will become the internal and external genitalia are undifferentiated. At this time the internal genitalia in an embryo of either genetic sex consists of two pairs of simple ducts or tubes. One pair, called the *Müllerian ducts*, will ultimately develop into the fallopian

tubes, uterus, and upper third of the vagina if the embryo is a genetic female (Fig. 4-2). The other pair, called the *Wolffian ducts,* will differentiate
into the sperm ducts, seminal vesicles, and epididymis if the embryo is a genetic male.

The external genitalia of both sexes initially consist of a *genital tubercle,* a
pair of *genital folds,* and a *genital swelling.* In a genetic female, the tubercle
becomes the clitoris, the folds form the labia minora, and the swelling develops
into the labia majora. In the genetic male, the tubercle differentiates into the
glans penis, the folds form the shaft of the penis, and the swelling develops into
the scrotum.

In nonhuman vertebrates and, theoretically, in humans, the development
of the internal and external genitalia depends on the presence or absence of
certain hormones in the fetus (Figs. 4-3 and 4-4). The fetal testes of amphibians,
rats, hamsters, and rabbits secrete (1) androgens, which are responsible for
stimulating development of the male structures, and (2) a second substance,
called the Müllerian inhibitor, which is important in suppressing development
of the Müllerian duct. Absence of these two substances results in Wolffian duct
degeneration and the development of female genitalia. Thus, in a genetic
female, hormones are not required for the genitalia to develop.

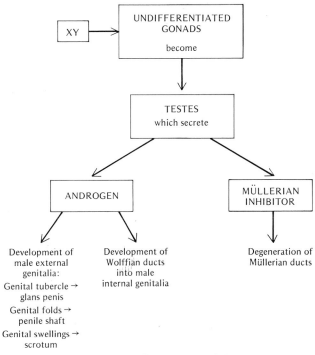

Figure 4-3 Differentiation of the male genital system.

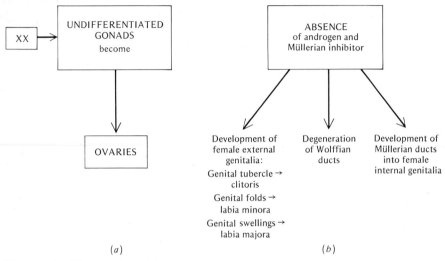

Figure 4-4   Differentiation of (a) female gonads and (b) female genitalia.

SEXUAL SELF-IDENTITY

Sexual self-identity has been defined as the feeling of how well one's characteristics correspond to his or her own concept of the ideal male or female (Kagan). The ideal, of course, is created by the society in which that person lives. Recently, other workers have distinguished between gender identity and gender role where *identity* involves a more private feeling of gender and *role* is "everything that a person says and does to indicate to others or to the self the degree that one is either male, or female, or ambivalent" (Money and Ehrhardt).

Many experimenters believe that gender identity as well as most "male" or "female" behavior is determined by the sex the person is officially assigned at birth. Assignment is made on the basis of external genitalia, and this role becomes fixed within a very short time and cannot be reversed (Hampson, 1964; Hampson, 1965; Money). Thus a genetic male with ambiguous but female-appearing genitals may be assigned a female role and reared as such. This person would then behave as a girl and would not wish to change even if the true identity were later discovered. Hampson and Hampson (1961) found that 23 out of a sample of 25 individuals assigned and reared in a sex role which contradicted the appearance of their genitalia eventually came to terms with the inconsistency and assumed the sex of their upbringing.

However, evidence is accumulating that many exceptions also exist (Diamond). Examples may be given of individuals assigned to one sex wishing to switch to the opposite sex, the desire for change often occurring at or near puberty. The inference from these latter examples is that, psychosexually, brains may have been primed or organized for one sex during early development, and despite assignment and upbringing in the opposite sex, this organization may take precedence.

Many new studies have been done. These include experiments to determine the effect of prenatal hormones on the later sexual behavior of nonhumans. They also include observations of measurable differences between male and female human infants. As a result, more scientists are reaching the conclusion that infants are definitely predisposed at birth toward one sex or the other in terms of gender identity and certain behavior. However, these predispositions can be modified by the child's social environment (Diamond).

Psychosexual Differentiation of the Brain

Unlearned Sexual Behavior in Nonhumans   In humans it is very difficult to distinguish between sexual behavior that is unlearned and that which is learned. Therefore, most of our evidence about the establishment of male or female sexual behavior at birth comes from nonhuman mammals such as rats, guinea pigs, rabbits, and Rhesus monkeys. Males of these species usually show acyclical sexual behavior during breeding seasons. That is, throughout the breeding season, male hormone levels in the blood are continuously high, and a consistent pattern of sexual behavior is exhibited. In male rats, these patterns include mounting without intromission (that is, mounting without penis penetration into vagina), mounting with intromission, and mounting with intromission and ejaculation. Female behavior is cyclical and changes constantly along with hormone levels in relatively distinct entities called *estrus cycles.* Ovulation occurs at the peak of such cycles either spontaneously (rats) or by a reflex initiated by intercourse (rabbits). During these peaks, female rats, for example, also show a very typical pattern of behavior: lordosis (back arching), ear wiggling, and hopping. Thus, in female rats, two components of sexuality are involved: estrus cycles and corresponding cycles in sexual behavior. Two components also exist in males: acyclic spermatogenesis and male sexual behavior. Occasionally, female behavior is shown by normal genetic males and vice versa. *This means that each sex possesses the neuromuscular apparatus for both male and female sexual behavior* (Whalen, 1968). What then determines which behavior shall predominate in any given individual?

Brain Differentiation in Nonhumans   Female rats that have their ovaries removed at birth and are given injections of estrogen and progesterone as adults will display female behavior (Whalen and Edwards). Male rats that have had their testes removed shortly after birth (before the tenth postnatal day) and given injections of estrogen and progesterone as adults also show female behavior (Grady et al.). When pregnant guinea pigs are injected with testosterone, the genetic female offspring show masculinization of structures and behavior. As adults these female offspring show a reduced responsiveness to female hormones but an increased responsiveness to male hormones and will perform mounting behavior (Phoenix et al., 1959). Testosterone has also been given a few days before birth to Rhesus monkeys that were genetic females. When these females matured, they showed malelike sexual behavior, as well as masculine behavior not directly related to sex, i.e., more rough and tumble play, aggressiveness, and play initiation (Phoenix et al., 1968). Implanting small quantities of testosterone into the brain has led to similar results. For example, Nadler and Wagner et al. implanted tiny quantities of testosterone in the hypothalamus of newborn female rats. As adults, these rats were sterile, did not ovulate, and failed to show cyclical fluctuations in the cornification of the vagina.

These experiments and many others have led a number of scientists to reach the following conclusions:

1 *Testosterone the "organizer"* (Fig. 4-5). Regardless of genetic sex, individuals will develop femalelike genitalia and display femalelike behavior as long as testosterone was lacking at certain critical times of fetal development. Testosterone produced from the fetal testes "organizes" the circuits of the brain controlling future male sexual behavior and acyclic sperm production but somehow "turns down" the circuits that would otherwise control female behavior and the estrus cycles. Estrogen does not play a role in the developing fetal brain but will later be involved in activating the adult female brain. Thus an individual of any genetic sex would become male if testosterone is present at a certain critical time when the brain is developing the circuitry associated with sexuality. In addition, a *strong* androgen such as *testosterone* from the *fetal testes* is required for fully male behavior; the weaker androgens produced by the adrenal glands are insufficient.[2] Male rats have been put under stress by rough handling both before and soon after birth. When the developing rats are exposed to stress, adrenal androgens appear in greater quantities in the blood than does testosterone. If more weak-type androgen than testosterone is present at the critical time of brain differentiation, the organizing ability of testosterone is reduced and the males will show increased femalelike behavior (Ward).

2 *Critical Periods.* Apparently testosterone must exert its influence on the brain at certain critical periods of development or it will not be effective in priming for male behavior and reproductive functioning. These periods appear to differ for various species: in guinea pigs, rabbits, Rhesus monkeys, and humans, the critical period occurs before birth; in rats, it occurs between 1 and 5 days after birth. The shortness of the critical periods has led some authors to imply that more problems can occur with male brain development than with female brain development, and they cite a higher incidence of transexuals, transvestites, and homosexuals among human males as examples (Bardwick).

It must be emphasized that organizing and subsequent activation of male and female circuits should not be construed as either an all-male or an all-female situation. It is highly probable that due to variations in hormonal

---

[2]All the androgens act like testosterone, but they vary in effective strength. The testes produce two and possibly three androgens, testosterone being the strongest. The adrenal gland produces at least five androgens, mostly with weak activity.

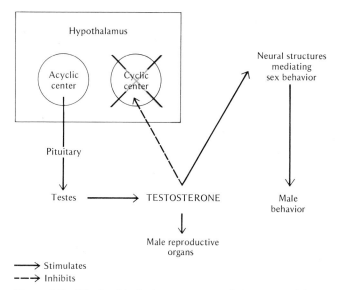

> Stimulates
--→ Inhibits

Figure 4-5 Effects of testosterone on neural structures of the newborn rat. In the hypothalamus testosterone impairs the further functioning of a cyclic center which is active in females. Testosterone also permanently modifies the neural structures mediating adult sex behaviour.

levels at critical times and/or to individual differences in the sensitivity of the responding brain structures, most individuals will have both circuits primed, but one circuit will be dominant. Thus the behavior of one individual can show elements of both sexes. In some extreme cases even the anatomy and physiology of the reproductive process is intermediate, and a person of this type would be classified as a form of intersex.

Some eminent sexologists do not entirely agree with the organizing effects of testosterone on male brains. R. E. Whalen (1968) states that lack of testosterone at the critical time during development leads to femalelike behavior in adult rats not because the brain lacks differentiation but rather because the penis fails to differentiate. He states that males castrated at the critical time of brain development show adequate mounting behavior (i.e., normal male motivation), but intromission and ejaculation are reduced (i.e., male performance is abnormal) because the penis is too short and not responsive to stimulation. Thus, the part of the brain controlling male motivation must be organized in some other way, and lack of testosterone at the critical time leads to poor penis development and thus poor male performance.

The final assessment of brain differentiation is yet to come. Evidence continues to mount that fetal testosterone or strong androgen is indeed the organizer. In a recent review of the subject, Gerall concluded that potential for masculine behavior in both genetic sexes (human and nonhuman) is fully developed when testosterone is present during critical periods of brain development. The female component is suppressed in direct proportion to the amount of strong androgen present. Large amounts completely inhibit female physiological and behavioral capacities. Smaller amounts during fetal life have varying effects that show up after the individual reaches puberty. It does become evident that even in a female fetus androgen may occur in varying amounts derived from the mother via the placenta or arising from the fetus's own adrenal glands. In humans, genetic females with a history of prenatal exposure to androgen, but with normal female genitalia, will show a higher incidence of lesbian behavior compared with genetic females without such androgen exposure (Money and Ehrhardt).

Human Sexual Distinctions at Birth

At birth boys on the average are larger, weigh more, and have more muscle mass than girls (Garn). They show greater motor activity and can raise their heads higher and earlier (Bell and Darling). Infant girls are more physically passive and show far greater sensitivity to a variety of stimuli; for example, girls will respond more to pain, touch, and pressure, and their skin has a greater ability to conduct electricity. Girls are also more irritable during a physical examination (Weller and Bell).

At 6 months of age, boys show greater attentiveness to a discontinuous musical tone. (Attentiveness has been measured by deceleration of the heart rate.) Girls are more attentive to a complex musical arrangement such as in a jazz concert (Kagan and Lewis). Also girls are much more capable of fixating on a visual stimulus such as a human face and show greater responsiveness and orientation to social situations (Lewis et al., Bardwick).

It appears that children are born with an already large number of characteristics originating in the genetic and hormonal milieu of fetal life. However, it is difficult to determine where heredity ends and learning begins. Some researchers claim that parents treat their male and female infants differently. For instance, the mother may babble more to her female infant and encourage a very close relationship between herself and the little girl; whereas she may foster greater independence in the tiny boy.

Social Environment and Sexual Behavior

The way an infant reacts initially to the environment is determined in part by the set of characteristics present at birth. This way of reacting as well as the assigned sex of the infant will elicit in turn a particular set of responses from parents and others which tends to strongly reinforce the original infant behavior. The child now learns those appropriate forms of activity which are most likely to produce positive and favorable responses from adults. The child tries out these activities by identifying with and copying members of his or her own sex and by acting as a counterpart to members of the opposite sex. The establishment of sex identity is most critical between the ages of eighteen months and four years, which is also the time of language acquisition. By the time the child is two years of age, it will be able to tell a male from a female. By the time the child is six years of age, an abstract concept of maleness and femaleness will have been conceived. When pairs of abstract designs were shown to six-year-olds, they invariably selected the larger, darker, more angular designs as representing something most like father, whereas the smaller, lighter-colored, less angular ones were selected as looking most like mother (Kagan).

Money and Ehrhardt, in one of the best analyses of gender differentiation, state, "Nature herself supplies the basic irreducible elements of sex difference which no culture can eradicate at least not on a large scale: women can menstruate, gestate, and lactate, and men cannot." As long as the child learns that these differences in sexual anatomy and functioning exist and maintains confidence in his or her future reproductive ability, then it makes little difference as to which optional characters of masculinity and femininity are exhibited by the parents. The mother could be a truck driver and the father a seamstress, but if each consistently gives the outward appearance of the appropriate sex in terms of anatomy and in terms of confidence in his and her own maleness and femaleness, the child will have few problems in developing his or her own sex-role identity.

In addition to a sexual self-identity, each person also develops a personal sexual, or erotic, style. The style includes the ability to satisfy one's sexual needs, the particular ways in which these needs are fulfilled, and the amount of sexual activity one exhibits. Development of a sexual style starts early in life, but it is highly influenced by the attitudes and information a person acquires at puberty from the family, peers, school, and the mass media. The qualities of the first sexual experiences also play a part. Evidence exists that when sexuality is explicit and openly discussed within the family and peer group, an individual will be prepared for high levels of sexual activity. However, individuals displaying the *highest* levels of sexual activity tend to be independent of both peer and family group and rely more heavily on their own sources of sex information, particularly the mass media—television, movies, magazines, books, and so on (Davis). There are two possible reasons for this, which may not necessarily be mutually exclusive: Even though sexual matters are freely discussed in the family, the parents may have trouble providing accurate information; consequently, the adolescent turns to books, television, and movies in order to find complete and reliable answers to questions. Alternatively, these individuals may for whatever reason be more oriented toward the media in the first place, and they may try to increase their understanding by reading books on sexuality and by viewing films that deal explicitly or implicitly with sexual relationships (Davis).

We come now full circle—back to the original question of the difference between maleness, femaleness, femininity, and masculinity. It should be apparent by now that there are no hard-and-fast definitions where exceptions would not apply. If definitions must be had, then they require much thought and care so as to avoid cryptic elements of sexism which occasionally slip into scientific explanations that should remain neutral. Some believe that concepts of feminine and masculine are totally derived from cultural models involving learned responses and having little or no basis in biology. Others believe that heredity and hormonal influences are like directors and producers setting the stage for a particular play. How the play eventually turns out is determined by the interaction between the actor and audience, that is, between the individual and his social environment.

BIBLIOGRAPHY

Armstrong, C. N. 1964. Intersexuality in man, in C. N. Armstrong and A. J. Marshall (eds.), *Intersexuality in Vertebrates Including Man*, pp. 349–389. Academic, London.

Bardwick, J. M. 1971. *Psychology of Women*. Harper & Row, New York.

Barr, M. L., and E. G. Bertram. 1949. Intersexuality, *Nature*, **163**:676–677.

Beach, F. 1969. It's all in your mind, *Psych. Today*, **3**(2):33.

Bell, R., and J. F. Darling. 1965. The prone head reaction in the human neonate: relation with sex and tactile sensitivity, *Child Dev.*, **36**(4): 943–949.

Brown, D. G., and D. B. Lynn. 1966. Human sexual development; an outline of components and concepts, *J. Mar. and Fam.*, **28**:155–162.

Cortes, J. B., and F. M. Gatti. 1970. Physique and propensity, *Psych. Today*, **4**(5):42–44.

Davis, P. 1974. Contextual sex-saliency and sexual activity: the relative effects of family and peer group in the sexual socialization process, *J. Mar. & Fam.*, Feb. Issue:196–202.

Diamond, M. 1968. *Perspectives in Reproduction and Sexual Behavior*, Indiana University Press, Bloomington.

Elger, W., et al., 1970. The significance of hormones in mammalian sex differentiation as evidenced by experiments with synthetic androgens and antiandrogens, in H. Gibian and E. J. Plotz (eds.), *Mammalian Reproduction*, pp. 33–44. Springer-Verlag, New York.

Ferguson-Smith, M. A. 1965. Karyotype-phenotype correlations in gonadal dysgenesis and their bearing on the pathogenesis of malformations, *J. Med. Genetics*, **2**:142.

Garn, S. M. 1958. Fat body size and growth in the newborn, *Hum. Biol.*, **30**:265–280.

Gerall, A. A. 1973. Influence of perinatal androgen on reproductive capacity, in J. Zubin & J. Money (eds.), *Contemporary Sexual Behavior: Critical Issues in the 1970's*, chap. 1. Johns Hopkins, Baltimore.

Grady, K. L., et al. 1965. Role of the developing rat testis in differentiation of the neural tissues mediating mating behavior, *J. Comp. Physiol. and Psych.*, **59**:176–182.

Hamburg, D. A., and D. T. Lunde. 1966. Sex hormones in the development of sex differences in human behavior, in E. E. Maccoby (ed.), *The Development of Sex Differences*, p. 24. Stanford, Stanford, Calif.

Hamerton, J. L. 1971. Sex determination and the significance of sex chromosome abnormalities in man and mammals, in J. L. Hamerton, *Human Cytogenetics*, pp. 169–195. Academic, New York.

Hampson, J. L. 1964. The case management of somatic sexual disorders in children; Psychologic considerations, in C. W. Lloyd (ed.), *Human Reproduction and Sexual Behavior*. Lea & Febiger, Philadelphia.

Hampson, J. L. 1965. Determinants of psychosexual orientation, in F. A. Beach (ed.), *Sex and Behavior*, pp. 108–132. Wiley, New York.

Hampson J. L., and J. G. Hampson. 1961. The ontogenesis of sexual behavior in man, in

W. C. Young (ed.), *Sex and Internal Secretions,* vol. II, pp. 1401–1432. Williams & Wilkins, Baltimore.

Hardy, K. R. 1964. An appetitional theory of sexual motivation, *Psychol. Rev.,* **71**(1):1–18.

Hook, E. B. 1973. Behavioral implications of the human XYY genotype, *Science,* **179** (4069):139–150.

Johnson, M. M. 1963. Sex role learning in the nuclear family, *Child Dev.,* **34**:319–333.

Jones, H. W., Jr. 1968. Development of genitalia, in A. C. Barnes (ed.), *Intra-Uterine Development,* pp. 253–272. Lea & Febiger, Philadelphia.

Jones, H. W., Jr., and T. A. Baramki. 1968. The basic forms of chromosomal aberrations, in A. C. Barnes (ed.), *Intra-Uterine Development,* pp. 327–361. Lea & Febiger, Philadelphia.

Jost, A. 1970. Hormonal factors in the sex differentiation of the mammalian foetus, *Philos. Trans. Soc. London,* Ser. B, **259**:119–131.

Kagan, J. 1969. Check one: male   female, *Psych. Today,* **3**(2):39.

Kagan, J., and M. Lewis. 1965. Studies in attention in the human infant, *Merrill-Palmer,* **11**:95–127.

Kirkendall, L. A. 1961. Sex drive, in A. Ellis and A. Abarbanel (eds.), *Modern Sex Practices,* pp. 172–191. *The Encyclopedia of Sexual Behavior* **1**:191. Ace, New York.

LaBarre, W. 1971. Anthropological perspectives in sexuality, in D. L. Grummon and A. M. Barclay (eds.), *A Search for Perspective,* pp. 38–53. Van Nostrand, New York.

Lewis, M., et al. 1966. Patterns of fixation in the young infant, *Child Dev.,* **37**(2):331–341.

Lynn, D. B. 1962. Sex role and parental identification, *Child Dev.,* **33**:555–564.

McFeely, R. A., et al. 1967. Chromosome studies in 14 cases of intersex in domestic mammals, *Cytogenetics* (Basel), **6**:242–253.

Mittwoch, U., et al. 1969. Growth of differentiating testes and ovaries, *Nature* (London), **224**:1323–1325.

Money, J. 1969. Sex reassignment as related to hermaphroditism and transexualism, in J. Money and R. Green (eds.), *Transexualism and Sex Reassignment,* pp. 91–113. Johns Hopkins, Baltimore.

Money, J. and A. Ehrhardt. 1973. *Man and Woman, Boy and Girl: The Differentiation and Dimorphism of Gender Identity from Conception to Maturity.* Johns Hopkins, Baltimore.

Nadler, R. D. 1965. Masculinization of the Female Rat by Intracranial Implantation of Androgen in Infancy, Unpublished doctoral dissertation, University of California Press, Los Angeles.

Overzier, C. 1963. Pseudo-hermaphroditism, in C. Overzier (ed.), *Intersexuality,* pp. 235–254. Academic, New York.

Phoenix, C. H., et al., 1959. Organizing action of prenatally administered testosterone propionate on the tissue mediating mating behavior in the female guinea pig, *Endocrinology,* **65**:369–382.

Phoenix, C. H., et al. 1968. Psychosexual differentiation as a function of androgenic stimulation, in M. Diamond (ed.), *Perspectives in Reproduction and Sexual Behavior,* Indiana University Press, Bloomington.

Polani, P. E. 1962. Sex chromosome anomalies in man, in J. L. Hamerton (ed.), *Chromosomes in Medicine,* pp. 73–139. Heinemann, London.

Romer, A. S. 1970. *The Vertebrate Body,* 4th ed. Saunders, Philadelphia.

Thompson, C. 1961. Femininity, in A. Ellis and A. Abarbanel (eds.), *The Nature of Sex,* pp. 43–54. *The Encyclopedia of Sexual Behavior.* Ace, New York.

Wagner, J. W., et al. 1966. Androgen sterilization produced by intracerebral implants of testosterone in neonatal female rats, *Endocrinology,* **79:**1135–1142.

Ward, I. L. 1972. Prenatal stress feminizes and demasculinizes the behavior of males, *Science,* **175** (4017):82–84.

Weller, G., and R. Bell. 1965. Basal skin conductance and neonatal state, *Child. Develop.,* **36:**647–657.

Whalen, R. E. 1966. Sexual motivation, *Psychol. Rev.,* **73**(2):151–163.

Whalen, R. E. 1968. Differentiation of the neural mechanisms which control gonadotropin secretion and sexual behavior, in M. Diamond (ed.), *Reproduction and Sexual Behavior,* pp. 303–340. Indiana University Press, Bloomington.

Whalen, R. E., and D. A. Edwards. 1967. Hormonal determinants of the development of masculine and feminine behavior in male and female rats, *Anat. Rec.,* **157:**173–180.

White, M. 1954. *Animal Cytology and Evolution,* 2d ed. Cambridge, New York.

Witschi, E. 1951. Embryogenesis of the adrenal and the reproductive glands, *Recent Prog. Horm. Res.,* **6**(1).

Zech, L. 1969, Investigation of metaphase chromosomes with DNA-binding fluorochromes, *Exp. Cell Res.,* **58:**463.

Chapter 5

Puberty

The body's physical condition has a strong influence on mood and thinking, and vice versa. This phenomenon is most clearly observed in the interaction between the mind and sexual functions. Thus the argument of whether genes or learning contribute more to sexual behavior makes little sense, for each bit of behavior is composed of both biological and psychological components in an ever-changing ratio that rarely involves continual dominance of one over the other. Herbert Marcuse in *Eros and Civilization* recognized the inextricable relationship of mind and body and called for a reduction in genital fixation and an "erotization" of the complete body, indeed the "entire personality" as an "instrument of pleasure." In his opinion, this would lead to a fusion of sexuality into our everyday lives, thereby eliminating the repression that has led to a preoccupation with sexual self-gratification. Whether you agree or disagree with this concept, learning about our sex organs in the context of a whole body and mind is indeed a valid approach.

Our sexuality develops from many sources, and it continues to develop throughout our lives. However, the physiological events that occur at puberty trigger a very rapid and noticeable phase of sexual maturation that we shall discuss in this chapter.

DEFINITIONS OF PUBERTY AND ADOLESCENCE

Prior to 1960, the simple acquisition of pubic hair was considered a sign of puberty. However, present studies define *puberty* as the sudden enlargement and maturation of the gonads, other genitalia, and secondary sexual characteristics that lead to reproductive capacity (Tanner, 1967). For females, important signs of puberty are breast development, appearance of pubic and axillary (underarm) hair, menarche, enlargement of the labia, and a sudden increase in height (Table 5-1). In males, signs of puberty include an increase in body height and enlargement of the penis and scrotum as well as growth of pubic and axillary hair (Table 5-2). Besides growth and changes in body proportions, there are modifications in the heart, blood vessels, and lungs that increase the ability to prolong muscular activity. At the base of all these alterations, and usually preceding them, are changes in the brain-hormonal system that controls the onset of puberty. Puberty ends when the person is physically capable of reproducing children—a condition that usually precedes legal adulthood by several years.

Adolescence is a socially defined developmental period. In the United States, a person is considered an adolescent from about the age of twelve or thirteen until one is able to assume full responsibility for oneself. Adolescence is a period of intensive learning, during which a person becomes able to cope with the practical realities of being an adult in a modern technological world. The period of adolescence tended to be shorter in our grandparents' time. And

Table 5-1 Sequence of Pubertal Changes in Girls

Characteristic	Age of first appearance, yr	Major hormonal influence
1 Appearance of breast bud followed by growth of breast	Breast bud, 8–13	Pituitary growth hormone, estrogen (maturation of milk glands), progesterone (maturation of milk ducts), thyroxine, etc.
2 Growth of pubic hair	8–14	Adrenal androgen
3 Body growth	9.5–14.5	Pituitary growth hormone, adrenal androgen, estrogen, etc.
4 Menarche	10–16.5	Hypothalamic releasing factors, FSH, LH, estrogen, and progesterone
5 Axillary (underarm) hair	Begins approximately 2 years after appearance of pubic hair	Adrenal androgens
6 Oil- and sweat-producing glands	Coincides approximately with axillary hair growth. Acne produced from clogged oil-producing glands	Adrenal androgens

Source: Modified from Tanner (1967) and Committee on Adolescence (1968).

Table 5-2 Sequence of Pubertal Changes in Boys

Characteristics	Age of first appearance, yr	Major hormonal influence
1 Growth of testes, scrotal sacs	10–13.5	Pituitary growth hormone, testosterone
2 Growth of pubic hair	10–15	Testosterone
3 Body growth	10.5–16	Pituitary growth hormone, testosterone, many others
4 Growth of penis	11–14.5	Testosterone
5 Changes in voice (growth of larynx)	Coincides approximately with penis growth.	Testosterone
6 Facial and axillary hair	Begins approximately 2 years after the appearance of pubic hair.	Testosterone
7 Oil and sweat glands	Coincides approximately with axillary hair growth. Acne produced from blocked oil-producing glands.	Testosterone

Source: Data modified from Tanner (1967) and Committee on Adolescence (1968).

in many tribal societies no adolescence exists—the child becomes an adult upon reaching puberty and performing certain tasks or initiation rites.

GROWTH

Following birth the velocity of body growth increases sharply until the end of the third year of life. At this point, rate of growth levels off and increases only slightly until puberty, when a marked acceleration occurs. In the United States, this accelerated growth usually begins two years earlier in girls than in boys but is less pronounced (see Fig. 5-1); however, considerable overlap does exist. Accurate predictions of adult height can be made by age eight, using information on height, chronological age, skeletal age, and prediction tables developed by Bayley and Pinneau.

The average maximum velocity of body growth for girls averaging 12.1 years of age has been recorded by Tanner at 9.0 cm/year and by Young at 7.0 cm/year. Boys show a peak velocity of 10.3 cm/year at the average age of 14.1 years (Tanner, 1967). Latest statistics show that the average height attained is 5 ft 9.9 in and 5 ft 6.6 in for an adult American male and female, respectively.

Girls, on the average, are ahead of boys in many aspects of maturation. Even in fetal life, females show an earlier hardening of the structures that become bones. The Y chromosome is known to contribute somehow to this relatively slow start among males. Children with XO (lacking one sex chromosome) resemble normal girls in their rates of growth; whereas children with XXY resemble normal boys (Tanner et al., 1959). A few areas of maturation find the male developing before the female. For example, boys are fertile

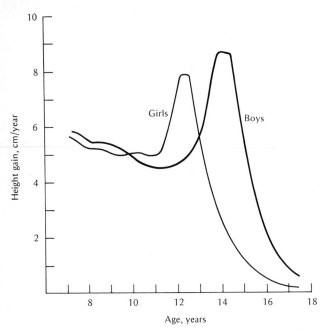

Figure 5-1 Adolescent spurt in height for boys and girls. The curves are from subjects who have their peak velocities within the age limits 12 to 13 years for girls and 14 to 15 years for boys. (*Marshall, 1970.*)

sooner than girls because the female usually does not release ova with any regularity until several years after menarche. In addition, boys, on the average, masturbate and experience coitus at younger ages than girls.

PROPORTIONS

Changes in bodily shape take place during puberty because various parts of the body grow at different rates (see Fig. 5-2). In boys, bone and muscle volume increase rapidly and under-the-skin fat decreases. Females, on the other hand, gain fat and accumulate less muscle and bone than boys do (Marshall). Thus, at puberty, boys appear taller and thinner than girls.

The male grows for a longer period of time, which accounts for his greater height and longer appendages relative to his trunk. In addition, differing patterns of growth lead to wider shoulders among males; whereas females develop broader hips, a more prominent rump, and thighs that show a greater angle of convergence from hip to knee. Position, shape, and size of the pelvic girdle account for most of these latter effects.

The pelvic girdle is composed of the lower portions of the backbone and the two hipbones; together, these structures form a casing around the lower trunk that protects the internal organs and provides the support necessary for

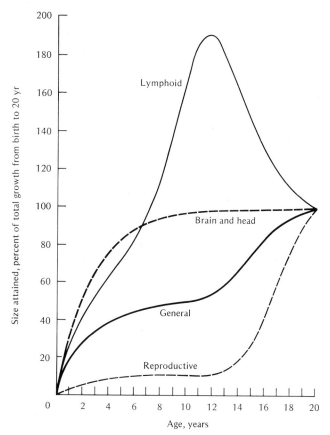

Figure 5-2 Growth curves of four major components of the body. Size at age 20 is 100% on the vertical scale. (Lymphoid tissue is involved in antibody production; it is found in the tonsils, in numerous special vessels and nodes, and in a number of other organs.) (*Tanner, 1967.*)

upright posture. If you look at Fig. 5-3, you will note that the hipbones are connected to the sacrum, which is a portion of the lower backbone. They then extend around the sides of the body and curve frontward, forming the bony ridge that you can feel underneath the pubic hair. At the midpoint of this ridge lies the pubic symphysis, a piece of cartilage that forms the joint between bones. During childbirth, the symphysis pubis stretches and thereby widens the pelvic cavity, through which the birth canal descends. Below and a little behind this front ridge lie the sockets that hold the ends of the thighbones.

    The pelvic architecture is an adaptive compromise among the mechanical demands for support of body organs in an upright posture, forces generated by lower limbs during upright walking, and the structural requirements of a birth canal in females. While a person is standing, the body weight is transmitted to the sacrum, from the sacrum to the hipbones, and thence to the thighbones. The

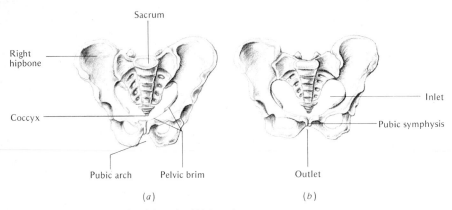

Right
hipbone

Sacrum

Coccyx

Pubic arch   Pelvic brim

Inlet

Pubic symphysis

Outlet

(a)   (b)

Figure 5-3 Human pelvis: (a) male; (b) female.

reciprocal force exerted upward on the girdle by the legs tends to squeeze the side walls of the pelvis together; however, the fusion of the two bones at the pubic symphysis prevents an inward collapse of the entire girdle. These two functions of the pelvic girdle occur in both sexes.

However, the requirements of birth are correlated with sex differences in pelvic shape; some of these are already present in the fetus, and others develop at puberty under the influence of hormonal and nutritional factors.

Looking at Fig. 5-3, notice that the *pelvic inlet* is the part of the pelvic cavity that is bounded along the front and sides by the pelvic brim and at the back by the sacrum. Below the inlet lies the *pelvic outlet,* which is located between the lowest parts of the hipbones and the coccyx, which is the bottom tip of the backbone. Since the birth canal lies inside the pelvic cavity, the pelvic inlet and outlet must be large enough to accommodate the head of a baby. At birth, females already have wider pelvic outlets, but there is hardly any sexual difference in the dimensions of the pelvic inlet, which in both sexes can be characterized as apelike. During female puberty, estrogen apparently stimulates growth of a newly formed center of bone located in the area where the hipbones connect with the thighbones (Tanner, 1967). This growth results in a wider pelvic inlet as well as broader hips in females. The female pelvis also tilts forward, which contributes to the protruding buttocks, the more pronounced lower back curve, and greater abdominal bulge which are characteristic of the female (see Table 5-3). Because the female's hips are wider, the thighs converge at a greater angle toward the knees.

There are variations in pelvic shape within each sex. Identification of those differences among adult females is particularly important because of possible problems associated with giving birth. The most important dimension is the pelvic inlet. Caldwell and Moloy have classified pelvic girdles according to this characteristic (see Table 5-4); inlet shapes other than gynecoid may lead to problems during childbirth.

Table 5-3 Characteristics of Adult Male and Female Pelvises

Characteristic	Male	Female
Bones	Massive, heavy, bumpy	Lighter in weight, thinner
Pelvic inlet	Narrow, heart-shaped; dimensions smaller than female	Generally gynecoidlike with greater dimensions than in male; occasionally android, anthropoid, or platypelloid (see Table 5-4)
Pelvis	Tilted backward	Tilted forward
Pelvic height	Tall	Shallow
Pelvic canal	Walls narrow and tend to converge	Walls wide and tend to diverge
Sacrum and coccyx	Placed forward	Placed backward
Pubic arch	Narrow; Gothic style; distance between forefinger and index finger	Wide; Roman style; distance between outstretched thumb and forefinger

PHYSIQUE AND TEMPERAMENT

Within both sexes, differences in proportions ultimately result in varying types of physique sometimes called somatotype, body habitus, or constitution. Cortes and Gatti report that although no cause-and-effect relationship can as yet be described, a correlation does exist between body build and temperament. A boy with a strong, powerful physique tends to develop an outgoing,

Table 5-4 Variations in Female Pelvic Girdle

Type	Description of inlet	Incidence
Gynecoid and gynecoidlike	Round	59%
Android and androidlike	Wedge or heart-shaped	22%
Anthropoid and anthropoidlike	Long oval	18%
Platypelloid	Flat	1%

relaxed personality; whereas a boy who is frail and has difficulty fending for himself tends to become inhibited and tense. These differences tend to be magnified if the family, teacher, and peers expect boys to prove their worth on childhood battlefields. By contrast, the differences can be ameliorated if children are taught to stand up for their rights in other ways.

Many researchers (Hamburg and Lunde) have indicated that the changes in physique associated with early and late puberty might have certain psychological consequences. In these studies, early-maturing girls appeared to be more submissive, socially indifferent, and ranked low in popularity. On the other hand, early-maturing boys seemed to enjoy high prestige among their peers. That these psychological differences may carry over and affect adult behavior has been well documented (Jones). Evidence also indicates that earlier puberty in females is correlated with obesity in childhood (McNeill and Livson); whereas in males it may be correlated with the presence of a well-developed, broad-shouldered, powerful physique. Tall and lean children tend to be late maturers.

PHYSIOLOGICAL CHANGES DURING PUBERTY

Increased growth and changes in proportion are accompanied by alterations in breathing, blood circulation, and body energy production (see Table 5-5). The development of differences in physical strength between the sexes also begins at puberty. Strength in males is greater than would be expected from the relative increase in muscle, and thus other contributing factors are important—a greater ability to transport oxygen to the tissues (more red blood cells per volume of blood), more hemoglobin per red blood cell, and higher blood pressure. Statistics from the U.S. Department of Labor indicate that the average adult male is exactly 57 percent stronger than the average adult female. Strength refers only to ability to pull against a weight. It does not include muscular endurance, agility, and speed.

Females of all ages tend to resist diseases and withstand extremes in temperature, humidity, and lack of water and food better than males (Potts). Although exceptions exist, males are more susceptible than females to infection by worms, bacteria, viruses, and fungi (Goble and Konopka). Death rates for both sexes are lowest in the ages ten to fourteen; however, at this time as well as at all others, males run the higher risk of death. Physiological factors contributing to these differences are poorly understood.

One hypothesis claims that females generally have a greater ability to resist or fight disease due to a better antibody-forming mechanism than that found in males (Washburn et al.). *Antibodies* are specific types of proteins formed by the body in response to invading foreign substances. The invading substance, called an *antigen*, is located on a disease-producing organism. The function of the antibody is to combine with the antigen and render it inactive until it is broken down by the body. It should be mentioned that each kind of antigen requires a different kind of antibody to subdue it. Apparently each X

Table 5-5 Physiological Functions in Relation to Sex and Puberty

Age	Sex	Blood pressure as heart contracts, mmHg	Heartbeats/ min	Breaths/ min	Mouth temperature, °C	Millions, ml plasma, red blood cells	Energy burned, cal/h/m² of body surface	No. of acid units in stomach
Prepuberty								
4	F	—	88	23–30	37.1	4.45	51	13
4	M	—	86	23–30	37.1	4.45	53	15
Puberty								
15	F	105.5	66	20–25	36.4	4.70	36	27
15	M	110.0	62	20–25	36.6	4.90	41	37
Adult								
21	F	110.0	65	16–18	36.6	5.40	—	33
21	M	120.0	61	16–18	36.1	4.60	—	50

Sources: J. M. Tanner, 1962; Iliff and Lee, 1952; Rothenberg, 1962.

chromosome has located on it genes responsible for the manufacture of certain antibodies that help resist disease. Women with their two X chromosomes have more of these genes and thus more of the antibodies. If the hypothesis is true, then one would expect women with the XXX genotype to have even larger quantities of antibodies than XX women. A recent study comparing 28 women with the triple-X syndrome to equal numbers of age-matched XX women found that the triple-X members of the study indeed have the highest level of a type of antibody called immunoglobulin (Rhodes).

CONTROL OF PUBERTY

What causes puberty? Possibly, intensification of an interaction between the hypothalamus, pituitary gland, and gonads. Throughout childhood, the hypothalamus secretes FSH and LH releasing factors. The pituitary responds by secreting FSH and LH, which, in turn, stimulate estrogen and testosterone production by the gonads. As in the adult, a negative feedback system is in operation; however, the puberty control center, or "pubostat," in the hypothalamus may be set so that only small amounts of sex hormones are secreted—so small, in fact, that they have little, if any, effect on sexual maturation (Fig. 5-4). Apparently the hypothalamus at this time is very sensitive and is strongly inhibited by minute levels of circulating sex hormones from the gonads. According to Donovan and Ten Bosch, the hypothalamus gradually matures throughout childhood, and at a certain point it becomes emancipated from this inhibition and begins secreting much larger amounts of the releasing factors. The brain, therefore, triggers the onset of puberty by raising the "set" level of stabilization—more releasing factors, more gonadotropins, and more sex hormones are secreted. Thus sexual maturation begins.

A great unsolved problem remains: Why does the timing of puberty differ from person to person? Children all over the world have been reaching puberty much earlier than did their ancestors. One hundred years ago the median age of menarche for girls in the United States was sixteen—today it is twelve. Indeed, since 1830, menarche has been occurring earlier by about 4 months every decade (Tanner, 1962). At the same time, when scientists compare cultures today, the onset of sexual maturation varies widely. For example, the earliest median menarcheal age reported for a culture is nine years six months for the Somali of Somaliland, and the latest is sixteen years reported for the Tanala of Madagascar and the Wogeo of Melanesia (Whiting). Even within populations, individual variation is great—breasts can begin growth at anywhere from eight to thirteen years of age in girls living in the United States. Heredity, diet, climate, stress, and socioeconomic factors have all been implicated as contributing to the trend toward earlier puberty as well as toward the widespread variation seen within and among cultures.

Hypothetically, genetic constitution could influence the rate of maturation of the hypothalamus and thus control the resetting of the "pubostat." Evidence for the importance of genes comes from very few studies. Identical twins reach

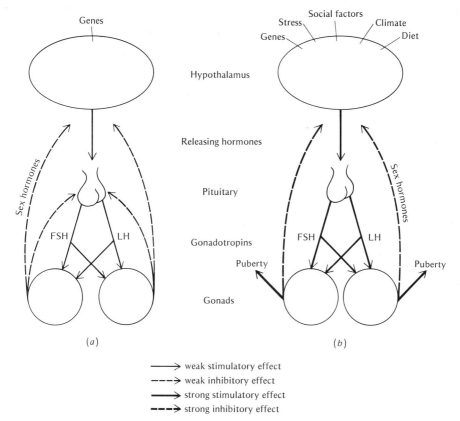

Figure 5-4 Puberty turned on by factors influencing the brain. (a) Before puberty, feedback mechanism is turned down; (b) at puberty, feedback mechanism is turned up.

menarche between 2 and 3 months of each other; whereas, nonidentical twins show a difference of 8 to 12 months (Petri, Tisserand-Perrier). One study by Reynolds and Schoen indicated that all of the signs of puberty were reached at exactly the same time by members of one set of triplet boys. Type of physique prior to puberty is partially controlled by genes. Tanner (1962) has shown that plumpness in girls and high muscle volume in boys before puberty are correlated with earlier maturation.

The effects of diet on the timing of puberty are controversial. The trend toward earlier maturation has been attributed to more and better food. With improved health and nutritional standards, children are able to reach certain critical weights, for example, 105.5 lb for girls, much earlier than ever before. The theory further claims that attainment of a critical weight leads to a change in the rate of bodily chemical reactions, which in turn causes a resetting of the "pubostat" (Frisch and Renelle).

However, according to some researchers, diet may not be as important as social stimulation or interaction between members of the opposite sex during childhood. Based on experiments with mice, Vandenberg concludes that quality of diet as a factor (high protein) accounts for only 5 percent of earlier maturation, whereas social stimulation accounts for 47 percent. Whiting could not find any relationship between menarcheal age and the average number of calories eaten or the amount of protein in the diet of close to 50 cultures.

Vandenberg has shown that if female mice are raised with other females but no males, puberty occurs at about 57 days of age. This age can be reduced by 17 days if the female is raised in isolation and by 29 days if the female is raised with one young male and no females. Thus, odor from the male or lack of odor from females may affect the "pubostat," stimulating an earlier maturation. These experiments should not be extrapolated to the human condition; however, they do suggest the need for new studies. Can interaction between siblings of the opposite sex cause earlier maturation in humans?

Whiting found strong correlations between infant stress and menarcheal age in a cross-cultural study of 50 societies. Certain cultures practiced customs which caused infant stress. Stress-producing practices included mother-infant separation and pain caused by the application of ornamentation, reshaping of a limb, exposure to extremes of temperature, administration of emetics, scraping with objects, subjecting to loud noises, and so on. These events usually occurred during the first two weeks of life and were defined as stressful if the children screamed or were obviously in pain, or if any wound failed to heal within 2 weeks. The average menarcheal age for societies without infant stress was 14.0 years. When either mother separation or painful stress was present but not both, menarcheal age was 13.6 years. When both forms of infant stress were practiced, the average age was 12.75 years. How stress at such an early age might influence puberty several years later was not discussed.

It is apparent that the onset of sexual maturation is triggered by a multiplicity of factors, but exactly how the "pubostat" is turned up remains to be elucidated.

SOME PROBLEMS OF PUBERTY

Acne

The pubertal increase in testosterone (boys) and adrenal androgens (girls) is responsible for a condition provoking much worry and concern among adolescents (Hamilton). The condition is called *acne,* and it is characterized by clogged sebaceous glands which show up as pustules and blackheads located mostly on the face and to a lesser extent on the chest and back. Sebum, the oil produced by these glands, acts as a lubricant. During puberty it is produced in large quantities and can irritate and block the hair follicles, causing redness and blackheads. The condition is more common in boys than in girls and affects close to 30 percent of young males in the United States (Masland et al.). Acne can be mild, a few blackheads scattered here and there, or severe with great ropelike lesions that may leave scars. Physicians recommend that young people affected by this condition wash the skin with a cleanser containing salicylic acid and sulfur a few times a day and avoid vigorous scrubbing. Severe acne may be treated with ultraviolet light and antibiotics. Acne patients should cut down on seafood, chocolate, nuts, and fried foods. It is also recommended that they get plenty of exercise, social activity, and sleep.

Frequently, a bumper crop of acne pimples is considered by the adolescent to be a result of masturbation. Reinforcement of such feelings may be derived from friends and parents who also believe that masturbation causes acne. The truth is, masturbation stimulates the same nerves and produces the same physiological effects on the body as does coitus, and coitus does not cause acne; nor does masturbation produce circles under the eyes, insanity, or any other adverse effect on the body. Masturbation techniques are commonly used by couples during sexual play, and we shall discuss this subject in some detail in the chapter on precoital stimulation.

Obesity

Significant overweight, called *obesity,* is a common problem during puberty, especially for girls. A person gets fat when more calories are taken in than are used up in daily activity. However, the tendency toward obesity may be genetic and/or may be related to food habits during infancy. Infants who are fed on whole cow's milk and solid foods during the first month or two after birth tend to develop more fat tissue than do babies fed on mother's milk or nonfat cow's milk. This large quantity of fat tissue accumulates and retains fat even in the face of a program of rigorous weight reduction. Steep weight gains during infancy may thus mean obesity in adolescence, which is difficult to overcome.

Other studies have shown that the patterns of weight gain for children resemble those of the natural parents rather than those of adoptive parents. This is not positive proof of inheritance but does suggest a genetic influence.

Motion picture studies of adolescents at summer camps have confirmed that obese girls and boys tend to exercise less and economize on such activities as walking, running, and swimming. However, before treatments with a regimen of exercise and diets are provided, a physician should exclude any possibility of metabolic or hormonal defects.

Episodes of overeating can be regarded as a typical adolescent response to the ambivalence and conflict of growing up. However, overeating is typical only if it is of short duration, does not lead to excessive weight gain, and ceases at the adolescent's own initiative rather than by parental coercion (Steele). If these criteria are not met, then the adolescent may be attempting to cope with a serious emotional conflict that requires counseling.

TERMINATION OF ADOLESCENCE

Attainment of adulthood depends more upon the idiosyncracies of the person doing the defining than on the characteristics of the person being labeled. There are legal, moral, biological, psychological and cultural definitions of sexual maturity and these rarely coincide. "Today you are a man," cry the relatives of a Jewish boy just turned thirteen. Regardless of level of growth and sexual maturity, the bar mitzvah is a *rite de passage* conferring adult status on the boy, making him totally responsible for all the religious duties of a man. Bar mitzvah literally means "man of duty." The counterpart for girls is the bas mitzvah, introduced over 40 years ago by conservative congregations in the United States.

Legally, however, one cannot achieve adulthood all at once. A legal minor is anyone below the age of consent, which averages about sixteen in the United States and ranges from seven years in Delaware to eighteen years in about 20 other states. If the age of consent has been reached, a person is legally capable of giving permission for sexual intercourse, and in most states a girl may marry without parental consent. A boy, however, must in most cases wait until twenty-one before he can marry without consent from his parents. Legal responsibilities for medical care are not delegated simultaneously—minors in California who are twelve years of age and older may agree without parental consent to treatment for venereal disease but not for a broken arm. In many states, minors fifteen years of age or older managing their own financial affairs and living independently of parents are called "emancipated." They are fully responsible for all medical, surgical, and hospital care for themselves (Gatov). According to the Welfare Reform Act, even unemancipated minors fifteen years and older can obtain family planning services, which include contraceptive treatment and follow-up, without getting permission from their parents. The minimum age for a driver's license is sixteen in most states, but a person cannot get a job until the age of eighteen without obtaining a work permit. Also, the person cannot enter into a legally binding contract until the age of twenty-one, except for services involving the performing arts (Strouse). In many states young people can vote and enlist at eighteen and go to a bar at twenty-one. If a minor commits a "crime against nature" (fellatio, anal intercourse) which may be a felony in many states, he or she will be treated as a juvenile delinquent rather than as a criminal. This means that the record will be sealed and considered confidential—in other words, no criminal record. Between the ages of consent and twenty-one, a person may be treated as a criminal for the same offense unless he or she is determined to be a "youthful offender" or "wayward youth" (The Handling of Juveniles from Offense to Disposition). A "youth" is considered, by the court, too old to be a delinquent and too young to be an adult and is usually a person with a good record.

These legal definitions do not necessarily coincide with sexual maturity in the biological sense—that is, when a person is capable of having children. Also they do not always coincide with adulthood in the moral sense as defined by Richard F. Hettlinger: "Sexual maturity is the capacity to enjoy sexual union as an expression of love for the partner, without needing to demonstrate one's power by dominating the other, and without doubting one's identity and worth as a sexual being." Finally, The Committee on Adolescence stresses responsibility toward one's family as a criterion of adulthood: "Socio-economic responsibility for children rather than sexual reproduction per se, would seem perhaps the ultimate criterion of adult status in most of the world."

BIBLIOGRAPHY

Bayley, N., and S. R. Pinneau. 1952. Tables for predicting adult height from skeletal age: Revised for use with the Greulich-Pyle hand standards, *J. Pediatr.*, **40**:423–441. (Erratum corrected in *J. Pediatr.*, **41**:371.)

Caldwell, W. E., and H. C. Moloy. 1933. Anatomical variations in the female pelvis and their effect in labor with a suggested classification, *Am. J. Obstet. Gynecol.*, **26**:479.

Cortes, J. B., and F. M. Gatti. 1970. Physique and propensity, *Psych. Today*, **4**(5):42.

Donovan, B. T., and J. J. Van Der Werff Ten Bosch. 1965. *Physiology of Puberty*. E. Arnold, London.

Frisch, R. F., and R. Renelle. 1970. Height and weight at menarche and a hypothesis of critical body weights and adolescent events, *Science*, **169**:397.

Gadpaille, W. J. 1968. Homosexual experience, adolescence, *Medical Aspects of Human Sexuality*, vol. II, pp. 29–38.

Gatov, E. (ed.). 1973. *Sex Code of California*. Graphic Arts of Marin, Sausalito, Calif.

Goble, F. C., and E. A. Konopka. 1973. Sex as a factor in infectious disease, *Trans. N. Y. Acad. Sci. Series II*, **35**(4):325–346.

Hamburg, D. A., and D. T. Lunde. 1966. Sex hormones in the development of sex differences in human behavior, in E. E. Maccoby (ed.), *The Development of Sex Differences*. Stanford, Stanford, Calif.

Hamilton, J. B. 1941. Male hormone substance: A prime factor in acne, *J. Clin. Endocrinol.*, **1**:570–592.

Hettlinger, R. F. 1970. *Sexual Maturity*, p. 66. Wadsworth, Belmont, Calif.

Iliff, A., and V. A. Lee. 1952. Pulse rate, respiratory rate, and body temperature of children between two months and fifteen years of age, *Child Dev.*, **23**:237–245.

Jones, M. C. 1964. Psychological correlates of somatic development, Presidential Address, Division 7, Amer. Psychol. Assoc.

Kelch, R. P., et al. 1972. Studies on the mechanism of puberty in man, in B. Saxena et al. (eds.), *Gonadotropins*, pp. 524–534. Wiley, New York.

Kinsey, A. C., et al. 1948. *Sexual Behavior in the Human Male*. Saunders, Philadelphia.

Kinsey, A. C., et al. 1953. *Sexual Behavior in the Human Female*. Saunders, Philadelphia.

McNeill, C. A., and N. Livson. 1963. Maturation rate and body build in woman, *Child Dev.*, **34**:25–32.

Marcuse, H. 1955. *Eros and Civilization*. Beacon Press, Boston.

Marshall, W. A. 1970. Sex differences at puberty, *J. Biosoc. Sci. Suppl.*, **2**:31–41.

Masland, R. P., et al. 1956. Some comments on acne vulgaris in adolescents, *J. Pediatr.*, **49**:680–684.

Masters, W. H., and V. E. Johnson. 1966. *Human Sexual Response*. Little, Brown, Boston.

Normal Adolescence. 1968. Committee on Adolescence, Scribner, New York.

Petri, E. 1935. Untersuchungen zur Erbbedingtheit der menarche, *Z. Morphol. Anthropol.*, **33**:43–48.

Potts, D. M. 1970. Which is the weaker sex? *J. Biosoc. Sci. Suppl.*, **2**:147–157.

Raboch, J. 1969. Men's most common sex problems, *Sexology,* Nov. Issue, pp. 60–63.

Reynolds, E. L., and G. Schoen. 1947. Growth patterns of identical triplets from 8 through 18 years, *Child Dev.,* **18:**130–151.

Rhodes, K., et al. 1969. Immunoglobulins and the X-chromosome, *B. Med. J.,* **3:**439–441.

Rothenberg, R. E. 1962. *Medical Dictionary and Health Manual.* Signet Book, New American Library, New York.

Sheldon, W. H. 1940. *The Varieties of Human Physique.* Harper, New York.

Steele, C. I. 1974. Obese adolescent girls: some diagnostic and treatment considerations. *Adolescence,* **9**(33):81–96.

Strouse, J. 1970. *Up against the Law.* Signet Books, New American Library, New York.

Tanner, J. M. 1962. *Growth at Adolescence,* 2d ed. Blackwell, Oxford.

Tanner, J. M. 1967. Puberty, in A. McLaren (ed.), *Advances in Reproductive Physiology,* vol. II. Logos Press. Academic, New York.

Tanner, J. M., et al. 1959. Genes on the Y chromosome influencing rate of maturation in man: skeletal age studies in children with Klinefelter's (XXY) and Turner's (XO) syndromes, *Lancet,* **2:**141–144.

The Handling of Juveniles from Offense to Disposition, vol. 1, 1967. GPO, Washington.

Tisserand-Perrier, M. 1955. Etude comparative de certains processus de croissance chez les jumeaux, *J. Genet. Hum.,* **2:**87–102.

Vandenberg, J. 1972. Implications of hurried puberty, *San Francisco Chronicle* (Aug. 13).

Vidal, G. 1966. *Sex, Death, and Money.* Bantam, New York.

Washburn, T. C., et al. 1965. Sex differences in susceptibility to infections: References on bacterial meningitis and septicemia. *Pediatrics,* **35:**57–64.

Whiting, J. W. M. 1965. Menarcheal age and infant stress in humans, in F. A. Beach (ed.), *Sex and Behavior,* Wiley, New York.

Young, H. B. 1970. Adolescence, in E. E. Philipp et al. (eds.), *Scientific Foundations of Obstetrics and Gynecology.* Davis, Philadelphia.

Chapter 6

Dimensions of Sexual Motivation

Sexual motivation is the urge for sexual activity. For our purposes this motivation can be considered synonymous with libido, sex drive, sexual desire, and sexual urge. The intensity of sexual motivation fluctuates within each individual, and it also varies from person to person (Kirkendall). Therefore, we cannot even attempt to define "normal" levels of sexual motivation. Instead, we shall describe the conditions that must exist if sexual excitement is to occur and discuss the factors that determine the strength of sexual desire.

The status of the sex-drive concept is currently in a state of confusion primarily because sexual motivation is not essential to the person's survival, whereas other motivational drives, such as hunger and thirst, are. Indeed, sex drive does not seem to require fulfillment or satisfaction—"No genuine tissue or biological needs are generated by sexual abstinence" (Beach and Jordan). Hunger and thirst are related to a depletion of substances within the tissues; whereas sex drive is more a recovery from previous sexual activity.

There is a variety of opinion concerning the origin of the sex drive. Hardy claims that since so much of human sexual behavior is determined by experience, it is best to think of sexual motivation as a learned appetite rather than as an inborn drive. Hardy includes the direction of behavior (e.g., orientation toward a partner of the same or opposite sex) as part of the motivational state. On the other hand, Whalen (1966) feels that all the basic drives have a physiological foundation, but the direction the behavior takes is learned. Thus in his view, sex drive is determined by the physiological state of the individual, and orientation toward a particular partner, whether homosexual, heterosexual, or bisexual, is learned. Since both sex drive and sexual orientation contribute to sexual behavior, the problem is to separate them so that both can be experimentally studied under controlled conditions. This can be done by studying young animals before certain habits are established or by studying animals in which motivation can be kept constant while habit varies.

AROUSAL AND AROUSABILITY

It is useful to view the factors of arousal and arousability as interacting components of sexual motivation. *Arousal* is an individual's level of sexual excitement at a particular moment; it can range from zero to orgasm (Whalen, 1966). Arousal level may be determined from:

   1 Frequency of response per unit of time—e.g., number of orgasms per hour, masturbations per week, and so on (Whalen, 1966).
   2 Reaction time. The speed with which a male begins to copulate when a receptive female is made available (Almquist and Hale). These studies have been made on domestic animals.
   3 Probability of response. If several male rats are caged with a female, the male that has the highest arousal level will mount her first when she is in heat. The arousal level of a male is directly proportional to the probability that he will get to the female first. Probability is calculated on the basis of past performances.

   Arousability is the rate at which an individual changes from a lower to a higher arousal level. In other words, arousability is the speed with which sexual excitement mounts toward orgasm. Arousability can be measured in either of two ways: by graphing the total rise in arousal level produced by one sexual stimulus (Fig. 6-1) or by counting the number of sexual stimuli that are required

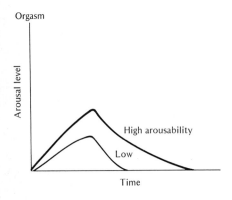

Figure 6-1 Changes in arousal level produced by a single sexual stimulus. Curves show high and low arousability individuals. (*Whalen, 1966.*)

to reach orgasm (Fig. 6-2). Note that arousal level must be measured before arousability can be determined.

These concepts have been derived from studies on rats and caution should be used in applying them to the complex behavior of humans. For instance, one person may, through past experience, come to associate a particular stimulus with sexual pleasure. This person will be highly aroused by the stimulus; whereas another individual may not even like it. In addition, we should be careful not to place high values on high arousability. Extremely fast orgasmic response may be desirable if the partner responds just as quickly. But would you consider it desirable for a man to reach orgasm within seconds of vaginal penetration? Would you say he has hyperarousability? On the other hand, would your conclusion be the same if his partner reaches orgasm at the same time? Contrary to popular belief, the reverse situation may exist. Would you consider extremely high female arousability desirable if coitus must be continued after it becomes tiring or uncomfortable for the woman?

VARIABLES INFLUENCING SEXUAL MOTIVATION

Capacity for arousal and arousability is regulated at least by the following factors:

1 Genotype
2 Hormonal levels—particularly androgen
3 Activity of brain, spinal cord, plus nerves leading to and from erotic zones
4 Sight, hearing, smell, taste, and touch
5 Prior sexual and social experience
6 The amount of time required to recover sex drive following orgasm
7 Age
8 Environmental factors—nutrition, disease, season, temperature, social interaction
9 Cultural influence
10 Stress
11 Aphrodisiacs or anaphrodisiacs

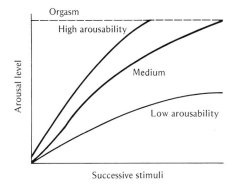

Figure 6-2 Increase in arousal level produced by several consecutive sexual stimuli. The high and medium arousability individuals reach maximum arousal level and orgasm occurs. (*Whalen, 1966.*)

Genotype

McGill and Blight, by crossing various strains of mice, have shown that the "male mouse genotype has a definite effect upon the time required to recover sex drive after an ejaculation." McGill has also indicated that other differences in arousability exist among many of the 200 genetically distinct strains and substrains of laboratory mice. Strain differences in sex drive also exist between many domestic animals (Fraser). At the present time, the relationship of genes to human sexual motivation is not clear, primarily because of the paucity of research in this area.

Chilton recently did a pilot study of psychosexual development in identical and fraternal human twins. Identical twins result from a single zygote that undergoes cell division and then splits into two separate groups of cells; both groups develop into fetuses. Identical twins, therefore, have identical heredities. Fraternal twins arise when two eggs are released at ovulation and are fertilized by separate sperm. Fraternal twins are no more genetically similar than are brothers and sisters who result from separate pregnancies. Chilton asked the twins the following questions, which are indices of sexual motivation: age at first orgasm; age when regular masturbation began; maximum number of times masturbation to orgasm had occurred in one day; age of first active genital stimulation by a member of the opposite sex. Identical twins almost always gave similar answers to these questions, whereas the fraternal twins did not. Although more research needs to be done before we can reach any conclusions, Chilton's results do show a striking degree of inherited sexual motivation. By the way, readers should not try to estimate their own arousability by answering these questions and comparing their results with those of their friends. Unless this type of experiment is carefully controlled, factors such as different moral upbringings, different opportunities, and tendencies to cover up or to brag will invalidate the conclusions.

Most experts agree that the tendency for low, medium, or high arousability is controlled by genes. Whether the tendency is realized depends on many factors: Genetic influence on physique, onset of puberty, neural and sensory capacity for learning and detecting environmental stimuli, and previous pleasurable or unpleasant experiences, will also influence arousability.

Hormonal Levels

Although contradictory statements exist in many textbooks, there is abundant evidence that sexual motivation in humans is definitely dependent upon hormonal levels, particularly upon androgens. Based upon a study of 102 men and women with low androgen production, John Money hypothesized that sexual desire is maintained by androgen in both men and women. A review of the literature led Richard Whalen (1966) to a similar conclusion: Men whose gonads are underactive or have been removed show reduced expression of sexual behavior. Whalen tentatively assumes that the reduced sexual activity reflects a reduced sexual motivation. Bremer found that sexual activity was reduced or abolished in varying amounts among 215 legally castrated males in Norway. (*Castration* means removal of both testes or both ovaries.)

Among females, menopause or loss of both ovaries reduces estrogen, but sex drive and activity seem to remain high in women who enjoyed sex before menopause or castration. However, loss of the adrenal glands, the source of most of the androgen in females, is definitely associated with a decrease in sexual motivation (Waxenberg et al.). Androgen was shown to increase the sensitivity of the clitoris and to enhance sexual desire and gratification, whereas estrogen expedites coitus by increasing lubrication and malleability of the vagina (Salmon and Geist).

Masica et al. interviewed ten genetic males (XY) with testicular feminization. Blood levels of testosterone are normal in these individuals, but their anatomy, psyche, and rearing are female. Experiments have shown that the tissues of these men are insensitive to testosterone; to be more exact, their tissues are not capable of converting testosterone to a substance called dihydrotestosterone, which appears to be for many tissues the active form of the male hormone (Masica et al.). The interviewees, when compared with normal females, reported lower frequency of sexual arousal from visual stimuli, less awareness of their sex drive, and decreased assertiveness and versatility in coitus.

Kinsey (1948) has indicated that human females appear to desire coitus more often during the 3 to 4 days just prior to menstruation than at any other time of the monthly cycle. Masters and Johnson (1966) have concluded that the fluid accumulation in the pelvic region, including the vulva, during the premenstrual days may cause neural stimulation leading to increased desire. Judith Bardwick believes that many women have a low feeling of self-esteem at this time and psychologically require human contact. It is interesting to note that preliminary investigations also indicate that androgen levels are highest in the blood during the premenstrual days of the menstrual cycle (Apostolakis et al.).

In one male subject, testosterone levels in blood taken during and immediately after coitus were significantly higher than those determined at other times (Fox et al.). No difference was found during masturbation, however.

Evidence from nonhuman mammals is also extensive. Castration in adult male rabbits, hamsters, rats, mice, and guinea pigs is followed within a few weeks by a complete loss of mating activity (Beach, 1970). This is true of both experienced and inexperienced males. Castration generally lowers testosterone levels, and injections of this hormone will restore full sexual activity as long as therapy is continued (Beach, 1970). In cats and dogs previous sexual experience influences sex drive during the short-term effects of castration. Experienced male cats (Rosenblatt and Aronson) and male dogs (Beach, 1970) maintain sex drive and sexual performance much longer after castration than do the above-mentioned species.

Among Rhesus monkeys, females with their ovaries removed are also affected by injections of testosterone. Herbert has shown that small doses of male hormone will enhance a female's willingness to mate, but her sexual attractiveness to males is dependent upon estrogen rather than testosterone. Herbert concluded that the estrogen was needed to stimulate production of vaginal odors which attract male monkeys, whereas testosterone acted on the female's nervous system, increasing her sex drive.

Beach and Levinson and Rosenblatt and Aronson suggested that, in males, reduced androgen levels affect the anatomy of the penis so that touch receptors located in the walls do not fully respond during coitus. In females, androgens cause growth of the clitoris and increase its sensitivity to touch (Dorfman and Shipley).

In addition, androgens appear to stimulate motivating centers in the brain. Tiny amounts of androgen can be implanted in the hypothalamus of male and female rats and rabbits. When the androgens are implanted in particular areas of the hypothalamus sex drive increases (Palka and Sawyer; Lisk, 1971). In another type of experiment, an unanesthetized rat is placed in a box containing levers, and electrodes are implanted at various points in the rat's brain. Electrical stimulation is delivered to these points whenever the rat presses a bar located in the box. The rate of bar pressing increases if the electrodes are placed at certain points; this indicates that pleasure centers are being stimulated. The rate of bar pressing decreases if the electrodes are moved to certain other points; this indicates the location of pain centers. If the electrodes are implanted in certain pleasure points in the hypothalamus and forebrain of a castrated male rat, the rate of bar pressing is slow. But if the male is then given injections of testosterone, bar pressing increases.

Radioactively labeled testosterone and estrogen have been found to accumulate in specific areas of the brain, particularly in the parts controlling sexual behavior (Stumpf).

Although much more research needs to be done, the following will summarize the present status of hormonal influence on sexual motivation:

1   Activation of sexual motivation requires the proper levels of hormones in combination with direct or symbolic erotic stimuli.

2   Androgen (particularly testosterone) may be considered the "libido" hormone in both sexes of many species including humans. It makes certain parts of the nervous system responsive to stimulation; these include the sexual motivation centers in the brain and the nerves directly associated with the genitals. In human females estrogens have a secondary importance because they facilitate vaginal lubrication and maintain the health of the vagina and vulva.

3   In certain mammal species (e.g., cats, dogs, and monkeys) experience retards the effects of low androgen but does not abolish them.

4   There appears to be an optimum amount of androgen beyond which no increase in desire occurs.

5   Present evidence has not directly related a given amount of androgen to a particular degree of motivation—for example, castration of male guinea pigs leads to a rapid depletion of testosterone but a slower decline of sexual

behavior (Resko). Resko believes that testosterone may somehow have long-lasting effects on the nervous system even after its disappearance from the blood.

6 It is not clear whether fluctuations in hormonal level cause alterations in behavior or whether certain forms of behavior stimulate changes in blood concentration of hormones. Evidence points to both possibilities. Rose et al. have shown that blood testosterone increased in male Rhesus monkeys when they had a dominant position in their group and had frequent copulations, but testosterone decreased when they were subjected to a decisive defeat in a battle with other males. The authors conclude that hormone levels are influenced by behavior and that these hormonal changes can, in turn, affect subsequent behavior.

Nervous System Activity

Sexual motivation is regulated by certain brain centers and also by nerves that arise from the genitalia and breasts (Diamond). In addition, stimulation of these parts of the nervous system can result in a wide variety of responses such as changes in heart rate, blushing, and sweating, all contributing to the sensation of sexual desire. These neural control centers are also involved in all other aspects of human sexual behavior—sexual intercourse, menstruation, childbirth, lactation, and so forth.

Aronson and Cooper partially desensitized penises in 14 sexually experienced cats by removing small portions of the dorsal nerve running along each side of the penile shaft. The cats then were no longer able to feel penis stimulation. The immediate result was a loss of orientation—the males got erections but failed to achieve intromission when mounting a female in heat. Subsequently, a total body disorientation occurred—a male would lie on his side, vigorously thrusting, and attempt to mount the female even though penis and vagina were far apart. The long-term effects included a decrease in sexual motivation resulting from the decline of sensory stimulation from the penis.

The same operation was performed on four male Rhesus monkeys (Herbert). In contrast to the cats, erection *and* intromission were successful; however, the smooth rhythm of thrusting became disorganized and irregular, mounting and intromission were prolonged (up to $1^{1}/_{2}$ hours), and ejaculation occurred rarely. Eventually a progressive decline in sexual activity was seen. Herbert concluded that sexual motivation probably decreased because the lack of sensation in the penis and failure to reach orgasm made sexual activity unrewarding.

The following summarizes our present but incomplete knowledge of the brain structures involved with sexual motivation. It is based mostly upon experiments with nonhumans, and partially upon observations of people with brain damage.

Temporal lobes   The largest portion of the brain is called the cerebrum (see Fig. 6-3). The cerebrum is divided into a number of lobes; two of these are the temporal lobes, which are located at the sides of the head underneath the

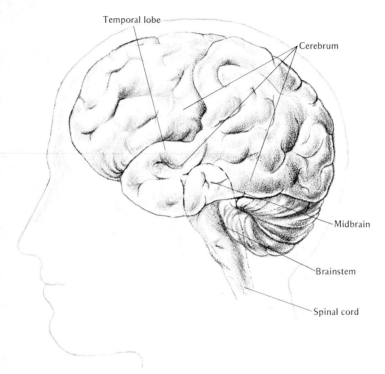

Figure 6-3   The exterior of the brain viewed from the side.

temple. Removal of both temporal lobes plus portions of the surrounding areas leads to a condition called the Klüver-Bucy syndrome. Symptoms include hypersexual behavior such as erections in the absence of erotic stimuli, changes in sexual orientation (new bisexual or homosexual interests), and copulation with inanimate objects. The fact that this condition is seen primarily in males supports the theory that separate areas of the brain control sexual behavior in the two sexes (Klüver and Bucy, Terzian and Dalle Ore).

Hypothalamus   Several sites in the hypothalamus (Fig. 6-4) appear to be important in the sexual motivation of both sexes (Stumpf).

Brainstem   The brainstem is often called the stalk of the brain. The bottom of the brainstem merges with the spinal cord, and its uppermost portion, called the midbrain, lies under the cerebrum (see Fig. 6-4). New evidence indicates that progesterone implants in certain parts of the midbrain may enhance lordosis or receptivity in female rats. Since it is known that progesterone can have certain androgenlike effects, this observation is not surprising. However, experiments on the midbrain need to be done in higher primates, and more studies of progesterone will also have to be undertaken. Farther down the brainstem lies the arousal center of the reticular activity core.

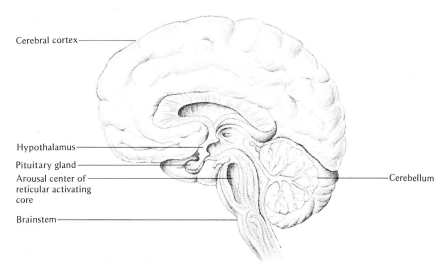

Figure 6-4   Sagittal section of human brain showing hypothalamus, pituitary, midbrain, and arousal center of reticular activating core.

When this site is exposed to the hormone epinephrine, the center increases neural responsiveness to all environmental stimuli. Thus a stimulated arousal center enhances the person's ability to detect the differences between closely related odors or to sense a light touch. Since sexual arousal is highly dependent on our ability to perceive sight, sounds, odors, and especially touch and pressure, stimulation of the arousal center can lead to initial increases in sexual motivation. Since epinephrine is released by the adrenal glands when the individual is under moderate to severe psychological or physical stress, theoretically, stress can increase sexual arousal. Later in this chapter we shall describe some of the sexually stimulating and inhibiting effects of stress.

All the brain areas mentioned above are influenced by each other, by the thought centers in the outer layer of the cerebrum, and by information coming in from sex organs as well as other receptors. It would appear, however, that the temporal lobes generally inhibit sexual motivation (particularly in males), the hypothalamus and midbrain stimulate it, and the reticular activating system influences the responsiveness of many of these neural structures.

Sensory Perception of Environmental Stimuli

Sensations of touch, sight, hearing, smell, and taste affect arousability. R. D. Lisk et al. have shown that destruction of the sense of smell in male hamsters leads to termination of sexual behavior regardless of prior experience. The sex drive of a male hamster is thus absolutely dependent upon the sense of smell, and odors emanating from a female in estrus lead to copulatory action. The female tends to be the more aggressive and will often fight the male if she is not in heat. The long-distance detection of estrus by the male probably tells him when it is safe to approach the female and protects him from getting injured or killed. In many other species, sexual motivation is dependent on a multisensory pattern where no one sense is indispensable. But in humans, the sense of touch is essential to arousability.

Previous experience is also important in many species. Beach (1942) experimented with experienced and inexperienced male rats. He desensitized the sense of touch in the snout, destroyed the sense of smell, and temporarily blinded them. When experienced rats were subjected to elimination of only one sense, they continued to mate readily, but when two or more senses were destroyed, they showed a marked decline in sexual motivation. Among the inexperienced rats, destruction of just one sense produced an immediate decrease in motivation and termination of all sexual behavior.

Among humans the physical condition of the individual and the context within which a sense perception occurs will determine whether a given sensory experience will be erotic. Obviously, a sensation will not usually produce a high level of arousal if the person is ill, extremely tired, preoccupied with some problem, or simply turned off by other aspects of the situation. In addition, a particular sensation tends to become more erotic if the person associates it with previous pleasurable experiences. If we are exposed to a given stimulus many times in a row, we can become positively or negatively conditioned to it. If touching an ear lobe with the tongue for the first time is positive and pleasurable, several times later it may become a sensuous act. When a certain perfume is related to a positive sexual experience, that specific fragrance becomes an erogenous stimulus and increases arousal level. At the same time, an odor can be associated with a negative event, and in this case it becomes an inhibitory influence. Most people would not be turned on by a skunk!

The highly arousable person is motivated by a greater number of positive stimuli than is the individual with low arousability. Indeed the techniques of therapy developed by Masters and Johnson (1970) include education and exercises that increase awareness of the positive influence of a wide variety of sensory inputs. Many of the couples who come to Masters and Johnson for treatment are unusually concerned about the quality of coital performance and tend to neglect erotic stimulation other than that produced by the friction of the penis against the walls of the vagina. Very often these people are too embarrassed to explore each other's bodies and restrict extensive touching to more "practical" activities such as giving a backrub or massaging a weary muscle. The therapist suggests that the couple avoid coitus for a short while and substitute another sensory experience, such as massages with a fragrant lotion. As the partners do these exercises, they become more relaxed about body contact, and they start to enjoy the feeling and touching. The fragrance adds to the pleasantness of the experience and may also be included in the repertoire of positive stimuli.

Previous Sexual and Social Experience

The pleasurable experience of sexual arousal increases the appetite for more such pleasurable experiences. The phenomena of genital and breast stimulation, arousal short of orgasm, and orgasm per se are all inherently pleasurable; once we have experienced these events we tend to reseek them. We also learn which factors enhance our ability to enjoy sexual activity. Girl and boy watching, hearing sounds of lovemaking, or viewing certain films become erotic because we associate them with the pleasure of genital stimulation.

In humans, hormones and parts of the nervous system set the stage for sexual motivation. But reinforcement learning plays a substantial role in determining what levels of motivation will be reached and what particular stimuli will be erotic. The term *positive learning reinforcement* means the following: If a particular way of behaving is encouraged by other people or is consistently pleasurable, a person will repeat the behavior again and again. For example, most children are naturally inquisitive and will frequently explore their bodies. Touching the genitals by accident leads to an intense feeling of pleasure. The child repeats this behavior, touching the genitals more often than other parts of the body because of the feeling of pleasure which serves as a positive reward or reinforcer. In addition, if the child repeatedly experiences a certain fragrance, sound, or fantasy while touching the genitals, these secondary factors will come to be associated with the pleasurable feeling derived from just touching the genitals alone. Eventually exposure to these other secondary stimuli may lead to the anticipation of pleasure and thereby to a higher level of arousal even though the genitals are not touched. The number of stimuli that increase arousal will be greater. Next, masturbation with its associated images and fantasies can be easily learned with orgasm acting as the positive reinforcer. As long as a secondary stimulus is periodically associated with touching the genitals, the stimulus will continue to increase one's sexual arousal level; otherwise, the stimulus will be temporarily eliminated from the erotic repertoire.

Negative reinforcement learning occurs if a certain behavior produces an unpleasant reward or simply no reward at all. Say a boy gets slapped once or twice while touching his genitals or his parents make clear to him in some other way that this behavior is shameful or naughty. As a consequence, whenever the boy touches his genitals he may feel guilt or fear that he will be disciplined or that he will disappoint his parents and lose their love. Sometimes the child will cease genital touching altogether. More often, he will repeat the activity because of its physical pleasure, but he will have a great deal of anxiety about being found out.

Learning to respond to stimuli associated with genital pleasure is further complicated by two other phenomena—generalization and discrimination. When a secondary stimulus such as scent becomes erotic, any similar stimuli are then capable of eliciting the pleasurable response. This is *generalization*. The strength of response is proportional to the similarity of the new stimulus to the original secondary one. The closer the similarity, the more likely generalization will occur. Thus people can become conditioned to whole classes of stimuli, not to just one. If touching the toe is erotic to an individual, massaging the entire foot or leg could become sensuous after repeated pairing of toe and foot touching. Increased sex drive in the presence of orange blossoms might lead to a positive response in the presence of all floral scents.

However, generalization is usually followed by some degree of discrimination. The term *discrimination* means that people can be conditioned positively to some stimuli but negatively to others, even though the stimuli are similar. Whereas generalization relies on our ability to associate stimuli with each other, discrimination relies on our ability to detect differences. Assume that two types of air freshener are constantly present in a home—essence of dill in the bedroom and eau de marjoram in the kitchen. A couple always has intercourse in the bedroom and becomes positively conditioned to the fragrance of dill. The couple never has intercourse in the kitchen; thus, marjoram is not reinforced by the pleasures of making love, but dill is. The couple may at first find eau de marjoram arousing because they associate herbal scent with sexual enjoyment. But since marjoram is not itself positively reinforced and since it is quite easily distinguished from essence of dill, it will eventually cease to be an erotic stimulus. Scents that smell almost identical to dill may, however, continue to arouse the couple, especially if dill is occasionally reinforced by coitus in the bedroom.

Age

Sexual motivation is not an all-or-nothing process that is suddenly switched on when the penis and clitoris reach a certain degree of development. The genitals with their attendant receptors exist before puberty, and the child can derive pleasure from stimulating them. Hardy, after surveying the literature, was impressed with the amount of cross-cultural data that showed extensive prepubertal sexual behavior, especially in permissive societies. Hormonal levels in the blood increase gradually many months before the physical manifestations of puberty begin. The hormones may activate portions of the nervous system so that adult sexual activity can start to occur.

There has been speculation about the ages at which males and females reach their maximum sex drive. Using evidence such as frequency of orgasm, masturbation, and erotic dreams, some researchers conclude that females, on the average, reach peaks of sexual arousal and arousability between the ages of thirty-six and forty; whereas males reach peaks during the late teens (Kinsey, 1948; 1953). However, these are estimated average figures, and widespread variations exist. Claims have been made that many women must overcome early anxieties, doubts, and fears concerning sex and that it may take as long as 10 to 15 years of experience to do this. In addition, females may be trained to be sexually aroused by fewer stimuli. For instance, women are not supposed to be aroused by pictures of male nudes or by the body lines of a passing male. Perhaps only after years of sexual experience does the average woman allow herself to enjoy these stimuli. One factor that has not been studied is a possible increase in the relative amounts of androgen compared with estrogen as a woman gets older. In other words, as a woman nears menopause estrogen production by the ovaries declines, but very likely androgen secretion by the adrenal glands remains the same.

More recent studies show that women are reaching high levels of arousal at earlier ages. This change may be partly due to an increase in sex education and to changing sex roles. Sex education may remove some of the guilt and fears about sexuality and reproduction and thereby make females more responsive to appropriate stimuli. And now that women are less and less expected to play a role of sexual unaggressiveness and innocence, they may be allowing themselves to feel and express a higher degree of sexual motivation.

Sense perception tends to decrease with age. The loss of sensory capacity in vision, taste, hearing, smell, and touch are well documented (Weiss). Newman reports a decrease with age in the ability to detect the difference between vibration and static touch on the glans penis. The decrease in sensitivity was gradual until the age of sixty-five, when it became precipitous. He also indicates a positive correlation between the amount of sexual activity regardless of age in healthy married couples and the ability of the male to differentiate between vibration and static touch—"Those with an active sexual life were significantly more sensitive to stimulus." (See Table 6-1). The reduction with age in all sensory capabilities has been attributed by Newman to such specific factors as:

1 Breakdown of the skin, which may distort the receptors.
2 Rigidity of the bones in the middle ear which amplify sounds by vibrating.
3 Yellowing and decreased functioning of the lens of the eye.
4 A decrease in the number of taste buds occurs with age, and this decrease is correlated with a reduced acuity in taste.
5 Increasing "sluggishness" of nerves. They need more powerful stimuli in order to transmit messages.
6 Decrease in the brain's ability to detect the differences between closely related stimuli; e.g., the brain may become less able to tell the difference between a vibration and a steady touch.
7 Circulatory disease of the aged—decreased flow of blood to receptors and to erectile tissue.

Secretion of sex hormones also decreases with advancing age. Blood

Table 6-1 Penile Threshold and Frequency of Coitus

Age group, yr	No. of subjects	Frequency of coitus within 1 yr	Penile threshold,* volts (low voltage = high sensitivity)
35–44	2	None	25.48
	12	Average of 109 times	4.90
45–53	2	None	13.62
	10	Average of 81 times	8.40
65–74	17	None	176.15
	13	Average of 22.4 times	39.40

*Low voltage is correlated with slight vibration; as the voltage is increased the amplitude of vibration is increased and the vibration becomes wider and more obvious. A low voltage means a person is more sensitive to slight vibration (has a low penile threshold). A high voltage means a person is less sensitive (has a high penile threshold).
Source: Newman, 1970.

levels of estrogen and progesterone drop precipitously beginning with menopause whereas testosterone levels in men decrease gradually. These changes in
hormones occur along with a reduction in the speed and intensity of physiologic response to sexual activity (Masters and Johnson, 1966). For instance,
muscles do not contract as quickly; blood congestion of erectile tissue occurs
more slowly; the vagina does not become as well lubricated. The key word,
however, is "reduction," not "elimination." As people age, they may reach high
levels of arousal more slowly, but erection and orgasm are possible far into old
age.

Many physicians believe that it is possible and even desirable for
individuals to continue sexual activity throughout their entire lives. Newman
and Nichols studied the attitudes and sexual activity in 250 subjects, including
black and white men and women ranging in age from sixty to ninety-three. All
persons reported a decline in sex drive when comparing their own youth with
old age. However, those who rated their sex drive as strong during youth
tended to rate themselves as moderate in old age; whereas when sex drive was
considered weak in youth it all but disappeared with old age. In addition,
regularity of sexual expression played a significant role. People who had
regular intercourse throughout most of their adult lives tended to continue
sexual activity far into old age. Those whose sexual experiences were sporadic
or infrequent during the middle years of life showed relatively little activity
during old age. Perhaps the less active people had always had a low level of
arousal. Or perhaps the regular positive reinforcement of sexual activity
maintains a higher degree of arousal. The importance of regularity is further
substantiated by Masters and Johnson (1966), who describe three women past
the age of sixty who maintained regular coital activity once or twice each week
despite thinning of vaginal walls and shrinking of labia majora caused by the
low postmenopausal estrogen levels. They concluded that "there is no reason
why the milestone of the menopause should be expected to blunt the female's
sexual capacity, performance, and drive." The waning sex drive in males has
been attributed by these authors to the general aging processes, chronic
infirmities, lack of regularity of sexual performance, and the psychological
factors of boredom, preoccupation with career, fatigue, over-indulgence in
food and drink, and fear of inadequate performance. However, as Newman and
Nichols conclude, if a couple remains in fairly good health they can and often
do have sexual intercourse in their sixties, seventies, and eighties.

Cultural Influence

The desire to have sex can in some cases be influenced by laws and moral
attitudes interacting with certain human characteristics. Charles Winick identifies the Godiva principle, which is the hypothesis that people seek out sexual
behavior in direct proportion to how illicit or illegal it is. Many people appear to
take deliberate chances because of one-upmanship or just to test the limits of
their tolerance. Thus, the titillation derived from the sexual portion of the
activity is added to the thrill of a novel experience. Conditioning can lead to

requiring a thrill whenever one desires sexual intercourse. Indeed some people believe that all this sex education, all this talk about sex, may somehow eliminate the risk, the cryptic subtleties, the mystery of getting involved in the unknown, thereby taking the edge off the capacity for sexual arousal and arousability. On the other hand, believing that too many laws might restrict the natural boundaries of sexual behavior, Marcuse and Brown called for a nonrepressive society and a resurrection of the entire body and personality as an erogenous instrument of pleasure. They believed that the theory if put into effect would place sex in proper perspective as part of our lives but not synonymous with our lives. It would reduce the preoccupation with sexual matters because the risk and thrill of doing something wrong would be gone. Their ideas have been partially put into effect and account for the development of encounter techniques, sensate focus exercises, and the increased concern about touching, pleasuring, and massaging. Throughout the United States perhaps even the trends towards physical fitness, diets, and sensuous good looks may be a part of this development. But the theory has not been totally implemented and many laws and repressive attitudes still exist. We, as a culture, are thus presently in the "crush"—on the one side, much of the risk is still available, but at the same time we are allowed to touch each other more often and experiment with expansion of sensual awareness. My feeling is that the "crush" or "stress" has led to our culture being more sexually motivated than at any other time in its history.

Social Interaction—Stress

An unusual or severe stress can activate the adrenal glands. Such kinds of stress are called *stressors*. Stressors may be viewed as immediate or possible future threats to the individual's body or to his psychological well-being. They include strong fear, anger, frustration, pain and cold, severe infections, and poisons and other noxious stimuli. The adrenal secretions activated by a stressor cause such physiologic changes as an increase in alertness and energy, greater sensitivity to stimuli, and increases in heart rate and output. These responses are the body's way of combating the stressor and, if possible, eliminating it. For instance, if the stressor is fear of an attacker, these physiologic responses may give the intended victim a strength he never knew he had. Severe loss of blood is another stressor; the adrenal-caused changes in the circulatory system can be particularly helpful in combating it.

Theoretically, stressors can increase sexual arousal because they increase sensitivity to stimuli (Fig. 6-5). In order to test this hypothesis, Calhoun studied the behavior of rats kept in crowded enclosures. Overcrowding acts as a stressor on many animals. Apparently some animals have a psychological need for a little physical distance between themselves and other members of their species, and overcrowding threatens this need. Calhoun identified four patterns of behavior exhibited by males in response to overcrowding. The behavior shown by these types was clearly outside that observed among rats in uncrowded populations.

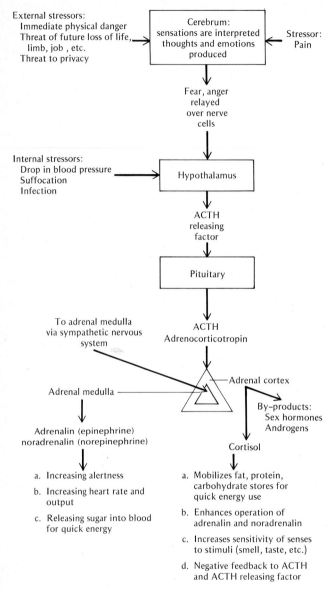

Figure 6-5 Diagram of the current concepts of the body's reaction to stressors.

1 Dominant males: Every natural population of rats has a few aggressive and dominant males on top of the hierarchy. These also existed in Calhoun's stressed population, but in this group the dominant males would periodically go berserk, biting the tails of other rats.

2 Pansexual males: These were generally below the dominant males in the status. They would make sexual advances toward other adult males, juvenile males and females, and females in heat as well as those not in heat. The males being mounted appeared to accept it without aggressive display. A certain amount of such behavior normally occurs in every natural population, but Calhoun quantified the pansexual activity in his population and concluded that it was extreme.

3 Probers: These males were considered hyperactive, cannibalistic, and rapists. They were always on the prowl for females in heat and upon discovery would pursue them into the nest box where copulation would take place without regard for signs of receptivity. Since the females were also disoriented, any offspring present from an earlier pregnancy often died from lack of suckling and were promptly devoured by the probers.

4 Somnambulists: A few males became very passive and nonsexual, were ignored by others, moved around only at night when the general population was asleep and looked extremely healthy because of a complete lack of aggressive encounter. Individual rats react differently to a given quantity of stress, and the somnambulists could be considered as reacting maximally with total inhibition of sexual motivation, aggression, and complete social disorientation.

Females in Calhoun's population became more physically aggressive, neglected their young, refused to build nests, and resisted the advances of males.

All the rats showed social disorientation, and four out of five groups showed a change in sexual motivation: The pansexuals and probers became hypersexual, and the somnambulists and females became hyposexual. Stressors, then, potentially increase arousability, but other aspects of the stress situation may override and inhibit sexual motivation. For example, extreme stress is known to inhibit testosterone levels.

Little research has been done on humans. But observations such as the following suggest that such research would be interesting. For instance, consider the classic case of the soldier who seeks sexual intercourse the night before he goes into battle. On the other hand, a person suffering from extreme frustration or anxiety over his job may exhibit decreased sexual motivation.

CONCLUSIONS

Although much more data is needed, present evidence would indicate that sex drive is influenced by multiple factors, some of biological origin and others from the socialization process. Factors of stress, earlier maturation, delay in psychological aging, use of birth control techniques, and rapid changes in cultural attitudes can all influence sexual motivation.

BIBLIOGRAPHY

Almquist, J. O., and E. B. Hale. 1956. An approach to the measurement of sexual behavior and semen production of dairy bulls, *III Int. Cong. Anim. Reprod., Artificial insemination papers for Sec. III,* 50–59 (74, 76, 106).

Apostolakis, M., et al. 1966. The effect of lynestrenol administration of testosterone, estrogen, pregnanediol and total gonadotropin excretion during the menstrual cycle, *Steroids,* **7**:146.

Aronson, L. R., and M. L. Cooper. 1968. Desensitization of the glans penis and sexual behavior in cats, in M. Diamond (ed.), *Perspectives in Reproduction and Sexual Behavior,* pp. 51–82. Indiana University Press, Bloomington.

Bardwick, J. 1972. Her body, the battleground, *Psych. Today,* Feb., pp. 50–54, 76, 82.

Beach, F. 1942. Analysis of the stimuli adequate to elicit mating behavior in the sexually inexperienced male rat, *J. Comp. Psychol.,* **33:**163–207.

Beach, F. 1947. A review of physiological and psychological studies of the sexual behavior in mammals, *Physiol. Rev.,* **27:**240–306.

Beach, F. 1970. Hormonal effects on socio-sexual behavior in dogs, in H. Gibian and E. J. Plotz (eds.), *Mammalian Reproduction,* pp. 437–466. Springer-Verlag, New York.

Beach, F., and L. Jordan. 1956. Sexual exhaustion and recovery in the male rat, *Q. J. Exp. Psychol.,* **8:**121–133.

Beach, F., and G. Levinson. 1950. Effects of androgen on the glans penis and mating behavior of castrated male rats, *J. Exp. Zool.,* **114:**159–168.

Bremer, J. 1959. *Asexualization.* Macmillan, New York.

Brown, N. O. 1959. *Life against Death.* Wesleyan, Middletown, Conn.

Calhoun, J. B. 1962. Population density and social pathology, *Sci. Amer.,* **206**(2):139–148.

Chilton, B. 1972. Psychosexual development in twins, *J. Biosoc. Sci.,* **4:**277–286.

Diamond, M. 1968. Genetic-endocrine interactions and human psychosexuality, in M. Diamond (ed.), *Perspectives in Reproduction and Sexual Behavior,* pp. 417–443. Indiana University Press, Bloomington.

Dorfman, R. I., and R. A. Shipley. 1956. *Androgens.* Wiley, New York.

Fox, C. A., et al. 1972. Studies on the relationship between plasma testosterone levels and human sexual activity, *J. Endocrinol.,* **52:**51–58.

Fraser, A. F. 1968. *Reproductive Behavior in Ungulates.* Academic, London.

Hall, C. S., and G. Lindzey. 1970. *Theories of Personality,* 2d ed. Wiley, New York.

Hardy, K. H. 1964. An appetitional theory of sexual motivation, *Psychol. Rev.,* **71**(1):1–18.

Herbert, J. 1968. Neural and hormonal factors concerned in sexual attraction between Rhesus monkeys, *Proc. 2d Int. Congr. Primat.,* **2:**41–49.

Kinsey, A. C., et al. 1948. *Sexual Behavior in the Human Male.* Saunders, New York.

Kinsey, A. C., et al. 1953. *Sexual Behavior in the Human Female.* Saunders, New York.

Kirkendall, L. A. 1958. Toward a clarification of the concept of male sex drive, *Marriage and Family Living,* **20:**367–372.

Klüver, H., and P. Bucy. 1939. Preliminary analysis of functions of the temporal lobes of monkeys, *Arch. Neurol. Psychiatry,* **42:**979–1000.

Lisk, R. D. 1962. Diencephalic placement of estradiol and sexual receptivity in the female rat, *Am. J. Physiol.* **203:**493–496.

Lisk, R. D. 1967. Neural localization for androgen activation of copulatory behavior in the male rat, *Endocrinology,* **80:**754–761.

Lisk, R. D. 1971. Hormonal basis of reproductive behavior, in V. G. Dethier et al. (consultants), *Topics in the Study of Life,* pp. 326–335. Harper Row, New York.

Lisk, R. D., et al. 1972. The influence of olfaction on sexual behavior in the male golden hamster, *J. Exp. Zool.,* **181:**69–78.

Marcuse, H. 1955. The self and the other: Narcissus, in *Eros and Civilization.* Beacon Press, Boston.

Masica, D. N., et al. 1971. Fetal feminization and female gender identity in the testicular feminizing syndrome of androgen insensitivity, *Arch. Sex. Beha.,* **1**(2):131–142.

Masters, W. H., and V. E. Johnson. 1966. *Human Sexual Response.* Little, Brown, Boston.

Masters, W. H., and V. E. Johnson. 1970. *Human Sexual Inadequacy.* Little, Brown, Boston.

McGill, T. E. 1965. Studies of the sexual behavior of male laboratory mice: Effects of genotype, recovery of sex drive, and theory, in F. Beach (ed.), *Sex and Behavior,* pp. 76–88. Wiley, New York.

McGill, T. E., and W. C. Blight. 1963. Effects of genotype on the recovery of sex drive in the male mouse, *J. Comp. Physiol. Psychol.,* **56:**887–888.

Money, J. 1961. Components of eroticism in man: The hormones in relation to sexual morphology and sexual desire, *J. Nerv. Ment. Dis.,* **132:**239–248.

Newman, G. and C. R. Nichols. 1960. Sexual activities and attitudes in older persons, *J. A. M. A.,* **173:**33–35.

Newman, H. F. 1970. Vibratory sensitivity of the penis, *Fertil. Steril.,* **21**(11):791–793.

Palka, Y. S., and C. H. Sawyer. 1966. The effects of hypothalamic implants of ovarian steroids on oestrous behavior in rabbits, *J. Physiol.* (London), **185:**251–269.

Pavolov, I. P. 1960. *Conditioned Reflexes.* Dover, New York.

Resko, J. A. 1971. Micromethods for estimating sex steroids in plasma: One method for investigating hormone action. *Am. Zool.,* **11**(4):715–723.

Rose, R. M., et al. 1972. Plasma testosterone levels in the male Rhesus: Influences of sexual and social stimuli, *Sci.,* **178:**643–645.

Rosenblatt, J. S., and L. R. Aronson. 1958. The decline of sexual behavior in male cats after castration with special reference to the role of prior sexual experience, *Behaviour,* **12:**285–338.

Ross, J., et al. 1971. Short latency induction of estrous behavior with intracerebral gonadal hormones in ovariectomized rats, *Endocrinology,* **89:**32–38.

Salmon, U. J., and S. H. Geist. 1943. Effects of androgens upon libido in women, *J. Clin. Endocrinol.,* **3:**235–238.

Skinner, B. F. 1948. *Walden Two.* Macmillan, New York.

Stumpf, W. E. 1971. Autoradiographic techniques and the localization of estrogen, androgen, and glucocorticoid in the pituitary and brain, *Am. Zool.,* **11**(4):741–754.

Terzian, H., and G. Dalle Ore. 1955. Syndrome of Klüver and Bucy reproduced in man by bilateral removal of temporal lobe, *Neurology,* **5:**373–380.

Vander, A. J., et al. 1970. *Human Physiology: The Mechanisms of Body Function.* McGraw-Hill, New York.

Waxenberg, S. E., et al. 1959. The role of hormones in human behavior: I. Changes in female sexuality after adrenalectomy, *J. Clin. Endocrinol. and Metab.,* **19:**193–202.

Weiss, A. D. 1959. Sensory functions, in J. E. Birren (ed.), *Handbook of Aging and the Individual,* pp. 503–542. University of Chicago Press, Chicago.

Whalen, R. E. 1966. Sexual motivation, *Psychol. Rev.,* **73**(2):151–163.

Whalen, R. E. 1972. Gonadal hormones, the nervous system and behavior, in J. L. McGaugh (ed.), *The Chemistry of Mood, Motivation, and Memory.* Plenum, New York.

Winick, C. 1969. The desexualized society, *The Humanist,* December Issue.

Winokur, G. 1963. *Determinants of Human Sexual Behavior.* Charles C Thomas, Springfield, Ill.

Chapter 7

Courtship and Nonmarital Intercourse

EVOLUTION OF COURTSHIP

Sexual behavior in many species, including our own, involves at least three steps: courtship, foreplay, and coitus—not necessarily in that order.

Courtship is the act of wooing. It means to pay particular attention to another in order to gain something in return, such as love, sex, marriage, security, companionship. Extremely widespread, courtship may be found in many diverse organisms from fruit flies to side-blotched lizards and must have evolved independently many times; that is, courtship has had many separate evolutionary origins among distantly related species. In nonhumans, courtship is often coupled with defense of a given area—a phenomenon called territorial behavior. Thus the physiological bases of aggression and courtship are probably closely related. In humans, courtship becomes more complex because the responses of courting individuals involve relatively more learning, are less predictable, and show degrees of intensity such as dating, going steady, and periods of engagement.

In many nonhuman animals, courtship consists of a complex series of steps that shows little variation among the individuals of the species. Lorenz calls such steretoyped behavior "fixed action patterns" because it appears to be "fixed" by the genes of the species. Courtship of the stickleback fish is an example of a fixed action pattern in a species that also demonstrates territorial behavior. Male stickleback fish directly attack other male intruders, and the fight is stimulated by the shape, size, and color, particularly red, of a full breeding male. A female stickleback entering a male's territory will in shape and size resemble other males and is rapidly approached as if being attacked. However, females lack the red color, and this appears to confuse the attacker, who then retreats. This has, in evolution, become ritualized or perfected into an invariant zigzag dance. The zig represents a tendency to attack, and the zag implies escape, but together they are recognized as courtship, each of the separate elements being suppressed. The ritualization and lack of variation in this sequence is highly adaptive—ambiguity of meaning is thus eliminated and the female is given clear, concise signs that mating is desired.

The neural and hormonal equipment controlling fixed action patterns is built in before birth, and the components of the behavior are activated at the time of puberty. Activation involves hormonal and neural readiness of the organism as well as the incentive to behave sexually. The incentive is derived from environmental stimuli such as the behavior, odor, or color of another individual. That coordinating mechanisms can be inherited is proved by experiments where juvenile individuals injected with activating hormones will show aspects of courtship without ever experiencing or observing them previously. Fixed action patterns of all types may be an adaptive mechanism in short-lived species where time for learning is lacking.

In birds and nonhuman mammals, it is generally believed that imitation, practice, and experience play an increasingly important role in courtship. In addition, birds and mammals can be conditioned to respond to a greater range of sexual stimuli. The stickleback male responds only to the presence of a stickleback that lacks the red color. In the wild, Japanese quail also show a fixed action behavior that is triggered only by recognition of a female quail. But Farris has shown that the male quail can be conditioned to respond sexually to other stimuli as well. When the sound of a buzzer is presented simultaneously with a female, and this is repeated many times, gradually eliminating the female, males will eventually learn to court the sound. As we move from birds to apes, the range of erotic stimuli increases as does the necessity of learning how to court and mate. In fact, zoos have discovered that apes raised in isolation where they cannot observe other members of their species courting do not know how to mate.

Because of the tremendous amount of learning that occurs among humans, human courtship can be distinguished from that of all other animals by its great variety and relative lack of predictable results. We can view the techniques of human courtship as methods of individually tailored persuasion tending to bring about a desired result, but because the results are rarely certain, people take a risk whenever they court. Hence a basic characteristic of humans is the tendency to preach that certain techniques are more valuable than others. This has led to a deluge of "how to do it" books and to advice to the lovelorn from thousands of professional and nonprofessional people.

FUNCTIONS OF COURTSHIP

The advantages and disadvantages of courtship have been discussed by a number of authors (Tinbergen, Bastock) and differ from species to species depending on the requirements of mating. Note that the showing of colorful adornments and the production of sounds and odors as well as the sequences of stereotypic behavior can be included under the heading of courtship behavior. These elements constitute advertisement or display of sexual readiness. But they can also attract predators; therefore the necessity of courtship must have been so overriding as to have facilitated its evolution in the first place.

The advantages include orientation to a specific location where coitus can take place, such as a nest, a burrow, or more precisely a genital aperature as in the brightly colored vulva of chimpanzees which may act as a guide to the male. Courtship also serves to synchronize mating activity and to identify those individuals who show sexual readiness. Only a female rat in estrus will arch her back, wiggle her ears, and hop about, signaling her status and causing a male to attempt copulation. Another advantage becomes evident when similar species live in the same habitat. Thus during early spring, the males of several species of frog enter a given pond, acquire a lilypad, and start calling. A few weeks later the females will be oriented to the pond because of the general chorus of sound, but once in the pond will be guided to their specific males by a combination of tone, rhythm, and pitch unique to the species.

In addition, there is an important element of sexual selectivity in courtship. When other males are displaying within a given population, there will be competition to attract females. The most attractive males who can also defend their territories most successfully against other males will mate with the largest number of females. Therefore the genes of the healthiest and strongest males will be passed on to the next generation.

Still another advantage, which is more applicable to humans, is advocated by Konrad Lorenz in *On Aggression*. Courtship tends to suppress nonsexual responses in the pair, particularly overt physical aggression. Lorenz claims that aggression or the desire to inflict damage on another is a natural, inherited drive. Others dispute the inherited aspect and contend that aggressive behavior is a learned response to frustrating influences (Montagu). The truth may be somewhere in between; that is, the propensity for aggression is inherited, but its realization depends upon environmental triggers (Goldstein et al.). The original function of aggression in animals was protection of territory. Individuals were spaced out within the environment for equal utilization of resources, and those who most successfully protected their slice of the pie were most likely to leave descendants behind. Behavior such as aggression that has been advantageous for so long must be considered part of human heritage.

Humans are definitely aggressive in the physically overt sense of fighting as well as in the more subtle form of manipulation, coercion, and persuasion. Our very language is imbued with aggressive phraseology—"I'll take a shot at it"; "Sharpen your wits"; "Attack that statement"; "Struggle with a problem";

"Keep a sharp lookout"; "Sink your teeth into it"; "I love you so much I could eat you up." This aggression in humans may be constructive, such as in intellectual assertiveness and in the minimal assertiveness required to find and attract a mate. Or it may be destructive, such as in fighting, exploiting, and manipulating. However, aggressiveness is not the only form of behavior that governs the interactions between people. Eibl-Eibesfeldt claims that altruism or behavior that supports and helps others is also deeply rooted in human evolution. Again, whether altruism is innate, learned, or both is not known. *What is significant is the role of courtship as a mechanism by which humans try to convince each other that altruism and not exploitation is the primary goal of the relationship.* Essentially, courtship functions to convey the thought that "we nice people" are compatible and share similar interpretations of society's rules and regulations. Ideally, any tendencies for destructive aggressiveness should be suppressed; that is, ideally because too often courtship is a tool used to cover up exploitive motives either unilaterally or reciprocally.

Attempts to reconcile nonaggression with aggression can lead to some rather interesting types of behavior, such as ambivalence and displacement. *Ambivalence* means that an individual cannot decide whether to approach or escape another individual, object, or situation. The behavior then becomes mixed, exhibiting a combination of approach-and-escape procedures. For example, in some species of gulls, courting individuals will stand back to back, but with their necks craned so that their heads are face to face. The posture supposedly is analogous to the zigzag dance of the male stickleback; the gulls' face-to-face posture represents the zig (attack), and the back-to-back posture represents the zag (escape). Although the posture now is courtship behavior, its evolutionary origin again appears to be steeped in the conflicting tendencies— to attack, to escape, or to be sexual. In this case again the ambivalent posture serves to inhibit attack-and-escape tendencies while enhancing the sexual interest (Tinbergen). The other type of behavior that may result from conflicting desires is displacement. *Displacement* means to replace difficult-to-handle feelings or behavior with something that seems totally irrelevant to the situation. For instance, courting ducks vigorously preen their feathers and show an intense interest in pulling grass. It is believed that the desire to approach and the desire to escape are both so strong that the animals cop out by becoming overly interested in feathers and grass. The preening and grass pulling is the displacement behavior, and it has become a ritualized part of courtship.

Are these patterns recognizable in human courtship? Although precise extrapolation from nonhuman animals to humans can be dangerous, the following vignette summarizes the possibilities: A young man enters a room full of strangers and initially positions himself in one corner—chest out, stomach in, straining to appear taller and more muscular than he really is. He peers at his watch, cleans his glasses, strokes his beard, and blows his nose even though he has not had a cold for four months. After shaking hands with the host, he receives a drink and lights up a cigarette. A young woman approaches, and he further attempts to appear larger than life. They exchange glances, and he says "hi" in a voice an octave above his natural tone. They murmur sweet nothings and pleasantries until the nervousness and hesitation are reduced. They eventually leave together. From this true-to-life story, it can be seen that ambivalent postures, displacement, and appeasement behavior are all part of human as well as animal courtship behavior.

SOCIAL ASPECTS OF HUMAN COURTSHIP

The functions of courtship as set out in this chapter apply to all cultures, but the precise patterns of behavior vary widely from society to society and between subgroups within a culture.

Differences between Countries

Evidence from a variety of sources indicates that the dating behavior and the attitudes of unmarried college students tend to be far more liberal among the English and Norwegians than among similar populations in Canada and the United States (Luckey and Nass). German students appear to be the most conservative in attitude and restrictive in behavior. The term *liberal* in these studies means that students more often participate in a wider range of sexual activities during courtship, from tongue kissing to intercourse. Thus English students are more prone to be involved in general petting, nude embrace, and coitus; whereas students in Canada tend to restrict their activities to casual and light petting (Luckey and Nass). Females tend to be more conservative than males in all countries.

Christensen further contrasts the sharp differences between Danish and American dating patterns. All forms of sexual intimacy are made a central part of the courting process in Denmark, where petting and coitus are regarded as part of belonging together. Danes tend to approve of starting petting and coitus earlier in the relationship. This is not to imply that Danish youth are loose or promiscuous. On the contrary, dating does not occur casually but usually in an arrangement of going steady with a strong commitment toward a future marriage. Courtship among many white middle-class American youths appears more random, casual, and frequent, at least initially. The field is gradually narrowed to fewer prospective mates as sexual intimacy increases, but coitus may be delayed until after marriage. In both countries, fidelity rather than promiscuity is the rule.

Differences between Some American Subcultures

Adolescents   The American pattern described above is only one among many of the courtship styles practiced in the United States. Rosenberg and Bensman studied courtship patterns among Appalachian, black, and New York Puerto Rican adolescents. The initial pairing of individuals for dating purposes occurs at local parties called "sets" for Puerto Rican youth, at high school dances for blacks in Washington, and at drive-in theaters for Appalachian youth. Double-dating in Appalachia is common not only for friendship's sake but often for simple protection against other guys starting trouble (Rosenberg and Bensman). Within all three groups, and contrary to popular belief, courtship patterns did not involve unrestrained sexual activity or widespread promiscuity. However, the double standard seemed to be very much in evidence. The males felt that sex with a willing female was permissible for the sheer "pleasure" of it—the "friction of two membranes." The affirmation of masculinity by counting "victories" was common and often occurred at the expense of the female who became an unequal partner. Females who performed nonmarital coitus usually did so because of peer pressure or obligation.

Young Working People   Among young single working people, courtship patterns vary with upbringing, geographic location, whether the person is living at home or not, and so on. Roebuck and Spray made an intensive study of the interactions within the setting of an upper-middle-class cocktail lounge. These authors found that young unmarried women ranging in age from twenty to thirty-five (median age: twenty-four) came to the bar primarily to "enjoy sex and companionship in pleasant and discreet circumstances without having to play a competitive, exploitive courtship game." This was often performed with older married men who were professionally and economically successful. Female behavior within the lounge setting served to postpone, consciously or subconsciously, the detection and location of suitable partners for marriage.

Counterculture   A number of authors have identified a group variously called the Counterculture, New Left, or Humanist Youth in which the traditional forms of courtship have been replaced by affairs of living together and "sex without courtship" (Salisbury and Salisbury). The counterculture consists of highly transitory and heterogeneous groups centered mostly on the East and West Coasts. These people believe, with good evidence, that science and technology have brought the world close to total destruction with bombs and pollution and that little concern for humanity is shown. They wish to be spontaneous and nonjudgmental with respect to sex—"Do your own thing" is the motto, as long as no one gets hurt. In this way, self-denial and elitist attitudes are at least theoretically reduced, and there is opportunity to experience a variety of life situations in the search for self-identity. Thus sex, including intercourse, is experienced freely whether in a short-term experience, extended trial marriage, or just for its own sake. But, except for the latter, fidelity is still supreme: "It may not matter how fast one relationship follows another, but one should remain faithful to whomever he is sleeping with at the time" (Salisbury and Salisbury). A positive result of such "gut feeling" philosophy is the attempt at breaking down "false fronts" set up between two individuals. In order to appear ultramasculine and superfeminine, we often mask those characteristics that might not fit into the larger society's definition of these categories. On the negative side, the counterculture ideal does not always work out in reality. A couple may feel free to jump into sexual activity before the personal relationship is well established. Yet, like most people, the partners usually have emotional needs for a close, stable pairing and become dependent on each other. If it turns out that they are poorly matched or not ready for a long-term relationship, they sometimes try to pretend that the affair is more than it is and have trouble ending it.

SIGNS OF DIFFICULTY IN COURTSHIP

No matter which pattern of courtship a couple chooses, certain danger signals can generally be recognized that could lead to early problems in a future marriage (Landis). Temporary breakups occurring frequently during a couple's engagement imply a lack of confidence in the relationship. Agreement on values and goals as well as the approval of friends and family are other important criteria to consider. Young, inexperienced couples generally have little basis for judging whether a relationship is solid and thus frequently make mistakes. Being able to reevaluate the total relationship and easily detect the signs of possible trouble will contribute significantly to interpersonal success.

INTERCOURSE OUT OF MARRIAGE

The term *nonmarital intercourse* describes intercourse out of marriage. Unfortunately, this term suffers from a lack of information about the individual situation, for it includes categories of people who do not even share the same problems and concerns. An unmarried adolescent girl, age fifteen, for example, would certainly have a different set of values than a recently divorced forty-five-year-old woman. The term *premarital intercourse* narrows the definition to intercourse occurring sometime between puberty and the first marriage. However, even this term is confusing since it does not take into consideration the fact that intercourse often occurs between individuals who are not planning a future marriage. Also it describes little about the intensity or quality of a sexual relationship. Thus, a couple might have had intercourse once before marriage but little else in terms of foreplay, mutual masturbation, and so on, whereas another couple may be deeply involved, utilizing a variety of sexually arousing techniques but stopping short of coitus. However, most people, regardless of subcultural influence, are concerned and at times preoccupied with the pros and cons of premarital coitus. Therefore we shall direct most of our attention to actual penile entry into the vagina among adolescent and college-age unmarried people. Older single, divorced, and widowed people generally have developed sexual styles with which they feel morally and emotionally comfortable, and so they usually find it easier to make decisions about their own sexual activities. Furthermore, contemporary American society tends to be more permissive toward these somewhat older people as long as they conduct their sexual affairs discreetly.

Premarital Intercourse

Claims that a sexual revolution has been occurring in this country are based primarily on individual observations that premarital intercourse has drastically increased since the early 1960s. Scientific data gathered over a long period of time that can be used to establish a basis of comparison are at a minimum. In addition, people often assume that an increase in premarital sex invariably results in a breakdown of standards; however, little evidence has been collected. Ira Reiss (1968), after many years of studying the problem, suggests that responsibility for sexual behavior during courtship has gradually shifted from parents to the young people themselves. Adolescents have gained a greater independence in the decision-making process about sexual matters. Gallup polls taken in 1969 and 1970 provide evidence that a difference in attitude does indeed exist between parents and young people. A majority (68 percent of persons over thirty years of age) believe that premarital sex is wrong, whereas only one college student in four says that the person you eventually marry should be a virgin. However, other evidence indicates that people who have adolescent children are most conservative; whereas people who have either very small children or adult offspring are more permissive (Reiss, 1971).

Has this change resulted in an actual increase of premarital intercourse? Prior to 1960, evidence indicated that little change had occurred since Kinsey published his surveys in 1948 and 1953. New data collected since 1960 and coming from a variety of sources indicate a significant increase in premarital coitus for high school and college women but not for men. In 1953 Kinsey did a national survey of adolescents between thirteen and fifteen years of age. He reported that 3 percent of the girls and 40 percent of the boys had experienced coitus. Twenty years later Sorenson (1973) surveyed the same age group and reported 30 percent for girls and 44 percent for boys. Another recent study based upon interviews with 4,240 teenage females showed an incidence of premarital coitus of 14 percent for fifteen-year-olds and 46 percent for nineteen-year-olds (Kanter and Zelnick, 1973). These authors suggest that premarital intercourse is being experienced at a younger age than ever before but that most of it is still experienced with one partner. Among the fifteen-to-nineteen-year-olds interviewed, an average of 60 percent had only one sexual partner. Kanter and Zelnick's findings confirm Sorenson's statement that premarital intercourse, among many adolescents, is a method of communicating affection, friendship, and kindness. Exploitation of another for strictly physical release is strongly frowned upon. Sorenson reflects that "sex is a means by which young people can be themselves in what they feel is a sea of impersonality and inhumanity."

Kanter and Zelnick also point out that the sexually active adolescent female in their study did not use the more reliable contraceptive devices such as the diaphragm, IUD, or pill. More than one-half did not use any contraceptive, and most of the remaining group relied on coitus withdrawal, rhythm, douche, foam, or condoms. This evidence casts doubt on the often-expressed fear that availability of the pill will lead to a drastic increase in sexual intercourse among adolescents (Guttmacher). Also, the increased incidence of coitus does not reflect a greater knowledge or enlightenment about sexual matters on the part of the girls in the sample. Almost one-half felt that intercourse during the menses would carry the greatest risk for pregnancy. Thus many believed that ovulation occurred at the time of the menstrual flow.

Lack of knowledge about the more effective contraceptives is not the only reason why adolescent girls fail to use them (Sorenson). Many feel that using the pill, for example, makes intercourse appear planned. According to them, it should appear spontaneous and natural as an act of love. Still others desire the feeling of being carried away by passion in order to protect themselves against the guilt of having planned it all. Some girls claim to be actively rebelling against the restrictive attitudes of their parents and feel consciously or unconsciously that getting pregnant would be a very good way of punishing their families.

For nineteen-to-twenty-year-old college women, estimates of premarital coitus prior to 1960 vary from 13 to 25 percent. Kinsey et al. (1953) reported an average of 20 percent for the same age group. More recent studies indicate a significant increase in sexual activity for females in this age group but none for males. Kaats and Davis (1970) reported a premarital coital rate of 41 percent for nineteen-to-twenty-year-old women at the University of Colorado in the spring of 1967. Conversely, males were not experiencing any difference in rate of premarital coitus (60 percent when compared with that which was reported at the turn of the century).

Reliance on the more effective contraceptives tends to increase with age. However, a phenomenon that is becoming more common is the unmarried woman who plans a purposeful pregnancy in order to raise a child in single parenthood. Reduced ostracism against unmarried mothers and growing financial independence of many women have created a cultural climate conducive to pregnancies out of wedlock.

Despite claims of positive consequences, the popular press frequently expresses the idea that mostly negative effects result from premarital coitus. An overemphasis on the sexual aspects of a relationship is often mentioned as a negative result.

Numerous authors have attempted to measure the effects of premarital intercourse on marital happiness, adjustment, and female orgasmic rates. Evidence about these effects, however, is contradictory. In one study, sexual satisfaction during the wedding night and honeymoon (first two weeks of marriage) was high among couples who had experienced premarital intercourse. Virginal couples appeared, however, to "catch up" with a relatively rapid sexual adjustment shortly following the honeymoon (Kanin and Howard). Another study found a low, positive correlation between premarital virginity and predictions of high marital happiness (Shope and Broderick).

These authors suggest that conventionality and strength of conviction are characteristics of the women who choose to remain virgins prior to marriage. The strength of conviction rather than virginity may be contributing naturally to future marital happiness.

Rates of orgasm have been shown to be higher among married women who have also experienced orgasm in premarital coitus (Burgess and Wallin). Many experts agree that coital experience can contribute to the attainment of orgasm; however, careful thought must be given to the actual cause-and-effect relationship between them. It is possible that women with the highest sexual motivation seek out premarital experiences that will produce orgasm and are most likely also, because of the high motivation, to attain orgasm easily in marriage (Fisher).

Other studies have concluded that the consequences of premarital coitus depend upon the emotional stability of the partners and the degree of parental restrictiveness (Kirkendall). In families where a highly permissive environment exists and freedom of choice in sexual matters is taught as a way of life, premarital coitus rarely leads to guilt and shame on the part of the young people involved. On the other hand, negative effects are many for young people coming from a home life where strong restrictions against any form of premarital intimacy are practiced (Christensen and Gregg). It has been suggested that "less generational conflict will occur if parents know less about the sexual activities of their children" (Bell). Many adolescents engaging in premarital intercourse seek close relationships with strong commitments to fidelity. They feel that the search for intimacy is not something easily shared with parents. In the search for self-identity and a true sense of worth, they must identify the concepts of acceptance and altruism found in warm interpersonal relationships. They often rebel at the idea that a license can suddenly, overnight, give them this sense of security and confidence. Only time and practice are supposed to contribute to the attainment of stability and dependability. Yet economic security is not available to most adolescents, and marriage must be postponed until such time as independence is obtained. The question is: Have moral or legal restrictions against sexual needs and desires been effective in retarding premarital intercourse without undue side effects? The answer must be left to the judgment of the reader.

Two medical reasons against premarital intercourse are well known; these are, of course, unwanted pregnancy and venereal disease. A less well known reason is a possible increase in the risk of cervical cancer among women who experienced coitus with multiple sexual partners during early adolescence. For instance, Rotkin has found evidence that suggests a positive correlation between early premarital intercourse among adolescents and cervical cancer. And Pereyra has found a positive correlation between multiple sexual partners early in life and later development of cervical cancer. No one knows exactly why this correlation exists. But having multiple coital partners probably increases the possibility of contacting a male who could be the source of a cancer-producing irritant.

People who find themselves unmarried because of divorce, separation, or death face a set of problems that are different from those of the never-married adolescent. They have been having intercourse on a regular basis and suddenly find themselves without means of sexual gratification. Little scientific investigation has occurred into the sexual problems of the postmarried, perhaps because of conflicting values. We tell our young premarrieds intercourse should occur only in the context of a marital unit made legal by a license. Within this unit, sex is of primary importance in helping to maintain the pair bond. Suddenly a dissolution of the unit occurs. What can the individuals do now? Shift back to the moral values held a long time ago before they were married, or seek out relationships that may result in sexual intercourse? Evidence indicates that the second road is more commonly taken. The majority of men and women while divorced, widowed, or separated become involved in relationships where intercourse will take place, and this occurs within one year after dissolution of the marriage (Gebhard). How does society view this? "The escape from this dilemma is the usual one: ignore and minimize the problem as much as possible, but if forced to take a position then condemn publicly and condone privately" (Gebhard).

Very little is known about the older never-married person. But it would seem that older singlehood is a rather heterogeneous group that includes low-arousability people as well as quite a few medium- and high-arousability people who defer or avoid marriage for various other reasons. For instance, with the availability of contraceptives, the anonymity provided by large cities, and the increasing career options for women, perhaps fewer people are rushing to the altar to satisfy needs for sexual gratification, social status, or female economic security. Marriage may be deferred until an extremely satisfying relationship evolves and/or the couple is ready to have children. Other people may have financial obligations to parents or siblings that preclude early family planning; for some of these people the obligations preclude early marriage as well. Others may have a close homosexual relationship that is not legally recognized. Still others cannot or do not want to take on the emotional responsibilities of a long-term relationship. Individual observations imply that many of the single people who live on their own in large cities have sexual life styles that are similar to those of the formerly married. Unfortunately, we do not have any scientifically researched data.

BIBLIOGRAPHY

Bastock, M. 1967. The physiology of courtship and mating behavior, in A. McLaren (ed.), *Advances in Reproductive Physiology*. Academic, London.

Bell, R. R. 1972. Parent-child conflict in sexual values, in R. R. Bell and M. Gordon (eds.), *The Social Dimension of Human Sexuality*. Little, Brown, Boston.

Bell, R. R., and J. B. Chaskes. 1970. Premarital sexual experience among coeds 1958–1968, *J. Marr. & Fam.*, **32**:81–84.

Burgess, E. W., and P. Wallin. 1953. *Engagement and Marriage.* Lippincott, Philadelphia.

Christensen, H. T. 1966. Scandinavian and American sex norms: some comparisons with sociological implications, *J. Soc. Issues,* **22:**60–75.

Christensen, H. T., and C. F. Gregg. 1970. Changing sex norms in America and Scandinavia, *J. Marr. & Fam.,* **32:**616–627.

Christopherson, W. M., et al. 1965. Relation of cervical cancer to early marriage and childbearing, *N. Engl. J. Med.,* **273:**235–239.

Eibl-Eibesfeldt, I. 1961. The fighting behavior of animals, *Sci. Amer., vol. 205, Dec. Issue, p. 112.*

Farris, H. E. 1967. Classical conditioning of courting behavior in the Japanese quail *Coturnix coturnix japonica, J. Exper. Analysis Behavior,* **10:**213–217.

Fisher, S. 1973. *The Female Orgasm.* Basic Books, New York.

Freedman, M. B. 1965. The sexual behavior of American college women: an empirical study and historical survey, *Merrill-Palmer Q. of Behavior and Development,* **11:**33–48.

Gebhard, P. 1970. Postmarital coitus among widows and divorcees, in P. Bohannan (ed.), *Divorce and After,* pp. 81–96. Doubleday, Garden City, N.Y.

Goldstein, B. 1968. Population dynamics of the lizard, *Uta stansburiana hesperis,* Unpublished master's thesis, San Francisco State College.

Goldstein, B., et al. 1970. On aggression by Konrad Lorenz—a discussion, *Calif. Elem. Adm.,* Suppl. May Issue.

Guttmacher, A. 1973. Are we in the midst of a sexual revolution? *Planned Parenthood–World Population Newsletter,,* 68, New York.

Kaats, G. R., and K. E. Davis. 1970. The dynamics of sexual behavior of college students, *J. Marr. & Fam.,* **32**(3):390–399.

Kanin, E. J., and D. H. Howard. 1958. Postmarital consequences of premarital sex adjustments, *Amer. Soc. Rev.,* **23:**556–562.

Kanter, J., and M. Zelnick. 1973. Sexual contraception and pregnancy experience of young unmarried women in the U.S., *Planned Parenthood–World Population,* 1352, New York.

Kinsey, A., et al. 1953. *Sexual Behavior in the Human Female.* Saunders, Philadelphia.

Kirkendall, L. A. 1961. *Premarital Intercourse and Interpersonal Relations.* Julian Press, New York.

Landis, J. T. 1970. Danger signals in courtship, *Med. Aspects Hum. Sex.,* **1**(1):34–46.

Lorenz, K. 1965. *Evolution and Modification of Behavior.* University of Chicago Press, Chicago.

Luckey, E. B., and G. D. Nass. 1969. A comparison of sexual attitudes and behavior in an international sample, *J. Marr. & Fam.,* **31**(2):364–379.

Montagu, M. F. A. (ed.). 1968. *Man and Aggression.* Oxford University Press, London.

Pereyra, A. J. 1961. The relationship of sexual activity to cervical cancer, *Obstet. Gynecol.,* **17:**154–159.

Reiss, I. L. 1968. *How and Why America's Sex Standards Are Changing,* Trans-action Inc., New Jersey.

Reiss, I. L. 1969. Premarital sexual standards, in C. B. Broderick and J. Bernard (eds.), *The Individual Sex and Society: A SIECUS Handbook for Teachers.* Johns Hopkins, Baltimore.

Reiss, I. L. 1971. Premarital sex codes: The old and the new, in D. L. Grummon and A. M. Barclay (eds.), *Sexuality: a Search for Perspective,* pp. 190–203. Van Nostrand, New York.

Roebuck, J., and S. L. Spray. 1967. The cocktail lounge: a study of heterosexual relations in a public organization, *Amer. J. Sociology,* **72**(4):388–395.

Rosenberg, B., and J. Bensman. 1968. Sexual patterns in three ethnic subcultures of an American underclass, *Annals of the American Academy of Political Science and Social Science,* **376**:61–75.

Rotkin, I. E. 1967. Sexual characteristics of a cervical cancer population, *Amer. J. Ped. Health,* **57**(5):815–829.

Salisbury, W. W., and F. F. Salisbury. 1971. Youth and the search for intimacy, in L. A. Kirkendall and R. N. Whitehurst (eds.), *The New Sexual Revolution,* Chap. 13. Donald W. Brown, New York.

Shope, D. F., and C. B. Broderick. 1967. Level of sexual experience and predicted adjustment in marriage, *J. Marr. & Fam.,* **29**(3):424–427.

Sorenson, R. C. 1973. *Adolescent Sexuality in Contemporary America.* World Publishing, New York.

Tinbergen, N. 1954. The origin and evolution of courtship and threat display, in J. Huxley et al. (eds.), *Evolution as a Process.* pp. 271–290. Collier Books, New York.

Chapter 8

Precoital Stimulation

For many individuals, sexual intercourse is preceded by a variety of activities which serve to increase sexual arousal. Such activities involve interaction with stimuli, symbolic and real, which are received via the senses of sight, hearing, smell, and touch. Previous conditioning must have occurred for a person to interpret a particular stimulus as an erotic one. The sense of skin contact contributes to feelings of pleasure, and its important role in sexual arousal apparently extends beyond the human to other animals where numerous species cuddle and huddle.

SKIN CONTACT

This is the skin some babies feel
replete with hippo love appeal,
Each contact, cuddle, push, and shove
elicits tons of baby love.

H. F. Harlow
The Hippopotamus

Touch has a positive influence on the way many animals behave. This behavior may take the form of orientation under a rock, in a narrow crevice, or in a close huddle with others of the same species. The adaptive value of contact behavior involves requirements for food, protection, and warmth, and in the case of some monkey species is an important prerequisite for survival of the newborn. Harlow (1965) has shown that many Rhesus monkeys raised on the bare floor of a wire mesh cage and isolated from their mothers die during the first 5 days of life. If a wire mesh cone covered with terrycloth is introduced into the cage, many more of the baby monkeys survive. Harlow also found that baby monkeys spend more time clinging to surrogate mothers made of cloth than to surrogate mothers made of wire, even though both types were rigged up to give plenty of milk. These data suggest that infant primates have a strong need for intimate physical contact, as strong perhaps as the necessity for food. "Contact comfort" may indeed be another of the basic drives similar to hunger, thirst, and sex.

Physiology of Skin Contact

The skin has five basic senses: pain, touch, pressure, warmth, and cold; each of these senses is detected by a different type of receptor. Tickle, itch, and pain are produced by stimulation of the same receptors. The particular sensation depends on the intensity of stimulation. For example, a mild stimulation of the skin with a finger causes a tickling sensation, rather pleasurable, sometimes provoking laughter or sexual arousal (Kepecs). Kinsey reports that some women even reach orgasm by having their ears or eyebrows tickled. Of special interest, ticklish people seem to show their emotions easily, laughing and crying with comparatively little provocation. Moderate stimulation of the skin causes an increase in the firing rate of the nerve endings and in the total number of nerve cells activated. This greater stimulation is usually detected as a combination of pain and pleasure—a sensation known as itch. Many people have been observed to scratch an itchy spot on the skin as long as it is "erotically gratifying" and until it becomes painful. Kepecs claims that masochists attempt to obtain as much pleasure as possible by staying in the "tickle-itch" end of the tickle-pain series and also by approaching the painful end without making it extreme. Extreme stimulation of the skin will, of course, cause extreme pain.

Receptors for touch and pressure differ from those involved in the tickle-pain series. For one thing, nerve cells associated with touch and pressure receptors conduct impulses to the brain more rapidly. For another, the touch and pressure nerve cells quickly adapt to continuous stimulation by becoming less responsive. The last point is of considerable importance. Pain is produced by noxious stimulation and would lose its "warning" quality if its associated nerve cells adapted quickly. In the case of touch and pressure, it may be more important for an organism to detect *changes* in stimulation rather than continuous sensation. Vertebrates that carry their young and others that may live in confined areas possess receptors that adapt quickly, little concern being given to the physical contact occurring in this type of behavior. Indeed, clothes on the human body, unless unnecessarily tight, are simply "forgotten" within minutes or seconds of putting them on, owing to rapid adaptation of the touch and pressure receptors. Changes in contact with clothing, such as a slipped girdle, popped bra, or flipped zipper, would be of more concern to the individual and are more quickly detected than the same articles normally in place. An understanding of the rapid adaptation of touch and pressure receptors is important to those who wish to increase sexual arousal. Many marriage manuals prescribe direct, continuous contact with the clitoris, nipples, earlobes, and so on, in order to give sexual pleasure, but stroking these structures continuously only leads to numbness and even pain. Thus, changes in stimulation provided by moving quickly from place to place may be more appropriate than continuous contact.

Temperature reception by the skin is also important in sexual arousal. Some aphrodisiac creams and lotions activate not only touch and pressure receptors but also the "warm" or "cold" receptors, thereby giving a more nearly total sensation of physical contact.

Erogenous Zones

Two people touching one another can experience considerable pleasure; however, the feeling of pleasure may be independent of sexual arousal. How and when arousal and pleasure become interrelated in the development of an erogenous zone is dependent upon previous conditioning. An erogenous zone is any part of the skin containing numerous receptors that when stroked causes sexual arousal. Any portion of the skin can be erogenous. Whether the numbers of receptors located in a given area are correlated with how easily that region becomes erogenous is not known. The skin of the back, for example, contains touch receptors about 65 mm apart; in the finger, they may be more concentrated—only 3 mm apart. Evidence does indicate that there is wide consensus among members of one sex as to which parts of the skin are most erogenous. A questionnaire was given to 417 females and 370 males, mostly between the ages twenty to twenty-five, attending a human sexuality course at San Francisco State University in the spring of 1971. One of the questions asked was, "Indicate the most important erogenous zone in your body (other than genital) that when stimulated gives you the most sexual arousal." Results are shown in Table 8-1. As can be seen, a great deal of similarity exists between the sexes except for the most important zone. Almost 37 percent of the females in the sample rated the breast as number one; whereas approximately 32 percent of the males rated their thighs as number one.

Foreplay

Physical contact which purposely increases sexual arousal prior to intercourse is called *foreplay*, or petting. Foreplay serves to heighten and synchronize the arousal levels of the partners. A great deal of variation as to the amount of foreplay exists between cultures, but it should be stressed that the differences are more quantitative than qualitative. The time involved in foreplay varies

Table 8-1   Primary Erotic Zone Excluding Genitals

Zone	Males, %	Females, %
Back	4.9	4.3
Breasts	4.9	36.5
Chest	4.6	0.24
Ears	7.0	8.1
Lips	10.0	6.0
Neck	4.6	6.5
Stomach	5.2	6.7
Thighs	31.5	14.2
Other	6.1	3.4

Source: Results obtained from a questionnaire given to 370 males and 417 females.

more than does particular type of foreplay (Ford and Beach). Thus, the Lepchas of the Himalayas show minimum foreplay, although males may occasionally caress a female's breasts; while the Trobrianders of Eastern Melaneasia spend many hours in complex foreplay. In our own society, the duration and complexity of foreplay are highly variable.

Gebhard has accumulated evidence of a positive correlation between the duration of foreplay and rate of orgasm in married women. Close to three-fifths of a sample of 78 wives experienced orgasm almost always if intercourse was preceded by a period of foreplay lasting longer than 21 min (see Table 8-2). Shorter periods of foreplay were correlated with lower rates of orgasm. Blood, claiming that foreplay increases the possibility of a woman's orgasmic response only up to a point, believes that protracted foreplay beyond 21 to 25 min no longer increases the rate of orgasmic response and can reduce it by the onset of fatigue or boredom. Fisher's recent work, *The Female Orgasm,* suggests that no correlation exists between duration of foreplay and rate of orgasm.

In the United States, much of the sexual activity that occurs prior to sexual intercourse has been embodied with the concepts of the work ethic and professional sportsmanship (Lewis and Brissett). Operating under the premise

Table 8-2   Female Orgasm Rate and Duration of Precoital Foreplay in Intact Marriages

Percentage of coitus resulting in orgasm	Average duration of foreplay in minutes			
	0	1–10	15–20	21 plus
	Percentage			
0	(2 cases)	3.9	7.6	7.7
1– 39	(1 case)	19.5	12.6	7.7
40– 89	(1 case)	34.6	28.9	25.6
90–100	(2 cases)	41.9	50.6	58.9
Total cases	6	179	79	78

Source: Gebhard, P. H., 1966.

that sexual activity among humans functions as a source of fun and pleasure in addition to reproduction, marriage manuals, counselors, and psychiatrists are set up to give advice on how to get the maximum play value out of sex. But to many people, "to play" means "to work at it," and hard. Traveling to the mountains or playing table tennis becomes a "grim resolve" and is filled with determination to win. So it seems with sex. A period of intensive training is often suggested and required where a person learns how to "grip" with the vagina, "probe" with the penis, apply just the right pressure with the teeth, and stick the tongue into a shot glass. Following exhaustive training, many, instead of becoming excellent technicians at sex play, are candidates for a chiropractor!

The following report on the methods of foreplay will lack precise descriptions of how to best employ them, leaving their use up to the reader's inventiveness, originality, and skill at acrobatics. Table 8-3 shows methods of foreplay in decreasing order of frequency as seen in the United States.

Kissing A kiss can be defined as a "salute with the lips," involving at least the senses of touch, taste, and smell. Of interest, kissing for erotic purposes is uniquely human. And even though kissing appears universally among Americans, its presence in other parts of the world is not nearly as common as manual manipulation of, and oral contact with, the genitalia (Ford and Beach). Indeed, a map showing the distribution of kissing as a practice among cultures would contain large vacant spots. Kissing was not found originally among the Australian aborigines, Maoris of New Zealand, Papuans, Tahitians, South Sea Islanders, and Eskimos, although importation by missionaries has since occurred. Up until 15 years ago, there was no word for kiss in Japanese, and the native Chinese did not kiss for any reason.

Breast Stimulation Breast stimulation, for the purposes of sexual arousal, is confined to the human species. No comparative study has been made of the

Table 8-3 Methods of Foreplay Arranged in Order of Decreasing Frequency

1   General body contacts—hugging, body caress
2   Simple kissing
3   Tongue kissing
4   Manual manipulation of female breast
5   Manual manipulation of female genitalia
6   Oral stimulation of female breast
7   Manual stimulation of male genitalia
8   Oral stimulation of male genitalia—fellatio
9   Oral stimulation of female genitalia—cunnilingus
10 Oral stimulation of anal area—anilingus
11 Painful stimulation

Source: Based on Kinsey, 1953; Ford and Beach, 1951; Brady and Levitt, 1965.

neural sensitivity found in breasts of various mammal species; however, stimulation is almost totally lacking among nonhuman animals. This is surprising, since an intimate neural and hormonal relationship exists between breasts and uterus. It is well known that breast-feeding an infant causes secretion from the pituitary gland of a hormone, oxytocin, that is essential for the release of milk and also causes the contraction of the uterus. Sexual intercourse itself has been known to cause milk release in a lactating woman, which also infers oxytocin secretion. M. Heiman has described how "the feeling of sexual pleasure" can be derived from nursing a baby. Masters and Johnson (1966) found that three of their female study subjects could reach orgasm by breast stimulation alone. Many women relate that mouthing of nipples and sucking of breasts is correlated with obvious contractions in the pelvic region which can be highly pleasurable. Thus breast stimulation has been implicated as being responsible for the release of oxytocin which then acts on the uterus and possibly other genitalia, causing contraction. This certainly would improve sperm transport and is highly pleasurable reinforcing foreplay even without coitus or orgasm. Evidence indicates that breast stimulation and subsequent oxytocin release may cause testosterone secretion, which in turn raises the level of sexual arousal (Armstrong and Hansel). Oxytocin may also raise the blood pressure and cause smooth muscle contraction, which is responsible for pelvic sensations in both sexes. Thus the total body effects produced by breast stimulation are seen as functional primarily in humans where maintenance of high arousal levels in prolonged foreplay is critical to potential coitus and full sexual satisfaction.

Manual Stimulation of the Genitals   Manual stimulation of the genitals is a highly pleasurable form of foreplay and can in itself lead to orgasm. The fact that it falls in eighth and ninth place on the list of American foreplay methods might be attributable to common early negative reinforcement of masturbation. For this reason, we shall direct our discussion toward masturbation. But keep in mind that masturbation and reciprocal manual stimulation involve the same anatomy and physiology and that both phenomena are part of the sexual repertoire of experienced adults.

Masturbation can be defined as self-stimulation of the genitalia and/or other parts of the body in order to derive erotic pleasure. The contention that masturbation can harm you, physically and mentally, is still deeply ingrained in the beliefs of some Americans. This is so despite the fact that no form of injury has been directly attributed to masturbation. In fact, no statement has ever been made by any medical or psychiatric organization as to maximum or minimum standards of masturbation. Nevertheless, many people have conceptualized a maximum frequency beyond which potential injury could occur. Masters and Johnson (1966) thus reported that one man who masturbated once a month felt that three times a week was excessive and could lead to mental illness; whereas another man masturbating two or three times a day believed that five or six times a day was excessive and could result in a "case of nerves." None of the 312 men interviewed expressed concern that his particular frequency was extreme. Theoretically at least, the body would cease responding physiologically before damage due to masturbation would occur. Clinical evidence for this is limited but does exist. J. Raboch (1969) reports on the results of a medical examination performed on a twenty-seven-year-old Jewish man held in a Nazi concentration camp during World War II. This man, along with 20 others, was fed and clothed well but was forced to masturbate every three hours day and night for a period of 21 months. Despite this amount of activity, no evidence could be found of genital or psychological disorder in sexual matters. Fertility was normal, and potency was excellent.

The incidence of masturbation is high for Americans of both sexes—85 to 96 percent of males, and 50 to 80 percent of females have experienced masturbation to orgasm at least once in their lives (Kinsey et al., 1953). Ninety-two percent of all men who will ever experience masturbation will have done so by the age of twenty. On the other hand, females, as a group, take longer to discover masturbation so that by the age of forty-five approximately 62 percent of all women who will ever experience it have done so. Frequencies range widely from the claim of zero to several times a day.

Because of the structure of the male genitalia, boys and men show relatively little variety with respect to masturbation techniques (Masters and Johnson). Some use firm gripping and stroking methods focusing primarily on the glans or on the shaft. Others lightly touch and tug the skin around the frenulum. Uncircumcised males generally restrict manipulation to the shaft and rarely retract the foreskin so that the glans is exposed. As a male reaches sexual tensions close to orgasm, rapidity of manipulation increases. At the point of ejaculation, however, manipulation appears to cease or markedly slow down. This decrease in manipulation may also occur during intercourse and contrasts with the desire of many females to strongly increase pelvic movements at the time of orgasm (Masters and Johnson). This implies a physiological incompatibility for the attainment of simultaneous orgasms. Immediately following an ejaculation, males may express the feeling of hypersensitivity to touch or pressure around the glans penis. This may reflect the entrance into a physiological refractory period experienced by most men following orgasm. Receptors and nerves require a period of recovery, the basis of which is still unknown.

Note that the primary focus of erotic stimulation for the majority of males is the penis and not the scrotum. Some males have been known to use vaginal substitutes during masturbation. These "vaginas" are usually made of life-like inflatable plastic with real human hair distributed appropriately. Some vaginal substitutes come built into stretch pants whereas others come as part of a whole life-size "woman" made of inflatable latex or vinyl.

Techniques of female masturbation appear to show as much variation as the females themselves; however, some common activities have been observed. Females rarely stimulate the glans clitoris directly but rather concentrate on manual stimulation of the clitoral shaft by tugging on the tissue of the prepuce and labia. A very important technique used by many women is the application of various forms of pressure to the mons veneris. Muscular tension developed along the inner surface of the thighs and the buttocks may indirectly stimulate the vulva. Pressing the vulva firmly or lightly against pillows, bed sheets, or another person is commonly practiced. Some women manually stimulate breasts and other areas such as thighs and buttocks. Accessory methods such as fantasizing or use of vibrators are employed; whereas artificial penises, called dildos, are inserted into the vagina only rarely.

Oral-Genital Stimulation   Oral-genital contact is widespread among many species, including our own. Female kangaroo rats are known to lick the penis and scrotum until the male is aroused enough for intercourse. Male African lions will often lick a female's vulva which rapidly heightens her sexual receptivity. Humans define three types of oral-genital contact: *cunnilingus,* which comes from the Latin, literally meaning "vulva—to lick"; *fellatio—* derived from the Latin *fellare,* meaning "to suck"; and *soixante-neuf,* French for "69," which refers to simultaneous oral-genital contact between two individuals.

R. Athanasiou et al. (1970) reported the results of a questionnaire on sexual attitudes and behavior in *Psychology Today.* Out of 20,000 responses they found little difference between the sexes in the giving and receiving of oral-genital stimulation. About 35 to 40 percent of both sexes responded that they experienced oral-genital contact frequently. These percentages approach the results published by Kinsey almost 20 years ago for individuals with considerable coital experience, and therefore indicate either an extremely sophisticated readership of *Psychology Today* or an increase in oral-genital activity over the years. Of those responding in *Psychology Today,* a sizable number stated that they never had experienced oral-genital contact, either giving or receiving, but would like to have tried it (14 to 20 percent males; 6 to 9 percent females).

Methods of stimulation in cunnilingus involve a partner's tonguing, sucking, and kissing of the clitoris and labial structures all the while adding saliva to reduce friction. If a woman is ovulating, high estrogen levels cause an increase in the amount of sugar in the vaginal fluids and a sweet taste will be evident, although this is not a diagnostic test for ovulation. The only time cunnilingus can be medically improper is during pregnancy. At that time, many large blood vessels are located close to the surface of the uterus. If air is blown into the vagina, bubbles may enter the blood stream, causing air embolism and possible death.

Fellatio involves a partner's licking of the frenulum and glans penis, sucking of the glans while gripping the shaft, and sucking as much shaft as possible. Some men have claimed difficulty trying to ejaculate while being sucked, possibly because of pressures built up in the mouth. Mouth pressures certainly fluctuate, becoming lower than penile pressure during sucking and higher than those inside the penis during blowing phases of the act. Swallowing also increases the pressure within the mouth. When oral pressures exceed those necessary to force an ejaculation, a male may experience a temporary inability to reach orgasm.

Despite the prevalence of oral-genital manipulation, the act is considered a felony in many states. This means that it is a major crime along with murder and arson, and individuals convicted in California, for example, have been known to serve an average sentence of 41 months in state prison (McCabe). For comparison, the average sentence for manslaughter is 42 months and that for rape with great bodily harm is only 36 months. In many states, the laws against *sodomy,* or *crimes against nature,* include oral-genital contact, but California, until January 1, 1976, had on the books a law which specifically mentioned and called for prosecution of persons committing "oral sex perversion" (California Penal Code 288a). The statute was particularly severe on a "person 10 years older than his coparticipant" and if "force, violence, duress, menace, or threat of great bodily harm" were involved. Recently, a superior court judge in San Diego ruled the law unconstitutional on the grounds that married persons consenting to oral-genital sex in the privacy of their own homes are no business of the law. It follows that if married persons cannot be prosecuted because of the right to marital privacy, unmarried persons become the only segment of society which can. Since this appears to treat unmarried persons unnecessarily harshly, and may violate their rights of equal protection under the Fourteenth Amendment, Penal Code 288a and other laws like it can be considered unconstitutional. It must be stated that superior court decisions "apply only to the case on which the judgment was made and are subject to appeal or rehearing by higher courts" (Gatov); therefore, Penal Code 288a was not removed from California law until the State Assembly and the Governor passed another law legalizing oral and anal intercourse performed voluntarily and in private.

Anilingus   Anilingus is a general name given to oral-anal stimulation and is distinct from anal intercourse. Because of this distinction, it is difficult to say whether a statute concerns anilingus per se. In many states, however, since anilingus is not mentioned as such, it could be prosecuted under statutes governing "sodomy," "crimes against nature," and "indecent exposure."

The skin of the anal region is richly endowed with receptors and much of the neural circuitry is closely allied to that of the genitalia. Prior conditioning of a person is critical if pleasure is to be derived from anilingus. Two people would obtain a great deal of psychological satisfaction in a relationship that shows almost total lack of inhibition. Medically, the healthy skin around the anus or elsewhere, if kept clean, appears to have a natural self-disinfecting mechanism keeping pathogenic bacteria from invading it. Nevertheless, a long history of sexual restrictions and the association of the anus with the act of defecation makes the anal area an uncommon erogenous zone. Even the author of *The Sensuous Woman* expressed concern when she considered sexual activity with the anus as "optional" (J).

Painful Stimulation   Some people in American society become conditioned to a certain amount of "scratching, pinching, and biting" which can increase levels of sexual arousal; however, mildly painful stimulation has become a regular part of foreplay in relatively few societies. Ford and Beach report that the Apinaye women of Brazil bite pieces of eyebrow off their partners and spit them loudly to one side. The Siriono of South America may poke at each other's eyes while scratching and pinching the neck and chest skin. Trukese women of Oceania enjoy poking their fingers into their lovers' ears, which seems to add to the excitement of all involved. Trobrianders bite each other on the face and lips until blood is drawn. Few generalizations can be made about why some cultures and not others utilize mild pain as methods of sexual stimulation. However, in those that do, it seems that both partners invariably participate, which is contrary to most nonhuman species, where painful stimulation is performed mainly by the male. In addition, these societies allow for a considerable amount of sexual freedom among their children. How this relates to the development of techniques causing pain is not understood except that with freedom to experiment and explore, the human is capable of devising an almost infinite number of methods of sexual arousal.

THE OTHER SENSES

Any stimulus such as a perfume, a song, an advertisement, or a garment that is associated with a prior pleasurable sexual experience can produce a sexual response. Besides touch, we are thus capable of being turned on by things we see, smell, hear, or think that correlate with positive past experiences. Some psychologists believe that only touch has a physiological basis of pleasure and that we must completely learn positive associations with all the other senses if they are to be avenues of erotic stimuli. I cannot accept this, simply because no experiments have been done that definitely prove it, and there exists indirect evidence that is contradictory. Cows give more and better quality milk to the sounds of Brahms and Beethoven than to no sounds at all. To many humans there are certain sounds and sights such as the Grand Canyon which evoke sensations of pleasure even if they have never previously been heard or seen. What pleases a human is, of course, highly variable and a matter of taste—yet some consensus does exist. Many repeated tastings of fine wines often lead to a general consensus among a large group of people with a wide variety of tastes as to which few vintages are the most superb. Thus whether we must learn all or have some inherent ability to "know" things that give us pleasure and are esthetically beautiful remains to be discovered.

Vision

One of our most powerful senses is vision. Possessing parts of over a million nerve cells in both optic (eye) nerves, we can see a candle 15 miles away in the dark of night. Certain colors, changes in light intensity, the cut of a garment, the way a person walks or stands can all act as erotic stimuli through the sense of vision. Controversy exists about differences between the sexes in their responses to visual stimuli. Physiologically, the two sexes possess similar average arousabilities, but men are supposed to be more often aroused by the physical person, naked or clothed, whereas women are more often "turned on" by the total situation, the decor, the partner's attentions, and the romantic quality of the surroundings.

Despite these suppositions, few detailed experiments have been performed. One study has recently been published by a group of German scientists on sex-specific differences with respect to visual stimuli (Sigusch et al.). The study was highly significant because an adequate number of people were tested, 50 males and 50 females, and physiological measures of sexual excitement (vaginal lubrication, erection, and so on) were obtained along with data from extensive questionnaires. The participants were all shown a variety of pictures, some depicting intercourse, some showing people kissing, others of men or women in bathing suits or in the nude. All persons were asked to judge pictures in two ways: (1) Did they consider the picture favorable or unfavorable in a moral, emotional, or aesthetic sense? (2) How sexually arousing did they find the picture? When the experimenters compared the answers to the first question, they discovered that the pictures containing romantic themes such as embracing with affection and kissing were judged more favorably by women than by men. Pictures of coitus and petting were judged somewhat less favorably by women than by men, and those of nudes and seminudes much more unfavorably by women than by men. On the other hand, the answers to question two showed less differences between men and women. Both sexes claimed that the pictures depicting coitus and petting were the most sexually arousing. However, the arousal content of the romantic pictures was also ranked very high by women, but it was ranked quite low by men. It must also be stated that wide variation existed for all judgments within each sex as well as between them. The authors concluded that women are more "conditioned" to situations with romantic contact and react as expected, but are capable of reaching degrees of physiological arousal similar to men.

Clothing

Clothing can also be used to increase visual stimulation. Because public nakedness is frowned upon in American society, clothing has become an extension of our sexuality, symbolic of our wishes and dreams and, at the same time, an armor protecting us from insecurities. Skeletons made of cloth change us into instant heroes and heroines, communicating desirability to all who glance our way. Besides sexual attraction, clothes are worn for comfort, for being fashionable, to assert our equal rights, for individuality, and to protect us from the weather. Actually during much of human history, both sexes wore skirts, colorful silks, laces, girdles, earrings, and tall, curly coiffures emitting rich perfumes from deep within their interiors (U. Stanndard). High heels were a male invention developed to keep the foot in a stirrup while riding a horse. Cheesecake was evident back in 1340 when both sexes wore long shapeless gowns and men began to shorten them in order to reveal their legs. Not to be outdone, women began to lower their bodices—"So as men's skirts got higher, women's decolletages got lower" (U. Stanndard). Indeed there are portraits of Queen Elizabeth I with an absolutely bare bosom. Eventually, men's skirts got so short they were called tunics and exposed genitalia had to be covered up by a codpiece or crotch pouch. Competition became intense and codpieces got bigger and better—stuffed and padded until a few reached grapefruit size. Thus, what was meant to conceal became a center of attraction.

Historically, as U. Stanndard suggests, Victorian England by the mid-nineteenth century was a real aberration in terms of clothing. Styles for men and women diverged sharply. All feminine aspects disappeared from men's clothes, which became colorless, with straight coats and high, stiff collars. Women's skirts expanded into ever-widening circles, gaining layer after layer of protection against possible "sexual abuses." Antisexuality reigned, possibly because of medical beliefs that semen should be conserved as a vital natural resource, never wasted in masturbation or nonmarital coitus.

Modern styles once again are convergent between the sexes, which means that European and American societies have returned to the natural similarities that have existed throughout our history (U. Stanndard). In the late sixties and early seventies, at least two styles of clothing appeared to be prominently considered by many people as providing sex appeal. The first style can be called the *military type*, consisting of fatigues, epaulets, and metal buttons combining the revolutionary aspects of Che Guevara and the more elegant parade-ground neatness of West Point. The second style, derived from the old West's ruggedness and natural hardships, may be called the "cow person." This style consists of boots and tight-fitting jeans with wide belts and bright buckles. Shirts have snaps, numerous seams, and hug the body closely. Women's styles not only include the military and western cut but possess an extra "natural" look of rounded breasts and real or fake nipples poking from beneath special bras that are designed to give a braless look—a return to the pioneer days of tough but feminine existence. The greater freedom in dress and similarity between the sexes is symbolic of a return to nature with its concomitant spirit of sexual flexibility and liberation from restrictions. I say symbolic because clothing worn by a person in European and American society is often designed to evoke a fantasy of sexual receptiveness on the part of an onlooker while also acting as a status symbol for the person and the person's partner. Indeed "fashion has been called a game of hide and seek between seduction and prudery" (Stember).

Hearing

Music, poetry, and words are often used to enhance sexual excitement and pleasure. The natural rhythm of a heartbeat has been suggested as one of the most soothing and pleasing sounds one can hear. After all, we develop in a uterus for 9 months very close to the sounds of the maternal heart. Supposedly the fetus becomes conditioned to the beating rhythm which occurs simultaneously with the life-giving provisions of the ambient environment—thus what provides life also beats. The conditioning of a child and adolescent to soft singing, diminuendos and crescendos of a symphony, or the sensuous rhythms of rock music serves to prepare an individual for associations with sex. "Indeed, rock music reflects the sexual fantasies and uncertain sexual identity of many youth" (Winick). For the first time in history, a form of music (rock) has been developed specifically for youth by youth to express concern about the whole gamut of human disorganization—problems of self-identity, civil rights, political organization, and contradictions in human sexual behavior. Songs contain not only stimulating rhythms and beats but lyrics that deal directly or cryptically with sexual activity. Charles Winick describes "Pictures of Lily" as a song that infers a boy masturbating while looking at a picture of a girl named Lily. No inference is needed with the song "Wet Dreams," which claims that a young man had a wet dream after the prom. Only the least imaginative would doubt the meaning of the title "Great Balls of Fire," however vague its lyrics. Listening to the words of these songs can indeed raise the level of sexual arousal, not only for the obvious sexual reference but because of the implicit threat to the adult society, which supposedly views the whole esoteric lot with doubt and confusion. There is danger in threatening the establishment, and there is sex in danger.

The adult society is not exempt from the responsibility of producing its own sexual stimuli that can titillate the senses. People in the advertising industry recognize that many products sell only if people can be convinced that new sex appeal is gained by their use. The stimulation of sexual fantasies with the handsome man from Glad, virile Mr. Clean, mature Mrs. Olson, or liberated Virginia Slims appears to be part of a master plan for sales. The possible cure for sexual inadequacy is hinted at by a number of advertisements. The impotence that can result from gastric distress is quickly dispelled on the wedding night by drinking alkalizers. The purification of putrid mouth odor, elimination of underarm stains, and the dehydration of the "wet head" all supposedly lead to the possibility of success in sexual endeavors. Oriented primarily toward youth and "swinging singles," the advertisements generally depict the married situation as drab and mundane, with the high point in life the fact that a specific cleanser "turns blue." It is interesting to note that some people have defined pornography as "materials whose dominant purpose is exciting sexual desire" (Mathis). If this definition were applied to the advertising industry, most advertisements would be considered pornographic.

Smell

The only senses not significantly utilized by the media are smell and taste, which are closely related. There is a variety of evidence from animal species and humans that odor may play an important role in sexual arousal. The term *pheromone*, derived from studies on insects, refers to any chemical substance produced by one individual that changes the behavior of another (Bronson). For example, 90 percent of a sample of sows in heat will assume a copulatory posture when provided with the odor of a boar and pressure of a handler's hand. Only 51 percent will assume such a posture in response to hand pressure alone (Signoret and du Bisson). Ewes in heat will successfully discover a ram hidden from view. Thus an important function of odor is long-distance signaling of sexual readiness in natural populations.

The effects of pheromones on humans is not clear. Some believe that body odor may, up to a point, be inherently stimulating. The more intense the level of sexual arousal, the more effective is the stimulatory power of body odor. The adaptive value of underarm and pubic hair has been suggested as a "catchall of odor" for the purpose of causing arousal. Association of a person with certain odors and positive sexual experience leads to conditioning toward these odors. Scientists at Syntex Corporation are reportedly working on isolating a chemical constituent of human vaginal fluids which will possess aphrodisiac qualities when sniffed. There is little doubt that odors can have a variety of effects— sometimes being offensive and at other times pleasant, all depending on the concentration, the particular set of circumstances, and the level of sexual arousal.

SOCIAL CONDITIONS

We have been discussing many factors that contribute to sexual arousal short of coitus. Some workers have claimed that humans differ from other animals in that sexual arousal flourishes not on physiology alone. Just as we can be conditioned to a certain touch, sound, or odor, so we can to the qualities of kindness, courtesy, and warmth. That certain conditions should exist that increase the possibility of achieving full sexual satisfaction has recently been eloquently stated by a number of authors (May, Salisbury and Salisbury). The following is a list of suggested social factors that may enhance sexual arousal:

1 Variations can maintain the novelty of each sex act, but diversity requires energy, and humans tend to settle on a few preferred techniques.
2 Unrestrained responses—Uninhibited expression of affection can increase sexual excitement and cause total participation of a couple.
3 Capacity to perceive, listen, and communicate desires.
4 Patience.
5 Tenderness.
6 Perspective.
7 Honesty, truth, integrity.
8 Elimination of exploitation.

BIBLIOGRAPHY

Armstrong, D. T., and W. Hansel. 1958. Effects of hormone treatment on testes development and pituitary function, *Int. J. Fertil.*, 3:196.
Athanasiou, R., et al. 1970. Sex, *Psych. Today*, July Issue.
Blood, R. O. 1969. *Marriage.* Free Press, New York.
Brady, J. P., and E. E. Levitt. 1965. The scalability of sexual experiences, *Physiol. Record*, **15**:275–279.
Bronson, F. H. 1968. Pheromonal influences on mammalian reproduction, in M. Diamond (ed.), *Reproduction and Sexual Behavior*, pp. 341–361. Indiana University Press, Bloomington.
Fisher, S. 1973. *The Female Orgasm.* Basic Books, New York.
Ford, C. S., and F. A. Beach. 1951. *Patterns of Sexual Behavior.* Perennial Library, Harper & Row, New York.

Gatov, E. R. (ed.). 1973. *Sex Code of California*, Public Education and Research Committee. Graphic Arts of Marin, Inc., Sausalito, Calif.

Gebhard, P. H. 1966. Factors in marital orgasm, *J. Social Issues*, **22**(2):88–95.

Gebhard, P. H. 1968. Factors in marital orgasm, *Med. Aspects Hum. Sex.*, **2**(7):22–25.

Harlow, H. F. 1965. Sexual behavior in the Rhesus monkey, in F. Beach (ed.), *Sex and Behavior*. Wiley, New York.

Harlow, H. F. 1972. The nature of love, in R. Ulrich and P. Mountjag, *The Experimental Analysis of Social Behavior*, pp. 249–274. Appleton-Century-Crofts, New York.

Heiman, M. 1963. Sexual response in women: A correlation of physiological findings with psychoanalytic concepts, *J. Am. Psychoanal. Asso.*, **11**:360–385.

J. 1969. *The Sensuous Woman*. Dell, New York.

Kepecs, J. 1969. Sex and tickling, *Med. Aspects Hum. Sex.*, **3**(8):58–65.

Kinsey, A. C., et al. 1953. *Sexual Behavior in the Human Female*. Saunders, Philadelphia.

Lewis, L. S., and D. Brissett. 1967. Sex as work: A study of avocational counseling, *Social Problems*, **15**(1):8–18.

Masters, W. H., and V. F. Johnson. 1966. *Human Sexual Response*. Little, Brown, Boston.

Mathis, J. L. 1969. Psychology of "girlie" magazines, *Med. Aspects Hum. Sex.*, **3**(10):25.

May, R. 1969. *Love and Will*. Norton, New York.

McCabe, C. 1972. Sex offenders, the Fearless Spectator column, *San Francisco Chronicle*.

Raboch, J. 1969. Men's most common sex problems, *Sexology*, November Issue, pp. 60–63.

Salisbury, W., and F. Salisbury. 1971. Youth and the search for intimacy, in L. A. Kirkendall and R. N. Whitehurst (eds.), *The New Sexual Revolution*, pp. 169–182. D. W. Brown, New York.

Signoret, J. P., and F. du Mesnil du Bisson. 1961. Etude du comportement de la triue en oestrus, *Fourth Intern. Congr. Animal Reprod. Artif. Insem., The Hague*.

Sigusch, V., et al. 1970. Psychosexual stimulation: sex differences, *J. Sex Research*, **6**(1):10–24.

Stanndard, U. 1971. Clothing and sexuality, *Sexual Behavior*, **1**(2):24.

Stember, C. H. (Moderator). 1970. Sex and clothing, *Roundtable Discussion with B. F. Reiss, E. K. Schwartz, J. Trobeg, A. Wychoff, Med. Aspects Hum. Sex.*, **4**(9):144.

Winick, C. 1970. Popular music and sex, *Med. Aspects Hum. Sex.*, **4**(10):148.

Chapter 9

Coitus

Coitus can be one of the most physically stimulating and emotionally gratifying of all human experiences. The word *coitus* comes from the Latin *coitio,* meaning "a coming together," and refers to vaginal engulfment of the penis. In the literature, *coitus* will often appear with a modifying term signifying a variation of the act. Thus *oral* coitus refers to an act of fellatio or cunnilingus; *anal* coitus involves penile penetration of the anus; and *femoral* coitus refers to rubbing the genitals between the thighs.

A number of synonyms exist for the term *coitus. Copulation* comes from the Latin, meaning an act of "coupling or joining." *Intercourse* is derived from the Latin *intercursus,* referring to an act of "running between" and when used with the modifier "sexual" refers to coitus. Students who are taking courses in older literature may be interested in the two obsolete terms *swive* and *jape.* Swive, meaning "to copulate," is an old English term probably sharing the same origin as the word swivel—a simple coupling or fastening device—and appears for the first time in a song written in 1300 concerning the sexual exploits of Richard of Alemaigne: "Whil that he wes kyng, He spends al is tresour upon SWYVNG" (Murray et al.). Chaucer was the first major author to use "swive." Later, in 1680, a Scotch translation of the book of Genesis was written, and since this part of the Bible contains numerous references to acts of intercourse, it was entitled the "Buke of Swiving." Jape, meaning "to have carnal intercourse," has a more obscure origin. In 1572, Gascogne extolls Barth Withipoll about promiscuity when he says, "First in thy journey jape not overmuch" (Murray et al.). Of interest, jape also means "to trick, beguile, befool, and deceive" and was revised to be used as such in the nineteenth century. Today it is still used to mean "jest, joke, or jeer."

Although found commonly in the literature, *coitus, copulation,* and so on are replaced by most people in their everyday conversations with slang terms such as "score," "ball," and "fuck." "Score" is defined as "sexual intercourse especially as a man wins from a woman by being pleasing and convincing" (Wentworth and Flexner). The concept that a man "wins" a woman's favor by persuasion reflects on the other meanings of "score," which include "a victim" and "a successful instance of cheating." The term "ball" originated around 1895 mainly in the American underworld, where it referred to any object or person which added to one's pleasure (Wentworth and Flexner). "Balling" refers to a "wild party" or "having fun in coitus." "Goof ball" refers to a "sex orgy."

For centuries, the word "fuck" has been considered taboo, especially in literature. Its origin is unknown, but the word first shows up in some poetry written by Dunbar in 1503. Its meaning in Dunbar's poetry and subsequent pieces is "to copulate." In 1680, for example, Rochester wrote in *Poems for Several Occasions,* "Much wine had past with grave discourse, of who fucks who, and who does worse." Rochester, in the same poetry, gave additional meaning to fuck as the actual act of copulation when he wrote, "Thus was I rook'd of twelve substantial fucks." By 1922, the term was was used profanely as the coarsest equivalent of "damn" (Burchfield): "God fuck old Bennett!" as written by James Joyce in *Ulysses.* After the early 1920s, the term evolved meanings relating the sex act to fraud. Many of the slang offshoots of fuck were widely used in World War II by military personnel. Today it is common for some people to express frustration with "fuck it," confusion with "fucked up," and a waste of time with "fuck off."

Fornication, adultery, and sodomy are additional terms that refer to the coital act and are distinguished from each other by differences in legal interpretation and meaning. *Fornication* is voluntary coitus between an adult male and female who are unmarried. It is a misdemeanor, with penalties of not more than one year in a county jail and/or $1,000 fine in 37 states of the union (Kling). Fornication statutes, although rarely enforced, are occasionally used to secure defendants the police wish to apprehend for other offenses. *The New York Times* printed a story in 1969 about a man and woman convicted of fornication in New Jersey, the first case of its kind recorded in that state for nearly 150 years (Strouse).

Adultery refers to voluntary coitus between two people, at least one of whom is married to a third party. The married partner has committed adultery; the unmarried partner is guilty of fornication. If both partners are married to other people, the offense is technically called "double adultery." Adultery is against the law in many states of the union, but in some states requires special conditions to be considered a crime. For example, adultery may be a misdemeanor if it occurs along with *cohabitation*—living together with a sexual relationship (Gatov). Thus if one or both partners are married to other people and live and have coitus together for a variable length of time, they have committed a misdemeanor in some states.

Sodomy has numerous legal meanings. California law identifies coitus with animals or penis-anus intercourse between humans as sodomy. In other states, sodomy is often defined in a broader sense as any "crime against nature," which essentially is any sex act other than face-to-face coitus between a man and a woman. *Buggery* is often used synonymously with sodomy.

FUNCTIONS OF COITUS

Most people would agree that sexual intercourse has evolved in relation to reproduction. Yet the duration of ovulation, and thus fertility, is so short that human coitus actually takes place most often at times of nonfertility. This represents what some have called "sexual autonomy" and differs from the case of nonhuman primates, where coitus and ovulation generally coincide. That coitus is biologically one of the most important ways in which humans can play has always been known but not universally accepted (Comfort). The term *play* has multiple meanings but as used here refers to nonserious activity or simply having fun. It is when the "play" in coitus becomes competitive and filled with determination for success that fear of failure and sexual dysfunctions arise. The aspect of "play" does not exclude the seriousness and adaptive value of the numerous other functions of coitus. Two people, deeply in love, can communicate the highest form of humanity in an act of coitus where words need not be uttered but the meaning is crystal clear. Others may express in coitus a more casual relationship of friendship, and still others obtain only the thorough physical gratification of "the friction of two membranes." Coitus is also an opportunity to learn more about anatomy and complementary behavior from actual experience.

As coitus is so positive and pleasurable, it can also be used to exploit and manipulate the behavior of another. The uncountable times when coitus has been induced by coercion or promise of reward no doubt equal the number of times it has been denied pending acceptance of some bargain.

The intense physical pleasure gained during coitus and orgasm acts as a powerful reinforcer in conditioning the two participants to each other. The development of a pair-bond or a partnership based on care and affection depends upon this conditioning. Indeed, Newton believes that "conditioning, reinforced through coital pleasure, may be the biologic foundation upon which patterns of family life are built."

A remarkable parallelism in physiological response is found in two people having coitus. Bartlett studied several couples and discovered that heart rates and breathing patterns fluctuated almost in unison during coitus, some couples being more identical in these responses than others. The harmonious response in breathing rate may be explained by the fact that respiration is partially under voluntary control, and a couple could consciously or subconsciously attempt to match each other. Why there should be any type of similarity at all in heart rate is unknown, but perhaps along with breathing synchrony it aids in the conditioning process.

It is interesting to note that sexual activity can affect hormone level. For instance, whether or not a female rat can maintain a pregnancy depends upon the number of times a male places his penis in her vagina (intromissions) before ejaculation. The greater the number of intromissions, the higher will be the progesterone in her blood. Progesterone is known to maintain the pregnancy (Adler et al.). Results from a study of alpacas indicate that mounting and intromission are necessary to provide an adequate stimulus for ovulation to occur (Fernandez-Baca et al.). Whether similar interactions occur in humans remains to be elucidated. However, hormone levels in human males may correlate with coital activity. One of the major findings in a study of day-to-day changes of testosterone in one male was that the lowest level of this hormone was recorded at the time of his sexual partner's menses (Fox et al.). Since testosterone is important in sexual motivation, the low level at this time may have reflected the fact that this couple rarely experienced coitus during the menses.

Coitus produces not only physical but also psychological pleasure, since it implies acceptance by another human being and successful establishment of sex-role identities (Miller and Siegel). Thus, another primary function of coitus is its contribution to the development of a reciprocal love relationship. Romantic love, or *Eros*, can be defined in many ways. Psychologists such as Harry Harlow and B. F. Skinner see love as a response to obtain psychological and social reinforcement or as an attachment to a "source of self-validation." Further claim is made that once love is established, it can feed back positively and increase the original physical pleasure derived from coitus and orgasm (Miller and Siegel). However, no scientific evidence exists as yet to prove this most important point. Masters and Johnson (1966) found that female orgasms occurring in masturbation or by using an artificial glass penis were often more intense physiologically than orgasms derived from coitus. Experiments are definitely needed that would compare the human sexual response of couples claiming to be in love with those claiming not to be. These experiments might be technically difficult to design, since objective evidence of what constitutes love is not easy to obtain.

FREQUENCY AND PERIODICITY OF COITUS

In a survey of 1,438 people, roughly matching the demographic characteristics of the American population, marital coitus was shown to occur with a median frequency of 127 times a year for people seventeen to fifty-five years of age (Hunt). These statistics contrast with a median rate of 103 times a year in the

Kinsey survey taken about 20 years ago and indicate a marked increase in the frequency of marital coitus for American couples. In a less extensive study, Fisher found an average of 182 coital contacts per year for 280 middle-class married women and their spouses. These statistical averages and medians should not be construed by the reader as an indication of normalcy. Wide variation exists in coital frequency that provides sexual satisfaction for a particular couple. Unusual adherence by people to the normality of statistical averages can cause unnecessary anxiety. Coitus three or four times a week is fine if it is satisfying for a husband and wife, but not because it reflects society's average and therefore is "normal." The weakness of a too-rigid acceptance of the average is reflected in the following story: "Two statisticians in the Allies' frontline trench during World War I observed a German soldier rushing toward them with rifle cocked and bayonet fixed. When the first statistician fired and his bullet went to the right, the second statistician fired and his bullet went to the left of the onrushing German. The two statisticians dropped their rifles at this point and embraced each other happily—because 'on the average' they had him" (Vincent).

In women, the "preferred" frequency of marital coitus tends to match closely the actual frequency; however, men tend to desire more coitus than they are actually experiencing (Fisher; Levinger). In a study of 60 middle-class married couples from greater Cleveland, the wives tended to overestimate their husbands' preferences for coital frequency, whereas the husbands tended to underestimate their wives preferences (Levinger). Wives and husbands who were the most accurate in estimating their partner's preferences were significantly more satisfied with their sexual relationship and total marriage than other couples.

The actual frequency of marital coitus is influenced by subjective interpretation of the other partner's expectations and is only partially determined by one's own desires. Fisher found, for example, "that the greater a woman's intercourse frequency the more she specified that her husband's preferred intercourse rate exceeded her own." Fisher also found that the frequency of actual coitus was higher in those women who showed a greater orientation toward self-grooming and who were relatively less anxious about nudity. The same study revealed that the rate of actual coitus was positively correlated with how sexually responsive a female considered herself to be as well as with the average number of different coital positions the couple employed per month.

Some controversy exists as to the periodicity of human sexual responsiveness and coitus. No evidence is available as yet which shows a definite seasonality of intercourse; however, there is evidence for slight but significant seasonality of births (Cowgill). A higher number of births occur during the later summer and early autumn months in each hemisphere. The peak of births implies a peak of coital contact occurring during the winter months.

Scientists have determined via the use of questionnaires and surveys that the greatest sexual responsiveness or "desire" for coitus (not actual coital contact) among women occurred most often at the midpoint of the menstrual

commands a "privileged cultural status," this means she will usually have an opportunity to volunteer her participation in coitus. Female status of this type is found among the Crow, Hopi, Trobrianders, and Wogeo where the woman's sexual satisfaction is deemed as important as the man's, if not more so (Ford and Beach). Woman-on-top coital positions seem to predominate in such cultures. On the other hand, in cultures where the primary coital position is face-to-face, man-on-top, the female's social status may often be less privileged than the male's (Beigel). The man-on-top coital posture is the one most often practiced in our own culture as well as in at least 31 other societies found in the cross-cultural study of sexual behavior by Ford and Beach.

Changes in social status of the sexes in a particular culture are reflected by an increased variety of coital methods. Our own society, which is in the midst of reevaluating sex roles, shows a significant increase, compared to 20 years ago, in the variety of coital positions used by married as well as unmarried couples (Hunt). The extent of coital variation also depends upon a particular couple's imagination, agility, and the degree to which the partners are willing to abandon inhibitions.

There are a couple of possible explanations for the correlation of coital position with gender status. First of all, the person on top is psychologically in the more dominant position. Second, the woman-on-top position may provide more pleasure for the woman, and thus high female status may imply more concern for the woman's enjoyment. The on-top position is advantageous for both males and females because it allows the person to move more freely and thereby control the rate and angle of penile-vaginal friction. And, according to some researchers, the woman-on-top and the side-by-side positions have the additional advantage of providing more clitoral stimulation. The central focus of female erotic stimulation lies with the clitoris (Masters and Johnson, 1966), which serves to receive and transform stimuli of both psychic origin and physical manipulation. The accumulation of blood in the clitoris and its subsequent expansion is responsible for the subjective increase in tension or urgency and the ultimate desire of a woman for psychological release.

Some differences in opinion exist about the importance of coital positions that allow direct contact of the clitoral glans with the penis. Prior to the publication of *Human Sexual Response* by Masters and Johnson, much of the literature on sexuality emphasized the importance of a man making direct penile-clitoral contact by using an "overriding" coital position (Van de Velde). This required that a male ride high over his supine partner while placing his penis in her vagina as illustrated in Fig. 9-8. Some physicians continue to claim that when women are "taught how to maintain good contact between the clitoris and the shaft of the penis after intromission by their position and movements (rock and roll is good coital physiology), thereby continuing clitoral stimulation, they are then able to have orgasm and a satisfying sex relationship" (Kleegman). However, Masters and Johnson claim that the overriding position is awkward, particularly for a woman who does not have a flexible vaginal outlet. In this position, the penile thrust would be directed toward the

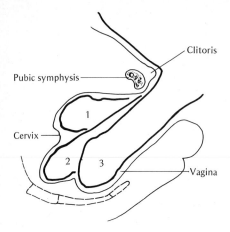

Figure 9-8 Axes of penile approach during face-to-face coitus. Approach 3 (male's body rides high over supine partner) is believed by some physicians to provide maximum clitoral stimulation; Masters and Johnson disagree.

back of the vagina and rectum rather than into the depths of the vaginal canal. Some women may have difficulty retaining the penis in this position without pelvic discomfort. In addition, at the height of sexual excitement, the clitoris involuntarily withdraws under its hood, reducing even further the possibility of penile contact. Masters and Johnson go on to say, "Only the female superior and lateral coital positions allow direct or primary stimulation of the clitoris to be achieved with ease." Indeed, these scientists believe that the clitoral response develops more rapidly and with greater intensity in the face-to-face, woman-on-top position than in any other coital position. What is meant here by "direct" stimulation in heterosexual intercourse is not actual contact between penis and clitoris but rather firm contact of the clitoral area with a male's pubic region (symphysis). Although the lateral and woman-on-top positions allow maximum stimulation, all coital positions provide indirect clitoral stimulation. According to the description by Masters and Johnson (1966), the thrusting of the penis into the vagina puts traction on the labia minora and clitoral hood, which tends to pull the clitoris downward. When the penis withdraws, the labia and hood are released from traction and the clitoris returns to its original position. This rhythmic up-and-down motion on the part of the clitoral shaft and glans, coupled with the active in-and-out stroking of the penis, produces significant indirect stimulation of the clitoris.

Coital Position and Insemination

The human vagina and uterus change shape and position relative to each other during sexual intercourse. These modifications increase the probability of pregnancy, especially in the face-to-face coital position with man on top, woman on the bottom. In the supine position, the vaginal barrel slopes downward at an angle of about 10 to 15° above the horizontal as seen in Fig. 9-9. The opening of the vagina is thus positioned at a higher level than the blind end, and this produces a natural gravitational tendency for semen to accumulate in the rear or cul-de-sac of the vagina following an ejaculation. As sexual

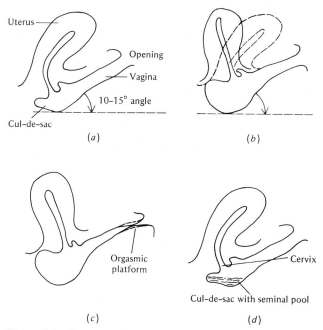

Figure 9-9 Changes in position and shape of uterus and vagina during man-on-top coitus. (*a*) Before intense arousal, (*b*) tenting effect during intense arousal, (*c*) orgasmic platform, (*d*) return to original position.

excitement increases, the inner two-thirds of the vagina expands and lengthens while the uterus shifts into a more elevated position above the vagina. Masters and Johnson have called these initial changes the "tenting effect," and it serves to increase the volume of the vaginal cul-de-sac and thus the space where semen can accumulate. As sexual tension mounts but before orgasm is reached, the walls of the outer third of the vagina become congested with blood (orgasmic platform), causing constriction of the vaginal opening and thereby reducing the possibility of seminal fluid leaking back out to the exterior of the body. Following the female's orgasm, the constriction of the vaginal opening and tenting effect are reversed and the uterus returns to its position prior to the onset of sexual stimulation. As the uterus resumes its original position, the cervix becomes immersed in any seminal fluid contained in the vaginal cul-de-sac. It is evident that compared with other coital positions, the man-above, woman-supine posture accompanied by the changes described above increase the possibility of pregnancy. However, Masters and Johnson cite certain situations that could reduce this possibility. A woman who has given birth may develop a less firm and somewhat wider vaginal opening compared to a woman who has never given birth. The constraining effect of the orgasmic platform on the seminal pool would be reduced in this situation. In addition, coitus with a woman on her back but in the knee-chest position would produce a seminal deposit in the front of the vagina rather than in the rear. Even if the female is totally supine, men who continue intercourse after ejaculation cause a flattening of the vagina which results in excessive loss of semen.

PHYSIOLOGY OF COITUS

Every organ system in the human body is affected by sexual intercourse. As bodily changes occur, they in turn modify the nature and intensity of the coital act. The influences of physiology on coitus and, conversely, of coitus on bodily change have been called the *human sexual response* (Masters and Johnson, 1966). Initiation of the sexual response is brought about by a combination of symbolic and actual stimuli that have become erotic through conditioning. Erotic thoughts originate in a person's cerebral cortex (the outer layer of the cerebrum), and the recognition of symbolic as well as physical sensation also occurs in the cerebral cortex. Information from the cortex is sent in the form of nervous impulses to other sexual arousal centers of the brain and thence to a group of nerves that are called the autonomic nervous system. The autonomic nervous system is responsible for the contraction and relaxation of involuntary muscles and for gland secretion—processes over which we have little conscious control. The system is divided into two components: the parasympathetic and the sympathetic. During most of our day-to-day life the parasympathetic division is the more active of the two. Parasympathetic activity is responsible for most of the restorative functions of the body, such as digestion, and for some of the bodily changes that occur during the sexual response—particularly during the early stage of sexual response. In contrast, the sympathetic division is highly activated by both severe stress and intense sexual arousal. It is not surprising, then, that a number of bodily reactions such as increases in heart rate, blood pressure, and breathing rate are typical of both the response to stressors and the response to sexual stimulation (see Table 9-1). These facts are particularly useful when one wishes to evaluate research on sexuality. For example, suppose that you want to evaluate an experiment that claims one sex to be more sexually aroused by viewing pornography than the other sex. If only heart rate and breathing rate are used as criteria, then the results can be judged invalid. The people in the experiment may have been responding with fear and anger rather than sexual arousal to the pornographic material. In general, increased genital secretion, tumescence of the genitals and breasts, dilatation of blood vessels (vasodilation), and rhythmic muscular movements are characteristics of sexual arousal alone (Zuckerman).

Masters and Johnson began their work on coital physiology rather obscurely in 1954 at the Washington University School of Medicine. Later they established the Reproductive Biology Research Foundation in St. Louis, Missouri. In 1966, they published their monumental work on the human sexual response, which contained information on 10,000 sexual response cycles derived from 619 females and 654 males. The authors have been criticized for emphasizing only physiology and not taking into consideration the effects of the psyche and for using a rather biased experimental group having similar

Table 9-1 Comparison of Bodily Changes Occurring during Anger, Fear, and Sexual Arousal

Change	Anger	Fear	Sexual arousal	Autonomic nervous control
Heart rate ↑	X	X	X	S
Blood pressure ↑	X	X	X	S
Hyperventilation	X	X	X	S
Adrenalin secretion ↑	X	X	X	S
Myotonia ↑ (muscle tension)	X	X	X	S
Gastrointestinal activity ↓	X	X	X	S
Skin temperature ↑	—	—	—	?
Color change (skin; labia)	X	X	X	?
Tumescence—clitoris; labia; breasts	—	—	X	P
Genital secretion ↑	—	—	X	P
Rhythmic muscular movement ↑	—	—	X	S
Orgasm	—	—	X	P and S
Vasodilation ↑	—	—	X	P
Electrical changes in skin	X	X	X	?
Erection—penis	—	—	X	P
Ejaculation	—	—	X	S (emission) P (expulsion)

Key: ↑ = increase   S = sympathetic   X = present
          ↓ = decrease   P = parasympathetic   — = not present
     Source: Data from Masters and Johnson, 1966; Zuckerman, 1971.

cultural backgrounds. To some extent these criticisms have validity, yet it is doubtful that the general aspects of coital physiology would differ greatly for other cultural groups. Actually, the work of Masters and Johnson is just a beginning, for although they reported modes and ranges of physiological reactions during coitus very little information was obtained on the amount of individual variation. Essentially they obtained averages of what hundreds of subjects experienced at different points during coitus, masturbation, and artificial coitus. Based on the results, the authors claimed that no difference exists between these three types of stimulation. Other researchers, although accepting most of Masters' and Johnson's conclusions, are not willing to accept this one (Fox and Fox, 1969). The physiological differences between artificial coitus using an electronic penis and regular coitus may not have been detected by the apparatus set up in Masters' and Johnson's laboratory. In addition, testosterone levels have been shown to be significantly lower during masturbation than during coitus (Fox et al.). Obviously, more work has to be done before conclusions can be made concerning the similarity of the sexual response in these various types of stimulation. The next decade may well see research that observes individual couples throughout the entire coital sequence repeated many times. These same individuals would then be observed in masturbation and artificial coitus and results compared. Also many improvements will be needed to reduce the artificiality produced by observations in a laboratory environment. A start in this direction was made by Cyril and Beatrice Fox (1969) when they studied their own sexual response while performing intercourse in the "habitual environment of their own bedroom." They were hooked up to an automatic recording apparatus and had no observers. They claim success in eliminating the inhibiting psychological artifacts of the laboratory environment.

Aside from anatomy, men and women show many similarities in human sexual response. Masters and Johnson have identified two basic physiological processes that underlie much of what happens during increased sexual arousal of both sexes. First, there is widespread pooling or accumulation of blood particularly in the genitals but also in the breasts, skin, earlobes, nose, and so on. This reaction is called *vasocongestion* and leads to the tumescence of the clitoris and penis. Second, there is an increase in muscular tension throughout the body; this is called *myotonia.* Limb movements become more rapid and irritable as muscle contractions increase both voluntarily and involuntarily in regularly recurring rhythms. Facial muscles contract, causing a person to scowl, grimace, or frown, and the neck becomes rigid. At orgasm, myotonia reaches its peak with involuntary rhythmic contractions of the penile muscles and orgasmic platform. The *orgasmic platform* is a swelling due to blood congestion of the outer third of the vagina. The swelling occurs just prior to orgasm, and its contractions are the only definitive sign that the woman has reached orgasm. The platform increases the friction on the penis and prevents leakage of semen out of the woman's body. In both men and women orgasm also brings about rhythmic contractions of the gluteal muscles located in the buttocks; and at peaks of sexual tension, spastic contractions of the muscles of the hands and feet called *carpopedal spasms* occur. Following orgasm both vasocongestion and myotonia are reduced to physiological levels similar to those which exist prior to sexual arousal.

Masters and Johnson characterized the sexual response cycle as having four successive phases—excitment, plateau, orgasm, and resolution. These arbitrary phases are convenient in describing anatomical and physiological events but should not detract from the fact that sexual arousal to orgasm is a continual process occurring in response to effective erotic stimulation. Figure 9-10 illustrates the rise and fall of intensity during the sexual response cycle. Note that the pattern of response is very similar from coitus to coitus in a given male and among different males. Major differences among males occur primarily in duration of the various phases rather than in intensity. In a female, the plateau to orgasm range will fall into one of three patterns; a given female may experience one pattern at one time and another pattern at some other time.

Excitement

The *excitement* phase involves a gradual increase in a person's sexual arousal level. The earliest signs are penile erection and vaginal lubrication occurring 3 to 15 seconds from the onset of stimulation. The excitement phase for the male also includes such parasympathetic effects as elevation, thickening, and flattening of the scrotum and size increase and elevation of the testes. The female experiences expansion and lengthening of the vaginal barrel, elevation and flattening of the labia majora, nipple and breast tumescence, changes in color of the labia minora (sex skin), and in about 25 percent of women early signs of a rashlike condition in the skin called the "sex flush." The sex flush becomes prominent in 75 percent of females and a lesser percentage of males. It begins characteristically in the skin of the abdomen and extends upward to the chest, neck, face, and back. The intensity of the color change in the skin depends upon the individual's level of sexual arousal and on the temperature of the room in which coitus is taking place—the higher the temperature, the more intense a given person's sex flush.

Plateau

If sexual motivation is maintained by adequate erotic stimulation, the excitement phase accelerates to the plateau phase. During *plateau,* the sexual excitement is intensified to levels approaching orgasm. Sympathetic influence becomes prominent in both sexes, accelerating the heart rate, blood pressure, breathing rate, and myotonia. In the female, Bartholin's gland secretion increases, and in the male, the Cowper's glands increase their secretions.

Orgasm

Orgasm is a highly pleasurable response involving the feeling of physiological and psychological release from maximum levels of sexual excitement. Orgasm is of short duration, lasting from 3 to 10 s, and is physiologically a response of the entire body. In the female contractions of the orgasmic platform, uterine muscle, and anal sphincter come rapidly and regularly every $8/10$ s. Similarly, rhythmic contractions of the penile muscles, seminal vesicles, prostate, and anal sphincter occur in the male. Heartbeat, breathing rate, and blood pressure all reach peak levels during orgasm.

On the average, a person at rest during a non-sexually aroused state has a heart rate of 69 beats per minute. At orgasm, a maximum rate of 180 beats per minute has been recorded in some people—a rate which approaches the maximum capacity of heart function. Exercise physiologists have shown that a heartbeat of 195 beats per minute lasting for 15 seconds can cause damage to the heart muscle.

The average breathing rate of a person at rest is about 12 breaths per minute, during which about 5 to 6 l[1] of air pass through the lungs. Just prior to orgasm breathing rates have been known to reach a maximum of 41 breaths per minute in a male with 30 to 39 l of air passing through the lungs per minute (Fox and Fox, 1969). The characteristics of female breathing rates differ somewhat from those of males. Immediately preceding orgasm a female shows a respiratory rate of 16 breaths per minute and temporary bouts of stoppage in

---

[1]One qt = 0.946 l.

breathing (Fox and Fox, 1969). Immediately following orgasm breathing rates of both sexes are similar—30 to 37 breaths per minute, which gradually decreases during the resolution phase.

The increased muscular tension throughout a person's body during orgasm causes a rise in blood pressure. Systolic blood pressure is the pressure in the arteries when the heart contracts, whereas diastolic pressure is the pressure in the arteries when the heart relaxes. In both sexes, systolic pressure rises sharply at orgasm, sometimes reaching a point almost twice as high as when the individual is at rest, and then drops sharply immediately following orgasm. Diastolic pressure is always less than the systolic pressure, but shows similar rises and falls in relation to orgasm.

A person's subjective awareness of orgasm is highly variable, but tends to focus on contractions of the genitalia. There is a general loss of sensory acuity in both sexes. Many men claim that they can sense when ejaculation is going to occur and can no longer be delayed (Masters and Johnson, 1966). Some men claim awareness of the first two or three contractions of the penile muscles which are highly pleasurable and powerful. The final contractions seem not to be as detectable. Many men claim sensitivity to the amount of seminal fluid passing through the urethra—the larger the volume the greater the feeling of pleasure.

In the female much greater variation exists both in the physiology of orgasm and in the subjective awareness of orgasm. Figure 9-10 shows three of the most common female patterns found in the study by Masters and Johnson. Pattern B shows a gradual increase in arousal during the excitement phase, a fluctuating plateau phase with small surges toward orgasm, and a slow return of physiological state to prearousal levels. This type of pattern has been called a "minor orgasm" by Judith Bardwick and occurs most often in young or sexually inexperienced women. Pattern A illustrates the multiple orgasmic response found in some women. This type of response reflects the lack of a physiological recovery period and thus the capacity of many women to have multiple orgasmic phases in one sexual response cycle. Six or seven orgasmic phases can be experienced by a woman, and as many as fifty have been reported by Masters and Johnson for one woman in their study. Pattern C shows a single orgasm of extreme intensity leading to a feeling of total physical release and physiological gratification. Many women primarily experience patterns of multiple orgasm or pattern C in masturbation.

Masters and Johnson suggest that after many coital experiences some women gradually change sexual response patterns; the developmental sequence beginning with pattern B (minor orgasm), changing to pattern C, and finally to multiple orgasmic responses. However, Bardwick claims that the developmental sequence begins with the "minor orgasmic pattern," changes to "multiple orgasms," and eventually leads to pattern C. The factors which cause changes in female patterns of human sexual response over time are unknown.

The subjective awareness of orgasm among females, although showing great variation, does include some consensus (Masters and Johnson). Individu-

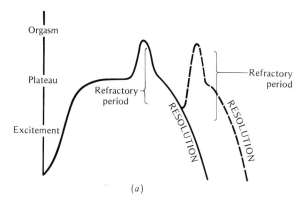

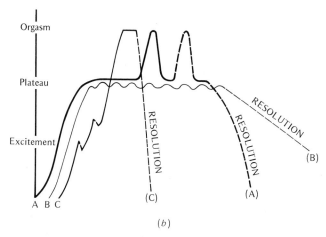

Figure 9-10 The sexual response cycle in (a) males and (b) females. *(From Masters and Johnson, 1966.)*

al statements describing a minor orgasm include the terms "tingly," "nice," "pleasant," and "affectionate gratification" (Bardwick). Pattern C has been described as feelings of "pure sensation radiating out from the pelvis" and "utter frustration if not achieved." Feelings of frustration are related to the anticipation of tremendous physical release in a woman who has experienced pattern C before. The vasocongestion occurring in the sex organs in this pattern is so great that failure to reach orgasm can lead to an uncomfortable feeling. Many women claim that orgasm patterns A and C begin with a sudden feeling of "stoppage" which is followed by an "intense sensual awareness" of the clitoris and a powerful feeling of "bearing down" or "expelling something from the vagina." Some women who have given birth relate that vaginal fluid is actually expelled and that orgasm does feel similar to the later stages of labor. Following feelings of "bearing down," many women feel a "suffusion of warmth" centered initially in the pelvic area and gradually spreading to encompass the entire body. This is followed by the awareness of "pelvic throbbing" coincident with the involuntary contractions of the vagina and uterus. Some women can even detect contractions of the rectal sphincter. The "pelvic throbbing" eventually is replaced by an awareness of a rapid heartbeat and fast breathing.

Female orgasm, regardless of pattern, is centered in the clitoris and involves the entire body. In a physiological sense, orgasms cannot be distinguished as vaginal or clitoral. Orgasms differ physiologically only in intensity. Psychologically, however, some women do distinguish between what they consider to be a vaginally centered orgasm and one centered in the clitoris (Fisher). The ability to detect the difference does not correlate with any level of maturity. That is, women who generally feel that their orgasms are centered in the vagina are neither more nor less "adult" or "mature" than women who claim clitoral orgasms.

Resolution

The *resolution* phase involves a physiological and psychological return to a non-sexually aroused state. Thirty to forty percent of men and women show a perspiration reaction during this phase. A thin film of sweat develops over most of the skin area in some people, whereas in others it may be concentrated only on the palms of the hands and soles of the feet. Many people are aware of a tremendous feeling of relaxation. Some may even laugh, others may cry, and still others want to sleep.

Immediately following orgasm most adult males experience reduced sensitivity to continued erotic stimulation. This is called a *physiological refractory period* and involves a temporary lack of receptor and nervous response to sexual stimuli. This refractory period is variable in duration and is a major difference in sexual response between the sexes. Because of the refractory period, most adult males are incapable of experiencing multiple orgasmic phases in the same cycle (Whitman). However, many adult males appear to recover rapidly from the refractory period, maintaining an erection following ejaculation. Evidence does exist that some preadolescent boys may experience multiple orgasms (without ejaculation) but this ability falls off rapidly following puberty (Whitman).

DISORDERS OF COITUS

"In many sexually inexperienced partners the delay of the female orgasm coupled with the rapidity of the male climax will constitute a sexual incompatibility" (Johnson). This statement, written by a senior lecturer in psychiatry at the University of Manchester, is significant in that it identifies two of the most common sexual concerns of men and women, namely premature ejaculation and a female's inability to achieve orgasm easily during coitus. It may be true that some couples will not consider either factor a problem if they feel satisfied with their relationship. Some couples may attain sexual gratification from means other than coitus, such as mutual masturbation or oral genital contact. But with the increase of books on sexual dysfunction and the availability of information about sex problems, more and more people are finding a need for sex counseling and therapy. Many couples learn to achieve rates of orgasm that produce maximum sexual gratification for them. Others do not. It has been conservatively estimated that more than half of the married couples in the United States have some sexual problem.

Premature Ejaculation

Most clinical definitions of *premature ejaculation* refer to a specified duration of penile-vaginal penetration: A man who cannot control his ejaculation for at least the first 30 seconds to a full minute after entering the vagina is called a premature ejaculator. However, Masters and Johnson (1970) have emphasized that this type of "stop watch" definition does not take into consideration the sexual satisfaction of the female partner. Occasionally, such short durations of coitus are quite satisfying to the female if she is highly aroused. These authors say that a premature ejaculator is better defined as one who cannot control ejaculation during penile-vaginal confinement for a sufficient length to satisfy his partner during at least 50 percent of their coital acts. However, even this definition suffers from the arbitrary designation of 50 percent satisfaction for the female. Perhaps the best definition for its brevity and conciseness is given by Vandervoort and McIlvenna: "A premature ejaculator is a man who wants to last longer but can't for a number of reasons."

The amount of concern expressed by a man about his premature ejaculation and his female partner's degree of frustration increases in direct proportion to the level of formal education achieved by each. Rarely do individuals who have completed only grade school report the existence of premature ejaculation. Often in these cases the man dominates in the sexual relationship and his gratification is of primary concern. Indeed the woman may welcome the rapidness of his orgasm so as to end the coital act as quickly as possible (Masters and Johnson, 1970).

The causes of premature ejaculation involve mostly previous conditioning and are rarely associated with biological disease. Masters and Johnson have described how early coital experiences in semiprivate conditions or other situations which encourage rapid orgasm easily condition one to later premature ejaculation. If the first few acts of coitus take place in the back seat of a car at a drive-in movie or in a house of prostitution where clientele turnover is rapid, the tendency is to ejaculate as fast as possible. Frequent repetition of these situations sustains the conditioning process.

Prior to the suggested therapy of Masters and Johnson, treatments and antidotes for premature ejaculation were generally ineffective. A man would often come to a psychiatrist or urologist without his spouse. Treatment included the use of an anesthetic such as a 1 to 5 percent Nupercaine solution to be applied on the glans penis just prior to intercourse. Some couples complained of total loss of feeling in the genitalia during coitus with use of this type of anesthetic. In addition, wearing three or four condoms all at once, drinking a few glasses of an alcoholic beverage, or masturbating prior to intercourse have all been prescribed as treatment. Some doctors have even suggested "thinking of other things" during the coital act as an antidote to premature ejaculation. Often this would turn out as an antidote for the entire act of coitus—the couple ending up "thinking of other things."

Masters' and Johnson's treatment involves development of a complex interaction between the partners in terms of increasing sexual communication and responsiveness and decreasing the demands of performance. During the first few days of therapy in a Masters and Johnson clinic, an intensive interview of the couple and medical examination of the male is made. On the third day of therapy, the couple is introduced to "sensate focus" exercises, which are concerned with experiencing and learning to enjoy the sensation of touch. A man and woman sit naked in the privacy of their room and take turns in feeling, massaging, stroking, and patting each other. Some couples use lotions, whereas others may use pieces of fur, velvet, or silk to rub on the skin. At first, the breasts or genitals are not involved. The general idea is to give and receive pleasure and to begin feeling sensuous without fear of an impending coital performance. The ability to receive pleasure without immediately having to reciprocate is also learned as part of the sensate focus exercises. After a few days, the couple is ready to begin stimulation of the genitals. Up to this point, the therapy is useful for many types of sexual problems, and it now becomes more specific. For premature ejaculation, the man lies on his back and the woman sits between his legs facing him with her feet on each side of his abdomen (see Fig. 9-11). This position allows the woman to massage and stroke the man's penis while he simply relaxes and enjoys it. Eventually he will attain an erection and soon will reach the "point of no return," or "ejaculatory

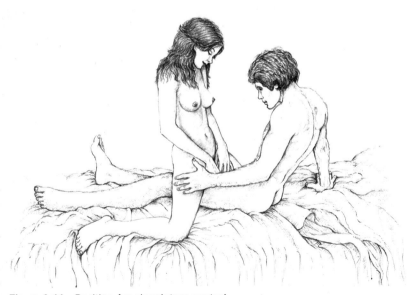

Figure 9-11   Position for ejaculatory control.

inevitability." Just prior to this point he signals that ejaculation is approaching. She now tries a "squeeze" technique that has been used for hundreds of years in many cultures but formally presented by James Semans and tested by Masters and Johnson (1970). She places her thumb on the frenulum of the erect penis and her first and second fingers on the opposite side above and below the corona (Fig. 9-12). With her fingers in this position she applies firm pressure to the penis for 3 to 4 s or alternately a less firm pressure for 8 to 15 s. Some sex counselors recommend instead that the base of the erect penis be gripped and squeezed for several seconds. Whichever method is used, the effect is to inhibit ejaculation and to reduce the erection. The woman can repeat manual stimulation of the penis, applying the squeeze technique each time her partner signals "ejaculatory inevitability." By prolonging the rate at which ejaculation takes place, a male can develop confidence and less fear of performance than ever before. The attitude of both partners can essentially change to a better understanding of their sexual behavior and greater sensitivity to each person's erotic desires.

Following the exercises mentioned above, the couple is ready for coitus. The face-to-face, female-above position is cited as excellent for treatment of premature ejaculation. The male in the supine position can permit the female full control over the rate of coital thrusting. She can begin by not moving at all, which gives the male time to adjust to a nondemanding situation and to enjoy the sensation of his penis in her vagina. For the man who "comes too soon," the first few minutes of penis penetration into the vagina are often the most critical, and if he can learn to prolong his response at that time, a major step toward cure will have been taken. At the "point of no return," the male removes his penis and his partner applies the squeeze technique. This procedure can be repeated for as long as the couple wishes.

A variant of the squeeze technique is suggested by some sex therapists. In any coital position, a man while thrusting can suddenly stop when he feels

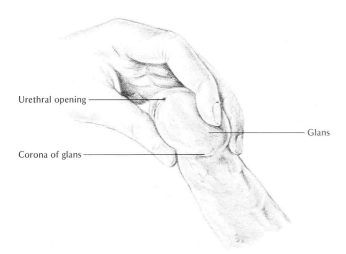

Urethral opening

Glans

Corona of glans

Figure 9-12   Demonstration of squeeze technique.

ready to come. He presses his pubic bone firmly against his partner's pubic bone for a few seconds until the urge to come is reduced. His penis will be deep in the vagina and he can concentrate on the sensation. This can be repeated following periods of thrusting as often as desired. Again, prolonging inter-course produces confidence and reduces the constant threat of failure.

Since publication of *Human Sexual Response,* there has been a tremen-dous boom in sex clinics designed to help couples cope with sex problems. Estimates run from 3,500 to 5,000 sex clinics in the United States as of 1974. Since sex treatments are relatively new, few standards of operation exist, and some clinics may simply be opportunistic in a scheme to "get rich quick." The reader is cautioned to check the credentials and background experience of clinic operators before embarking on a regimen of therapy for a sex problem.

Impotence

Another major concern of many men is *impotence.* The term comes from the Latin, meaning "lack of power" and is defined as the inability to achieve or maintain an erection sufficient for coitus to take place. The condition is called *primary impotence* if a man has never in his life achieved or maintained an erection for coitus (he may have for masturbation and during nocturnal and morning erections). If a man previously has had at least one successful coitus and then subsequent and chronic failure of erection occurs, his condition is called *secondary impotence.* Many men experience an occasional case of impotence which usually does not require therapy.

Some physicians have suggested that impotence is on the increase (Liddick). They further claim that female liberation and the increased demand for male performance are the primary causes of the increase, while other physicians and psychologists believe that numerous factors are involved. Much of the American society appears to be more open and candid about all aspects of sex. Men and women are likely to recognize and report their sexual problems in greater numbers than ever before. Many females are learning that their sex drives and requirements are as great as, if not greater than, those of males. In the past, many men did not accept the responsibility of sexually satisfying their wives or lovers. Today these attitudes are reversing. Men are assuming more responsibility for their female partner's sexual satisfaction, and fears of sexual inadequacy are therefore increasing. Fear of failure in coitus represents the most common cause of impotence in the United States (Masters and Johnson, 1970). Ninety percent of all cases of impotence are caused by psychological factors, including past inhibitory experiences and negative reinforcement leading to "fear of coital failure." Some recent evidence indicates that continued heavy use of marihuana or less frequent use of the more potent hashish may also cause impotence (Maugh). Heavy use of these drugs probably was far more common in the United States during the 1960s and early 1970s than in earlier decades. Some scientists also believe that alcoholism is increasing in the United States. In extreme forms of alcoholism, impotence occurs frequently and is correlated with cirrhosis of the liver, malnutrition, or disrupted nervous function (Levine).

Some cases of impotence (about 10 percent) are caused by biological diseases and malfunctions. Fifty percent of diabetic (mellitus) men are impotent, apparently due to the effects diabetes has on that part of the nervous system which controls both the urinary bladder and genital functions (Ellenberg). Other biological causes include a low testosterone level, disturbances in the circulatory and nervous systems, and abnormalities of genital anatomy.

Treatment of impotence depends upon the cause. Various devices have been used to treat biologically caused impotence. Ellenberg reports that in some cases of partial impotence a rubber band is wound around the base of the penis to help trap blood in the erectile tissues and thereby maintain an erection. Lash has used surgically implanted bags of silicone to help prevent buckling of the penile shaft during coitus. Impotence of psychological origin requires extensive restructuring of the male and female partner's attitude toward their sexuality. Sensate focus exercises and revelation of the causes can and do help (Masters and Johnson, 1970).

Impotence is a ground for annulment and divorce, as of 1970, in most states of the union except those that have adopted "no fault" divorce laws (Pilpel and Hunting). In most cases, impotence had to exist prior to the marriage in order to be used as a ground for divorce.

Orgasmic Dysfunction

Orgasmic dysfunction is broken down into two categories: identifying women who have never achieved an orgasm as *primary* and women who have experienced at least one orgasmic response through coitus or masturbation but who currently are nonorgasmic as *situational* (Masters and Johnson). Both primary and situational orgasmic dysfunction should not be confused with *frigidity*, which when used correctly refers to a woman with a low or undetectable sex drive. Unfortunately the term *frigidity* has been misused to define a number of female sex problems, including orgasmic dysfunction, and should therefore be abandoned.

Kinsey (1953) estimated that 30 percent of married women did not reach orgasm in coitus during the first year of their marriage, but only 10 percent remained nonorgasmic in coitus after 10 years of marriage. More recent statistics (Hunt, 1974) reveal that between 15 and 20 percent of women (both single and married) rarely or never achieve orgasm in coitus during their first year of coital experience. However, caution must be exercised when studying these statistics as some women may think that orgasm is supposed to be stronger or different from the orgasmic sensations they are experiencing.

Hormonal imbalance, excessive use of drugs and alcohol, aging, and anatomical abnormalities of the genitalia are responsible for a few cases of orgasmic dysfunction; however, most cases are of psychological origin. Considerable controversy exists as to which psychological factors are most contributory: a male partner's negative attitude and poor sexual technique, the existence of hostility or resentment of one partner toward the other, the fear and guilt a woman develops when she has been taught to suppress her sexual feelings, inability to lose control of mind and body during orgasm. Many women seem overly concerned about achieving the peaks of sexual arousal that modern society has told them they are capable of. Thus they too, like many men, develop fears of performance. Mary Jane Sherfey has suggested that when coitus is infrequent and of short duration, orgasm may not be easily achieved.

Seymore Fisher's conclusions about female orgasm have caused considerable stir in the medical field because they generally conflict with those of Masters and Johnson and other sex counselors. He has claimed that a woman's inability to reach orgasm is *not* due to her male partner's technique, parental attitudes whether liberal or conservative, sources of sex education, her level of sexual motivation, feelings about religion, degree of femininity, early traumatic sexual experiences, or general mental health. Rather he found orgasmic dysfunction most often in women whose childhood-paternal relationships were cool, indifferent, or nonexistent. The availability of a father who showed interest in the child's welfare and who set down guidelines, whether strict or liberal, were critical factors in the female's adult ability to achieve orgasm. In addition, if a woman lacked confidence in her personal relationships with her lover or husband, she often had difficulty achieving orgasm. A male partner's lack of dependability contributed primarily to irregular frequencies of coitus for a given couple, and this irregularity led ultimately to orgasmic dysfunction. Whether these or other factors are most important remains to be confirmed by additional research in the area of female sexuality.

Therapy involves a total restructuring of both partners' attitudes towards sex. Establishing the female's personal sex identity and recognizing the existence of her sexual desires are prerequisite to achieving orgasm. The partners identify any negative behavior patterns that may be inhibiting the sexual response. Perhaps a change in environment to more private conditions can help. Sharing of positive sexual experiences and not forcing enjoyment enhance the possibility of reaching orgasm. Sensate focus exercises help identify each partner's most erogenous zones and teach both partners that feeling sensuous through touch is necessary to produce full sexual enjoyment. The female-above coital position can be used to experience the feeling of vaginal expansion produced by her partner's penis. She can learn to experience and enjoy mutual nondemanding pelvic thrusting. The maximum clitoral stimulation in the female-above position as well as psychic acceptance of her potential for sexual response should ultimately lead to the ability to attain orgasm as often as desired.

Kegel has developed certain pelvic muscle exercises which help women increase their capacity to achieve orgasm. The muscle involved is the pubococcygeus muscle, which controls both urination and constriction of the vaginal barrel. This muscle contracts involuntarily during orgasm, and by increasing its tonus and strength, pelvic sensations can be enhanced. A woman can identify the muscle as the one which starts and stops the flow of urine. By contracting and relaxing the muscle at least 90 times a day, its tonus can be increased and the woman's response to sexual stimulation enhanced. If soreness sets in, the exercises can be temporarily terminated for one or two days. During the exercises, a woman can insert a finger into the vagina in order to provide some resistance to the contractions. She can practice bearing down as if in labor, which increases the blood supply to the vaginal area and subsequent capacity for vaginal lubrication.

Evidence exists that when one partner is cured of a sexual problem, the other may develop one. Therapy is thus often directed at establishing open and full communication between partners at all stages of treatment. Careful check of the partners' attitudes and behavior by a sex counselor during therapy is mandatory.

Vaginismus

Vaginismus is defined as irregular and involuntary contractions of the muscles surrounding the outer third of the vagina whenever there is an attempt at coitus. The effect is a closing of the vaginal opening before penile penetration. Even the thought of coitus can produce vaginismus. The condition is said to be a classic psychosomatic illness produced by certain types of prior conditioning. Masters and Johnson (1970) found that 12 cases of vaginismus out of 29 had a history of sexual inhibitions associated with strong religious family life. In other cases, traumatic sexual experiences such as gang rape or acts of incest may have caused the vaginismus. Some women show vaginismus following incidents of painful intercourse. Vaginal infection, torn pelvic ligaments, low blood estrogen, and psychological inhibitions are some of the factors that are known to cause painful intercourse. According to Masters and Johnson, a few cases of vaginismus occurred in homosexually oriented women who attempted to have heterosexual intercourse.

Besides sensate focus exercises and psychological restructuring, Masters' and Johnson's treatment for vaginismus involves the use of a series of graduated vaginal dilators. The male partner inserts a small dilator into the vaginal opening. When irregular vaginal contractions stop, a slightly larger dilator is inserted to replace the original one. The largest dilators are left in place for several hours. The procedure is repeated for 3 to 5 days or until spastic vaginal contractions have ceased. Coitus can now take place, although dilators may have to be used just prior to intercourse for a few weeks. Of 29 cases in the study by Masters and Johnson all were cured.

BIBLIOGRAPHY

Adler, N. T., and J. A. Resco, et al. 1970. The effect of copulatory behavior on hormonal change in the female rat prior to implantation, *Physiol. Beh.*, **5**(9):1003–1007.

Bardwick, J. M. 1971. *Psychology of Women.* Harper & Row, New York.

Bartlett, R. G. 1956. Physiological responses during coitus, *J. Appl. Physiol.*, **9**:469–472.

Beigel, H. G. 1953. The meaning of coital postures, *Int. J. Sex.* **4**:136–143.

Burchfield, R. W. (ed.). 1972. *A Supplement to the Oxford English Dictionary, vol. I, A–G.* Clarendon Press. Oxford.

Comfort, A. 1974. On sexuality, play and earnest, *The Human Context,* **4**(1):177–184.

Cowgill, U. M. 1969. The season of birth and its biological implications, *J. Reprod. Fertil. Suppl.,* **6**:89–103.

Ellenberg, M. 1973. Impotence in diabetes: A neurologic rather than an endocrinologic problem, *Med. Aspects Hum. Sex.,* **7**(4):12.

Ellis, A. 1967. Coitus, in A. Ellis and A. Abarbanel (eds.), *Modern Sex Practices,* pp. 101–119. Ace, New York.

Fernandez-Baca, S. D., et al. 1971. Effect of different mating stimuli on induction of ovulation in the alpaca, *J. Fert. & Steril.,* **22**:261–267.

Fisher, S. 1973. *The Female Orgasm.* Basic Books, New York.

Ford, C. S., and F. A. Beach. 1951. *Patterns of Sexual Behavior.* Perennial Library, Harper & Row, New York.

Fox, C. A. 1970. Measurement of intra-vaginal and intra-uterine pressures during human coitus by radio-telemetry, *J. Reprod. Fertil.,* **22**:243–251.

Fox, C. A., and B. Fox. 1969. Blood pressure and respiratory patterns during human coitus, *J. Reprod. Fertil.,* **19**:405–415.

Fox, C. A., and B. Fox. 1971. A comparative study of coital physiology, with special reference to the sexual climax, *J. Reprod. Fertil.,* **24**:319–336.

Fox, C. A., et al. 1972. Studies on the relationship between plasma testosterone levels and human sexual activity, *J. Endocrinol.,* **52**:51–58.

Gatov, E. (ed.). 1973. *Sex Code of California.* Graphic Arts of Marin, Inc., Calif.

Hunt, M. 1974. *Sexual Behavior in the 1970's.* Playboy Press, New York.

Jensen, G. D. 1973. Human sexual behavior in primate perspective, in J. Zubin and J. Money (eds.), *Contemporary Sexual Behavior—Critical Issues in the 1970's,* pp. 17–31. Johns Hopkins, Baltimore.

Kinsey, A. C., et al. 1953. *Sexual Behavior in the Human Female.* Saunders, Philadelphia.

Kegel, A. H. 1952. Sexual functions of the pubococcygeus muscle, *Western J. Surg. Obstet. Gynecol.* **60**:521.

Kleegman, S. J. 1969. Clinical application of Masters' and Johnson's research, in P. J. Fink and Van Buren O. Hammett (eds.), *Sexual Function and Dysfunction,* pp. 23–33. Davis, Philadelphia.

Kling, S. G. 1965. *Sexual Behavior and the Law.* Pocket Books, New York.

Johnson, J. 1968. *Disorders of Sexual Potency in the Male.* Pergamon, London.

Larsson, K. 1973. Sexual behavior the result of an interaction, in J. Zubin and J. Money (eds.), *Contemporary Sexual Behavior: Critical Issues in the 1970's,* pp. 33–51. Johns Hopkins University Press Bull., Baltimore.

Lash, H. 1968. Silicone implant for impotence, *J. Urol.,* **100**:709.

Levine, J. 1955. Sexual adjustment of alcoholics, *J. Stud. Alcohol,* **16**:675.

Levinger, G. 1970. Husbands and wives estimates of coital frequency, *Med. Aspects, Hum. Sex.,* **4**(9):42.

Liddick. B. 1972. Male impotence. Troubled sex—perform or panic, *S. F. Chronicle,* August 18, quoting Drs. G. L. Ginsberg, W. A. Frosch, and T. Shapiro.

Masters, W. H., and V. E. Johnson. 1966. *Human Sexual Response.* Little, Brown, Boston.

Masters, W. H., and V. E. Johnson. 1970. *Human Sexual Inadequacy.* Little, Brown, Boston.

Maugh, T. H. II. 1974. Research news: Marihuana: The grass may no longer be greener, *Science,* **185**(4152):683–685.

Miller, H. L., and P. S. Siegel. 1972. *Loving—A Psychological Approach*. Wiley, New York.

Money, J., and A. Ehrhardt. 1973. *Man & Woman, Boy & Girl*. Johns Hopkins, Baltimore.

Murray, J. A., et al., (eds.). 1919. *A New English Dictionary on Historical Principles. vol. V, part II, I–K*. Clarendon, Oxford.

Murray, J. A. et al., (eds.). 1919. *A New English Dictionary on Historical Principles, vol. IX, part II, Su-Th*. Clarendon, Oxford.

Newton, N. 1973. Interrelationships between sexual responsiveness, birth, and breast feeding, in J. Zubin and J. Money (eds.), *Contemporary Sexual Behavior—Critical Issues in the 1970's*, pp. 77–115. Johns Hopkins, Baltimore.

Pilpel, H. F., and R. B. Hunting. 1973. Impotency as ground for divorce, *Med Aspects Hum. Sex.*, **6**(4):57–58.

Semans, J. H. 1956. Premature ejaculations: a new approach, *South. Med. J.*, **49**:353–357.

Sherfey, M. J. 1966. *The Nature and Evolution of Female Sexuality*, vol. I. Random House, New York.

Strouse, J. 1970. *Up Against the Law*. Signet Books, New York.

Udry, J. R., and N. M. Morris. 1968. Distribution of coitus in the menstrual cycle, *Nature*, **220**:593–596.

Vandervoort, H. E., and T. McIlvenna. 1972. *The Yes Book of Sex. You Can Last Longer*. Multi Media Resource Center, San Francisco.

Van de Velde, T. H. 1930. *Ideal Marriage*. Covici, New York.

Vatsyayana. *The Kama Sutra*. Librairie Ostra, Paris.

Vincent, C. E. 1973. *Sexual and Marital Health*. McGraw-Hill, New York.

Wenger, M. H., et al., 1968. Autonomic activity during sexual arousal, *Psychophysiology*, **4**:468–478.

Wentworth, H., and S. B. Flexner. 1967. *Dictionary of American Slang*. Thomas Y. Crowell, New York.

Whitman, R. M. 1967. Multiple orgasms, *Med. Aspects Hum. Sex.*, **3**(8):52.

Zuckerman, M. 1971. Physiological measures of sexual arousal in the human, *Psychol. Bull.*, **75**:297–329.

Chapter 10

Pregnancy

The *gestation period* for humans is defined as the period of pregnancy, and averages 267 days in duration from fertilization or 280 days from the last menstrual cycle. The approximate date of delivery can be calculated by using *Naegele's rule:* Count 3 months back from the first day of the last menstrual cycle and add 7 days. To illustrate, let's assume that January 20 is the first day of the last menstrual cycle. Counting backward 3 months would bring us to October 20 and adding 7 days to this date would designate October 27 as the approximate date of delivery in the same year as the last menstrual cycle.

There are a number of physical and behavioral changes that indicate a woman is pregnant. Most of these changes can occur for reasons other than pregnancy, and self-diagnosis must be done with caution. A few changes are more definite and usually are determined by an obstetrician. These changes or "signs" of pregnancy can be categorized as presumptive, probable, and positive, depending upon their reliability. *Presumptive* signs indicate possible pregnancy. *Probable* signs are much more reliable but do not provide conclusive evidence of pregnancy. *Positive* signs are those which occur only if the woman is pregnant.

PRESUMPTIVE SIGNS OF PREGNANCY

The first evidence of pregnancy is *amenorrhea,* which is lack of menstrual flow. Unfortunately, the woman can miss a period for many other reasons: the stress of travel, a change in diet, worrying about pregnancy, studying for exams, or just having a case of nerves. Just as amenorrhea can occur for reasons other than pregnancy, so can bleeding or spotting occur during a pregnancy. Bleeding has been known to follow normal implantation of a zygote, and it can also occur if the pregnancy is ectopic, and in the presence of vaginal or uterine lesions. In addition, bleeding in a pregnant woman as well as irregular bleeding in a nonpregnant woman may indicate a disorder in the tissues of the vagina or uterus.

A number of *breast changes* such as increased fullness and an unusual tenderness around the nipples may be noticed very early in a pregnancy. The areolae and nipples become enlarged and deeply pigmented. The breasts appear swollen and show many prominent veins just below the surface of the skin. If, for any reason, a pregnant woman's breasts decrease in size, there is a good possibility of an impending problem that could lead to premature termination of the pregnancy. Breast changes are considered only a presumptive sign because they can occur for other reasons. For example, the breasts may enlarge and become tender when a woman is taking the pill.

Many women experience nausea and occasional vomiting during the early stages of pregnancy, and this has been called *morning sickness.* Actually, the term morning sickness is misleading because nausea and vomiting frequently occur at other times of the day and are especially common during the preparation of an evening meal. This may be due to the odors arising from cooking food coupled with an empty stomach, anticipation of eating, and end-of-day fatigue. The body may be adjusting, during early pregnancy, to increases in estrogens, progesterone, and other hormones. The basal metabolism (rate of body energy production) of a woman is lowered somewhat during the first 3 months of pregnancy; one of the results is a reduction in the normal contractions of the intestinal tract that propel food products toward the anus. All these factors may contribute to morning sickness, but the exact causes are unknown. Many physicians recommend eating small quantities of starches such as dry toast, crackers, or cooked cereals to help reduce mild forms of nausea. The first signs of morning sickness are usually experienced 2 weeks after the first missed period and generally disappear 6 to 7 weeks later. If nausea is severe or vomiting is frequent, the patient may have to enter a hospital for treatment. Since nausea and vomiting occur as symptoms of many diseases, they are considered only presumptive signs of pregnancy.

Many pregnant women experience an increase in urinary frequency sometime between the twelfth and sixteenth week following a missed period. During this time an increase occurs in the flow of blood to the walls of the urinary bladder. This stimulates contractions of the smooth muscle in the bladder and in turn increases a woman's desire to urinate. The frequency of urination decreases after the sixteenth week; but it increases again in the later stages of pregnancy because of pressure on the bladder arising from an enlarged uterus and fetus. Urinary frequency may also increase as the result of bladder infections and other diseases, and hence is only a presumptive sign of pregnancy.

During the first 3 months other presumptive signs may include bizarre food cravings, changes in color of the vaginal and cervical walls because of increased blood flow to those structures, development of stretch marks or abdominal striae, increased sugar in the urine, and formation of a dark pigmented line extending from the pubic hair to the umbilicus, called the linea nigra. Not all these characteristics will develop in the same woman, and some pregnant women show very few presumptive signs (Bookmiller and Bowen).

PROBABLE SIGNS OF PREGNANCY

Probable signs of pregnancy are more likely to be reliable, and are usually ascertained by an obstetrician (Barber and Graber). The earliest probable sign usually occurs by the second week. This is a softening of the uterus, most often seen first at the site of implantation. Around the eighth week, the uterus also softens between the cervix and the uterine body. Enlargement of the uterus is a probable sign and can usually be detected beginning with the third month of pregnancy. As the uterus enlarges, it also changes shape from a globular to an elongate form. Intermittent, painless contractions of the uterine muscles occur beginning with implantation and are maintained throughout pregnancy. They can be felt by placing two hands on the enlarged abdomen above the pelvic symphysis. "Quickening" or fetal movements usually begin around the fourteenth to sixteenth week. However, they are not positive signs of pregnancy because they can be difficult to distinguish from contractions of the bowel or gas.

POSITIVE SIGNS OF PREGNANCY

Fetal movements are considered a positive sign of pregnancy only when a physician feels these movements through the abdominal or vaginal wall (Reid et al.). The fetal skeleton can be positively identified with x-ray techniques by the sixteenth week following a missed period. A new ultrasonic sound technique has been used to positively determine the presence of one or more fetuses (Philipp et al.). Ultrasonic sound is bounced off the contents of a woman's uterus and the echoes are captured on a scanning screen. The technique is very much like sonar and is to soft tissues what x-rays are to bone and other hard tissues. So far, the method appears to have no side effects and has been used successfully to determine fetal heart rate and blood flow. The fetal heart rate can also be identified by a physician using a stethescope. Although the fetal heart starts to beat during the third week after conception, it cannot usually be heard until the fourth month. The physician must distinguish between the fetal heart rate, which ranges from 120 to 140 beats per minute, and the maternal heart rate, which ranges from 69 to 80 beats per minute. The physician holds the maternal pulse while simultaneously listening to the uterine contents with a stethoscope. While using a stethoscope, a physician can occasionally hear a soft murmuring sound coincident with the maternal pulse which is caused by blood passing through the uterine sinuses. In addition, occasionally a muffled sound called funic souffle can be heard, which is blood pulsing through a partially constricted umbilical cord.

A positive pregnancy test is generally 95 to 96 percent reliable and is thus considered a positive sign of pregnancy. Pregnancy tests are based on the ability to detect a pregnancy hormone in the urine called human chorionic gonadotropin or HCG. The developing placenta secretes HCG into the blood, and this hormone helps maintain the corpus luteum and thus the pregnancy. The hormone is excreted in the urine and is first detectable about two weeks after the first missed period. Formerly a small sample of a patient's urine was injected into an immature female animal. If HCG was present, it would stimulate production of eggs by the immature animal's ovary; this would be detected by killing the animal and performing an autopsy. Today, animals rarely are involved, and several types of immunological pregnancy tests are used instead. One test uses latex particles with HCG molecules attached to them. If antibodies against HCG are obtained and mixed with the latex particles, the antibodies would react with the HCG causing the latex particles to clump together. If a patient's urine sample containing HCG is added to some antibodies, a reaction occurs but cannot be seen with the naked eye. Most of the antibodies would have reacted with HCG in the urine. If latex particles with HCG attached are then added to the urine sample, the latex would not clump together since all of the antibodies would have already reacted with HCG in the urine. The lack of clumping means that the test is positive (HCG is present in the patient's urine) and the woman is pregnant.

MEASUREMENTS OF THE FEMALE PELVIS

An obstetrician generally performs a thorough examination on the pregnant woman several months before labor is to begin. The physician is interested in her general health and must determine the size and shape of her pelvis and the position of the fetus in the uterus. The size and shape of the pelvis can be determined indirectly through a vaginal examination. Two fingers of the physician's gloved hand are placed in the vagina. The physician checks first for the mobility of the tail bone or coccyx. If the tail bone is unusually rigid, it may snap back during labor, causing considerable pain. This difficulty is thus anticipated. The physician then checks the contours of the pelvic walls by circling his gloved hand around the vaginal canal. The slope of the pelvic walls is also determined. Then the physician will make an indirect measurement that will indicate something about the size of the pelvic inlet. The size of the inlet must be large enough if labor is to take place without complications. The physician brings the examining hand upward so that the first sacral vertebra (sacral promontory) can be felt through the vaginal wall with the middle finger (see Fig. 10-1). The hand is held flush with the lower end of the pelvic symphysis (front of the pelvic girdle) and this point is marked on the hand. The hand is then removed from the vagina and the distance between the tip of the middle finger and the marked spot on the hand is measured. Generally, 2 cm is subtracted from this measurement, and if the result is 11.5 cm or greater, the pelvic inlet is considered adequate for passage of the fetus.

POSITION OF THE FETUS IN THE UTERUS

Obtaining knowledge of the fetus's position in the uterus is necessary in order to prevent any complications of labor. *Attitude* or posture of the fetus refers to the relationship of one fetal part to another. The fetus usually shows an attitude of *universal flexion.* This means that the various parts of the body are flexed so that the arms are folded across the chest, the thighs are folded on the abdomen, the legs are bent on the thighs, and the chin touches the chest. Universal flexion generally means that an easy birth will take place and that the fetus has adjusted itself to the intermittent contractions of the uterus.

The relationship of the long axis (from head to foot) of the fetus to the long axis of the mother is called *presentation.* Just prior to birth, the most common presentation is *longitudinal,* where the long axis of the fetus is parallel to the long axis of the mother. The most common longitudinal presentation is *vertex,* where the back of the fetus's head is born first (shows up first in the vaginal opening). More rarely, the fetus's chin, face, or forehead emerges first. Sometimes the longitudinal presentation is *breech.* A breech birth refers to the fact that the fetus's buttocks or legs are born first. A breech birth generally does not increase the risk to the mother, but labor is prolonged, and a lack of oxygen to the fetus may be a problem; this can damage vital tissue, such as the brain. A *transverse* presentation means that the long axis of the fetus lies at an angle or crosswise with respect to the long axis of the mother.

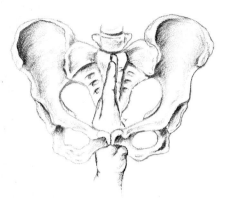

Figure 10-1 Physician's finger feeling the sacral promontory through the walls of the vagina. (*Redrawn from Reid, 1972.*)

Thus, the fetus first presents a shoulder, stomach, arm, or back, and this can lead to complications of labor. Often a transverse fetus is delivered through an incision of the abdominal and uterine walls—a technique called a *cesarean operation.*

COITUS DURING PREGNANCY

Physicians vary as to the advice they give regarding coitus during pregnancy. The most recent evidence from Masters' and Johnson's work indicates that sexual intercourse can take place throughout pregnancy except if there is vaginal discharge or abdominal pain. Most physicians state that intercourse should cease about 2 weeks before the due date because uterine contractions are increasing at this time. Pregnant women can reach orgasm, and no evidence exists that uterine contractions during orgasm lead to spontaneous abortion, that is, miscarriage.

LABOR

Labor, or *parturition,* is a group of processes responsible for the expulsion from the uterus of the fetus, placenta, and membranes of pregnancy. Labor is also called confinement, childbirth, and accouchement. There are three stages of labor: dilatation, expulsion, and placental.

During the first stage, which is called *dilatation,* muscular contractions pull the walls of the cervix outward until the opening between the uterus and vagina is large enough to accommodate the fetus's head. Dilatation begins when strong uterine contractions occur every 10 to 20 min, each contraction lasting about 25 to 30 s. This stage may last anywhere from 1 to 20 h, depending on how many previous pregnancies a woman has had. The greater the number of previous pregnancies, the shorter the duration of the dilatation stage. During this phase, a blood-tinged mucous plug is expelled from the cervix and this process is called "show." Also a membrane (amnion) immediately surrounding the fetus's watery environment ruptures and this has been referred to as "the water bag breaking." The dilatation phase ends when the cervix has fully dilated to about 10 to 11 cm in diameter from a previous 1 to 2 cm.

The expulsion phase starts as soon as a part of the fetus's body, generally the head, presents itself at the opening between the uterus and vagina. Uterine contractions now occur at 1 to 2 min intervals and last from 45 to 95 s. The baby is actually born during this stage, which can last from 2 min to 1 h, depending again on the number of previous pregnancies in the patient's history. As the baby's head moves slowly through the vaginal opening, it puts pressure on the tissue around the exterior vaginal opening. Sometimes the pressure is sufficient to cut off blood flow to the tissue or to cause it to tear. To prevent such complications, an incision is usually made in the vulvar skin extending from the lower edge of the vaginal opening back toward the anal opening. This procedure, which is called an episiotomy, is done under general or local anesthesia. Following delivery, the episiotomy is cleaned and sutured.

The *placental* stage of labor occurs after delivery of the baby and involves expulsion of the placenta from the mother's uterus. The duration of this phase ranges from 1 to 15 min.

CARE OF THE BABY

The baby will be held firmly by the ankles with head down so that drainage of mucus from the throat, nose, and mouth can take place. Sometimes a suction device will be used to suck out mucus that does not drain. The baby's arms and legs are then studied, fingers and toes counted, and sex determined from examination of the external genitalia. The baby is then usually placed on the mother's abdomen, and the umbilical cord is cut immediately after cessation of its pulsations. The physician gently massages the baby's feet or back, which usually elicits the characteristic loud cry and first breath. In many hospitals, a special scoring system called the APGAR Rating Evaluation is performed to obtain basic information on a baby's vital signs. It does not always provide a true picture, but does give a tentative and rapid diagnosis. A score of two points is given to the following five vital signs: heart rate must be over 100 beats per minute; crying must be strong, indicating healthy breathing; active muscle contractions must take place; reflexes must be strong—checked by placing a tube into the baby's nostril which elicits a cough or sneeze; color of the baby should be pinkish white or pinkish brown rather than blueish (a blue color indicates circulatory problems).

POSTPARTUM PERIOD

The *postpartum* period begins immediately following the placental stage of labor and ends when the woman's reproductive organs have returned approximately to the nonpregnant state. This period usually lasts about 6 weeks and includes the healing of the episiotomy and reduction of the weight of the uterus from 1,000 to about 50 g. The vaginal opening tends to gape right after birth. In time it gets smaller, but it rarely returns to the prepregnant state. However, if the woman routinely exercises the vaginal muscles used in manipulation of the penis, muscle tone will increase, and coitus will be just as pleasurable as it was before pregnancy. Following delivery, women experience a uterine discharge of mucus and blood originating from the former site of placental attachment. During the first few days of the postpartum period, the discharge is bright red, but by the fifteenth or sixteenth day, it becomes yellowish white and is diminished in quantity. Women who have had several previous pregnancies sometimes experience uterine contractions which are painful in the postpartum period. These "afterpains" usually disappear by the fourth or fifth day.

Breast-feeding generally begins with regularity on the third day postpartum. The fourth or fifth day the breasts begin to produce significant quantities of milk. The schedule for feeding is usually every 4 hours for the average-size baby. If the baby shows little or no weight gain following breast-feeding, he or she may not be getting any milk even though it is available, or the mother may be producing insufficient amounts. Assuming availability, failure of a baby to obtain sufficient milk is usually due to inverted or flattened nipples or to the presence of engorged breasts. Low-pressure pumping of the breasts for about 5 min using a breast pump usually softens the breasts and draws out the nipples. The continued secretion and production of milk depends upon the amount of suckling. A mother can expect to breast-feed for several months. Breast-feeding can inhibit ovulation but should not be used as a contraceptive technique, since many pregnancies do occur at this time. If a woman elects not to breast-feed, she is given hormonal medication after delivery to suppress the production of milk. In addition, some physicians recommend the application of ice packs and a breast binder to relieve discomfort associated with engorgement.

Mothers frequently experience a feeling of the "blues" usually between the second and fifth day of the postpartum period. For example, a mother begins to cry without apparent reason. In rare cases the woman may become extremely depressed, show periods of extreme quiet alternating with periods of shouting or singing, or refuse to eat and become quite suspicious of people around her. These severe symptoms are called *postpartum psychosis.* Generally the psychosis will disappear in time, but it may require psychiatric care.

Generally physicians ask couples to abstain from coitus for 4 to 6 weeks after delivery. During this time uterine and vaginal tissue is healing and is susceptible to infection. Penetration of the penis into the vagina could cause the wounds to reopen and bleed or could introduce infective organisms.

BIBLIOGRAPHY

Barber, H., and E. A. Graber. 1969. *Quick Reference to OB-GYN Procedures.* Lippincott, Philadelphia.

Bookmiller, M., and G. L. Bowen. 1967. *Textbook of Obstetrics and Obstetric Nursing.* Saunders, Philadelphia.

Philipp, E. E., et al. 1970. *Scientific Foundations of Obstetrics and Gynaecology.* Davis, Philadelphia.

Reid, D. E., et al. 1972. *Principles and Management of Human Reproduction.* Saunders, Philadelphia.

Chapter 11

Abstinence and Contraception

POPULATION GROWTH

"Growth Rate Down," "American Fertility Rate Dropping," "A Zero Birth Rate," and other similar headlines have appeared in various newspapers around the country since late 1971. Based upon data obtained by the Census Bureau and the National Center for Health Statistics, the fertility rate in the first nine months of 1972 was 2.08 children per family. This rate is even less than the Zero Population Growth suggestion of 2.1 offspring as the ideal average family size. During the last 16 years, the fertility rate has been cut almost in half, resulting in a much slower rate of population gain. Population growth will halt completely only when birth rate equals death rate and the rate of immigration matches emigration.

Various suggestions have been made in an attempt to account for the drop in fertility rate: (1) Young women, primarily between the ages of twenty and twenty-nine, are opting for an alternative way of life to motherhood. These women wish to remain single and to become economically independent—traveling, studying, working. (2) Some young couples have made decisions to adopt children and defer having their own. (3) The availability of effective contraceptive techniques and liberalized abortion laws contribute to the lowered rate. (4) Many young people are postponing marriage and using contraception when involved in nonmarital coitus. (5) There is much individual concern about the correlation between high population density and increases in pollution.

RESISTANCE TO BIRTH CONTROL

If these social changes have indeed caused the drop in the fertility rate, they become even more startling, because resistance to reproductive control lies deeply ingrained in all human society. The basic drive to reproduce is poorly understood but exists in all species. Among people, "glorification of mother-hood," "reverence for life," "fear of being left without heirs," "the need to prove one's virility," and the natural desire to love and raise children are but a few of the characteristics that resist the total acceptance of birth control (Rudel et al., 1973). A good example of conflict comes from public opinion surveys asking whether birth control services and education should be provided for nonmarried teenagers. As of August 1972, white Americans generally favored education about birth control but were more reluctant to actually provide birth control services for teenage girls (Blake). However, this contradiction may say more about acceptance of a young person's sexuality, especially that of a young "innocent" female, than about reproductive drive. A person may acknowledge the wisdom of preparing teenagers for married sex, but the same person may consciously or unconsciously find premarital coitus unacceptable. In addition, despite advances in birth control technology and increased sex education, "we have a substantial number of people in the United States using ineffective methods of contraception or using effective methods carelessly" (Ryder and Westoff). This has led to unwanted pregnancies occurring in more than one-third of women using contraceptives over a 5-year period. Of course, some of these women may never have received sex education; some unmarried women may be too embarrassed to seek prescription contraceptives; others may have been prescribed a contraceptive that is uncomfortable or conflicts with their personal lifestyle. And it has been shown that psychological conflict and lack of proper motivation can lead to more contraceptive failures than chemical and/or mechanical defects of the birth control method combined (Barglow and Klass). People who show a capacity to plan ahead, who feel they have control over their own futures, and who feel morally free to enjoy sexual intercourse for purposes other than procreation have been suggested as patients most likely to show success in family planning (Barglow and Klass). On the other hand, some moral values may provide a psychological block to desire for birth control. Intercourse for procreation purposes is a strong religious and racial value in many subcultures. Women with conflicts about handling their genitalia often develop fears about using spermicidal creams and diaphragms. Indeed, there is evidence that certain personality types may be more often associated with one particular contraceptive technique than with another. One study on 100 women found that 70 percent of those who were against using an intrauterine device (IUD) also found the idea of masturbation and premarital sex repulsive (Metzger and Golden). On the other hand, women using the IUD were more likely to have had premarital sex and to view all aspects of sexuality more positively than nonusers. More recent statistics indicate that there may be sound medical reasons for not using the IUD.

CRITERIA FOR SELECTION OF BIRTH CONTROL TECHNIQUE

Once the decision to control the rate of pregnancy is made, the type of technique to be used is a matter of individual choice. However, a thorough knowledge of effectiveness, methods of use, side effects, reversibility, expense, and religious acceptability are prerequisite to proper selection.

Birth control methods can be classified into four categories: *Abstinence*—which means that intercourse does not take place around the time of ovulation or does not take place at all. *Contraception*—this includes chemical or mechanical techniques that prevent conception or fertilization from taking place and are relatively easy to reverse. Some methods considered under this category, such as the IUD, actually do not prevent sperm from meeting an egg but instead inhibit an already fertilized egg (zygote) from implanting in the uterine wall. Technically an IUD should more properly be called a *contra-implantation* device. *Sterilization*—this generally involves surgical techniques which remove or block a portion of the reproductive tract preventing conception. Despite claims of reversibility, sterilization should currently be considered as permanent. *Abortion*—this involves induced expulsion from the uterus of the embryo or fetus before it weighs 500g. It does not include miscarriage since induction is lacking in this case.

EFFECTIVENESS AND SAFETY

Two basic questions continually asked by interested students are how effective and how safe are the various methods. The Federal Food and Drug Administration requires a specific series of test procedures before any drug can be marketed. Generally, these procedures are also used in testing mechanical devices such as the IUD. The first step in the series involves studies of toxicity and effectiveness on laboratory animals (rats, dogs, monkeys). If the method is safe and effective in the animals, it may then be tested on a small sample of highly motivated, fully informed human patients. Tests usually take the form of randomized double-blind experiments. In other words, the new contraceptive is given to only half of the experimental group; the other half is given a pill or injection containing some harmless substance or, in the case of mechanical devices, sham operations. Even the researchers do not know who got the fake and who got the real thing. If in these clinical trials major adverse side effects are lacking and if no more than one pregnancy is found, efforts to determine percent of safety and effectiveness among a larger number (at least 1,000) of patients will then be attempted. Frequently, new techniques and devices will be dispensed through a family planning agency or clinic, and extensive follow-ups on patients will be made.

Contraceptive effectiveness is usually expressed as the rate of pregnancy that would occur if a couple used a particular contraceptive during regular intercourse for 100 years. Of course, researchers can speed up the process by studying larger groups over a fairly short time, such as 100 couples for 1 year or 200 couples for 6 months. A pregnancy rate may be calculated using the Pearl Index (Pearl) as follows:

$$PR = \frac{P \times 1200}{W \times M}$$

Where PR = pregnacy rate
P = number of pregnancies
1200 = 1200 months or 100 years
W = number of women in study
M = number of months of exposure or cycles of therapy

The reader is urged to examine published pregnancy rates carefully in order to determine whether indices express failure of the method per se or failure due to irregularity and faulty use by couples as well as method failure (see Table 11-1).

Table 11-1   Rates of Pregnancy per 100 Women per Year in the United States

Method	Failure of method only*	Method and patient failures combined†
Combination pill	0.1	0.7
Sequential pill	0.5	1.4
Minipill	—	2.54[a]
IUD—large Lippes loop (pregnancy rate with device in place)	1.9	2.7
Diaphragm (with spermicidal jelly or cream)	2.6	14.4[b]; 12[c]
Condom	2.6	13.8[b]; 14[c]
Withdrawal	—	16.8[b]; 18[c]
Vaginal foam	—	28.3
Vaginal jelly or cream alone	—	36.8
Rhythm	—	38.5[b]
Douche	—	40.8[b]; 31[c]
Laparoscopy sterilization	0.6[d]	—

*Pregnancy rate based only on patients who follow recommended method perfectly.
†Pregnancy rate including those patients who use technique with some irregularity and error.
Source: Data from Guttmacher, 1973, except:
    (a) Information supplied by Ortho and Syntex.
    (b) Westoff et al., 1961.
    (c) Baunach and Baunach, 1964.
    (d) Rudel et al., 1973.

The pregnancy rates of various contraceptive and sterilization techniques can be compared with the rate reported for unprotected intercourse, which is between 70 and 100 pregnancies per 100 couples having regular intercourse for 1 year (Tietze et al.).

ABSTINENCE

Total

To abstain means to refrain from doing something—drinking, eating, smoking, or whatever. When we are talking about birth control, *abstinence* means avoiding coitus, either periodically or continually. Abstinence is 100 percent reliable if it is total, that is, continual. In the United Kingdom, giving up all intercourse to avoid conception was found in 1 percent of married couples with one child (Cartwright). Evidence is lacking concerning the effects of celibacy on physiological mechanisms. Compared to other bodily functions, such as feeding, drinking, urinating, defecating, and breathing, intercourse is the only one that can be and is totally suppressed and eliminated from the life-style of many people. No adverse side effects have been documented because, obviously, accumulation of such data is itself totally suppressed. Of interest, the Catholic church recognizes the difficulties of total abstinence and requires of all persons entering the religious life a testing period called postulancy and noviceship lasting a little more than two years. At the end of this period, if proper psychological foundations are set and if still celibate, religious vows may be taken by the novice.

Rhythm

Rhythm means abstaining from intercourse only during the fertile period of the menstrual cycle. Until about 1930 the rhythm method was almost totally ineffective because most people believed peaks of fertility occurred around the time of menstruation. Since 1930, however, scientists have been able to determine that ovulation occurs approximately 2 weeks before the first day of the next menstrual cycle. Nevertheless, time of ovulation is difficult to predict because signs of ovulation often go unnoticed, and the time of the cycle prior to its occurrence is highly variable. Some women with perserverance and care have been known to identify the time of ovulation. Often a combination of indices is needed:

    1 Mittleschmerz—This refers to pain in the lower abdomen occurring at the time of ovulation in some women. It may last from a few hours to a day or more. Some obstetricians have suggested that a "bounce test" may be used to bring on mittleschmerz in those women who do not naturally experience it (Shettles). A woman is to begin the process around the fifth day of her cycle and must bounce up and down on a couch or sofa several times in a row. This is done every day until mittleschmerz occurs.

2 Changes in Temperature—It has been substantiated that body temperature is relatively low during the first or preovulatory portion of the menstrual cycle (about 97.5°F). Researchers have postulated that immediately preceding ovulation the temperature drops 0.2 degree, but directly following ovulation the temperature rises again about 0.6 degree. The second or postovulatory portion of any menstrual cycle is thus associated with a relatively high body temperature (98.6°F, (37°C)) maintained by the increased levels of progesterone. It should be pointed out that many women do not show this shift in temperature or may show an increase at a time other than at ovulation (Loraine and Bell). Nevertheless, it is suggested that women can measure oral or anal temperatures at the same time each morning beginning with the ninth day of the cycle.

3 Tests for Vaginal Sugar and Acidity—Levels of glucose and acidity can be determined in the vagina by using special chemically treated paper. Generally, vaginal glucose is highest at ovulation whereas acidity is lowest. Tes-Tape, which may be purchased at any drugstore, is inserted in the vagina every day. When the yellowish tape turns deepest blue, glucose level is highest and theoretically ovulation is near. Similarly, using appropriate pH paper (acid range), the highest level of relative alkalinity which should be associated with ovulation, can be determined.

4 Intermenstrual Bleeding—A few women may show some spotting at the time of ovulation.

5 Cervical Mucus Test—Sometimes called the "stretch test," cervical mucus may be drawn out into long, thin threads between two microscope slides. The mucus threads stretch out the longest at the time of ovulation; this stringiness or "spinnbarkeit" is due to the high levels of estrogen present in the blood at ovulation. Some women have been known to perform this test on themselves by obtaining a sample of their own cervical mucus. A physician should be consulted prior to attempting this test.

In the future, it may be possible to simply dip a chemically treated paper into the cervical mucus and "read" the results. At ovulation certain enzymes (alkaline phosphatase, amino peptidease) are considerably reduced in the cervical mucus, and this could be detected using the special paper.

6 Saliva Tests—Also in the future it may be possible to test fluctuations in certain enzymes found in the saliva that correspond to the time of ovulation. The woman may simply hold a chemically sensitive strip of paper in her mouth each day and "read" the results.

Once the time of ovulation is determined, a woman can follow her menstrual cycles for at least a year. She determines the shortest and longest of her cycles. From the shortest cycle, she subtracts 18 days in order to determine the first day of her "unsafe" period. From the longest cycle, she subtracts 11 days to obtain the last day of her "unsafe" period. For example, a woman's "unsafe" period would last from day 8 to day 24 if her shortest and longest cycles were 26 and 35 days, respectively.

THE PILL

The "pill" generally refers to oral contraceptives, of which there are four types currently available: combination pill, sequential pill, minipill, and postcoital pill.

Combination Pill

The *combination pill* contains synthetic estrogens and chemical compounds called progestogens that act like progesterone and can be taken orally without destruction by the digestive system. The hormones are not synthesized from any animal material, and in fact, the progestogens are either modified compounds derived from Mexican yams (*cabeza de negro*) or manufactured from scratch. It is thus possible for a woman who is a vegetarian to use the combination pill without breaking any dietary rules.

How the Combo Pill Works   The synthetic estrogens decrease the secretion of FSH from the pituitary (Vorys et al.). This may occur by direct inhibition upon the pituitary and/or indirect inhibition on hypothalamic-releasing factors. This mechanism stops the maturation of follicles in the ovaries, and the lack of mature follicles means ovulation cannot take place. The progestogens are known to add to the antiovulatory effect by suppressing the midcycle surge of LH (Taymor). In addition, progestogens are known to inhibit the estrogen-controlled buildup of endometrial lining (Rudel et al., 1967). The endometrium does not thicken and may become inhospitable to implantation by a zygote. The reduced endometrial buildup also means that there will be a scanty menstrual flow, sometimes none at all. Progestogens also cause a thickening of the cervical mucus, which decreases the motility of sperm (Rudel et al., 1965). To summarize: *The combo pill primarily inhibits ovulation but can also make the endometrium inhospitable to implantation and the cervical mucus hostile to sperm.*

Regimen   The combo pill is taken for 20 to 21 days beginning with the fifth day of any given cycle. Some brands provide an additional seven pills of a different color containing inert ingredients. The menstrual flow should begin a few days following the last "active" (hormone-containing) pill taken. Five days following the onset of menses the pill is taken again daily for 20 to 21 days of the new cycle. If menses does not occur, which may be the case during the first few cycles, the woman is instructed to count seven days after her last "active" pill and begin taking the new pills just as if she had menstruated. To allow for gradual absorption by the digestive tract, each pill should be taken following the largest meal of the day—usually after dinner. If a pill is missed, it should be taken the following day with the next pill. If two pills are missed, they should be taken together with the third subsequent pill. It should be noted that omissions of one to five tablets can increase the pregnancy rate by a factor of 50 (Goldzieher).

Which Combo Pill to Use?   At present, there are 20 brands on the U.S. market containing one of two estrogens in combination with one of five major forms of progestogen (see Table 11-2). All the combination pills provide equivalent effectiveness but may differ with respect to side effects. The decision as to which brand to prescribe for a particular woman depends upon her physiological makeup and on the knowledgeability of her physician. This last point is important. If the physician bases his or her opinion on information derived from constant updating, the decision will be a better one than if based only upon clinical impressions. Evidence clearly indicates "that the clinical impression, even of seasoned practitioners, is apt to bear little relationship to the facts" (Goldzieher).

Many erudite physicians recommend "using the lowest-dose preparation that will provide excellent effectiveness while avoiding undesirable side effects as much as possible" (Tyler). However, the idiosyncracies of a particular woman's physiology can dictate some differences in prescription. For example, some women can be described as highly estrogenic. They normally show a heavy menstrual flow, have relatively large breasts, and frequently experience the premenstrual syndrome. These are indices of a relatively high estrogenic activity. Brands of the pill which contain the lowest dosage or chemical activity of synthetic estrogen plus a progestogen which shows little or no estrogenlike activity would be recommended for these women. Other women may show characteristics reflecting relatively low blood estrogen such as small breasts, scanty menses, sometimes a tall and thin figure, and a degree of malelike characteristics such as facial hair. For these women, a pill that contains a relatively high dosage of synthetic estrogen and a progestogen that acts like estrogen would be the drug of choice. Thus, the requirements of a woman may be balanced against the characteristics of a particular brand of pill.

Side Effects   Some side effects are caused by too little or too much of a specific hormone. Others involve interaction between the type of synthetic

Table 11-2 Some Low Dose Brands of Combination Pill Commercially Available

Brand	Manufacturer	Synthetic estrogen	Synthetic progestogen
Enovid-E	Searle	Mestranol, 0.1 mg	Norethynodrel, 2.5 mg
Demulen	Searle	Ethinyl estradiol, 0.05 mg	Ethynodiol diacetate, 1.0 mg
Norinyl	Syntex	Mestranol, 0.08 mg	Norethindrone, 1.0 mg
Norlestrin	Parke Davis	Ethinyl estradiol, 0.05 mg	Norethindrone acetate, 1.0 mg
Ortho-Novum 1/50	Ortho	Mestranol, 0.05 mg	Norethindrone, 1.0 mg
Ovral	Wyeth	Ethinyl estradiol, 0.05 mg	Norgestrel, 0.5 mg
Ovulen	Searle	Mestranol, 0.1 mg	Ethynodiol diacetate, 1.0 mg

hormone and the idiosyncracies of a specific woman's physiology. Still others may result from the particular ratio of hormones in a given preparation. Side effects appear also to increase simply by the power of suggestion. In one study, a group of women given oral contraceptives and a warning showed three times as many side effects as a group given oral contraceptives and no warning (Pincus et al.). Whatever the cause, some side effects may be considered as beneficial (Table 11-3) and others as detrimental. The adverse effects can be categorized into those which show an experimentally established association and those which have been reported but neither confirmed nor refuted (Table 11-4). As can be seen from Table 11-4, the synthetic estrogen has been identified as the causative agent in the case of many side effects. For example, too much synthetic estrogen may decrease the ability of the brain to synthesize certain neurotransmitters, particularly serotonin, a chemical required for transmitting messages between some nerve cells (Adams et al.). Normally vitamin B_6 is necessary for this synthesis, but estrogen blocks its action. A type of depression involving pessimism, crying, dissatisfaction, and tension is associated with low levels of this neurotransmitter. Vitamin B_6 therapy reduces this depression (Adams), and pills with the lowest level of synthetic estrogen would be recommended.

Progestogens are known to act on the body like progesterone, estrogen, or androgen (male hormone). The relative ability to act in a particular way depends upon the chemical structure. Thus, norethynodrel (see Table 11-2) acts more like estrogen and has the weakest progestational activity of any progestogen in a combo pill. If side effects are due to the influence of too much estrogen, a brand containing a progestogen other than norethynodrel would be recommended.

It can be seen that thorough knowledge of pill ingredients and their effects can help the physician make a more accurate decision as to the type of pill for a particular person.

At the present time, cancer is not known to be caused in humans by the combo pill. However, estrogen may stimulate growth of an already-present carcinoma, and the combo pill should not be taken in these cases. Recently, Provest, manufactured by Upjohn Company, was removed from the commercial market because of its association with the development of breast nodules in beagles (Anonymous).

Table 11-3 Beneficial Side Effects Reported by Women on the Pill

1 Relief of dysmenorrhea (menstrual pain)
2 Relief of premenstrual tension
3 Regulate menstrual cycles
4 Decreased menstrual flow
5 Relief of acne
6 Decreases in certain malelike physical characteristics; e.g., facial hair
7 Relief of mittelschmerz
8 Some report increases in libido; others decreases or no change
9 Some report increases in feeling of well being; others decreases or no change

Source: Peel and Potts, 1969.

Table 11-4 Adverse Side Effects of the Pill—Most Commonly Reported

Side effect	Confirmed	Suggested
Weight ↑		X
*Fluid retention		X
Engorgement and fullness of breasts		X
Breast tenderness and soreness		X
Headache	X	
Libido ↓		X
*Depression ↑		X
*Vitamin B₆ ↓	X	
Vitamin C ↓		X
*Nausea and vomiting	X	
*Discoloration of skin (chloasma)	X	
†Breakthrough bleeding	X	
Infertility after going off pill		X
Thrombophlebitis (inflammation of a vein causing obstruction of blood flow)	X	
Pulmonary embolism (obstruction of blood vessel in lungs with blood clot, air bubble, bit of sloughed off tissue from another vessel, etc. Obstructing material originates in another region of body. Obstructing blood clot or dead tissue may come from an inflamed vein.)	X	
Cerebral thrombosis (blood clot originating within a vessel supplying the brain and causing obstruction of blood flow to brain)	X	
*Blood pressure ↑	X	
Change in populations of vaginal microorganisms (bacteria, yeast, etc.)	X	

*Estrogen may need to be decreased.
†Progestogen activity or dose may need to be increased.
Key: ↓ = Decrease
↑ = Increase
Source: Rudel et al., 1973; Spellacy and Birk, 1972; Peel and Potts, 1969.

A serious and well-documented side effect of oral contraceptives is an increased incidence of blood clotting within the vessels. The clot may partially or totally obstruct blood flow at the place where it forms, in which case it is called a thrombus. Or it may be carried to a smaller vessel, where it plugs up flow; in this case it is a type of embolus. The relative risk of thromboembolism in women on the pill was 7 times the risk in nonusers in one British study (Vessey and Dall) and 4.4 times the risk of nonusers in a study done in the United States (Sartwell et al.). In an earlier study, researchers reported an average of three deaths per 100,000 users due to blood clots compared to 0.35 deaths per 100,000 nonusers (Inman and Vessey). Evidence indicates that synthetic estrogens in quantities above 0.075 mg are more apt to cause thromboembolism than lower dosages (Inman et al.). Thus, the Food and Drug

Administration has recommended against the use of oral contraceptives containing more than 0.075 mg estrogen.

It is of interest that women with blood type O rarely show blood clots caused by oral contraceptives.

People who are against birth control often use the statistics for increased thromboembolism as evidence why women should not use the pill. On the other hand, populationists compare this risk with that of pregnancy, illegal abortion, and so on, and in this case, "with tongue in cheek one could perhaps say that the oral contraceptives are as safe as the diaphragm" (Hellman) (Table 11-5).

Sequential Pill

The normal menstrual cycle is characterized by estrogen dominance during the first half and progesterone dominance during the second half. Attempts to create a pill that would mimic this normal physiology resulted in the *sequential pill.* Like the combo pill, sequentials are taken beginning with the fifth day of a given cycle. But unlike combos the first 15 sequential pills contain only a synthetic estrogen. The remaining five to six contain both estrogen and progestogen. The early estrogen therapy inhibits ovulation by retarding follicular development in the ovary. The progestogen given so late in therapy does not help to inhibit ovulation, but it does help prepare the uterus for a menstrual flow that resembles the normal menses in quantity. Because only one hormone is inhibiting ovulation, the sequentials are not as effective as combination therapy (see Table 11-1). Recently, C-Quens, manufactured by Eli Lilly Company, was removed from the commercial market because of its association with the development of breast nodules in beagle dogs (Anonymous).

Minipill

In a world of miniskirts, minicircuits, and mini mice, little wonder at the arrival of pills with the mini label. On January 3, 1973, two brands of *minipill*

Table 11-5 Comparative Risk of Death from Oral Contraceptives in the United States †

	Death rate/100,000
Oral contraceptives	3
Pregnancy	35.8 (based on live births)
Illegal abortion*	26.7
IUD	2
Diaphragm (from pregnancy occurring due to diaphragm failure)	3
Auto accidents	20.8

*Based on an estimated 1,000,000 illegal abortions per year.

†As this book goes to press the U.S. Food and Drug Administration is proposing the following additional warning labels for contraceptive pills: Women over the age of 40 should not take the pills because of increased risk of heart attack. A higher risk of spontaneous abortion is reported among women who become pregnant soon after going off the pills; it is recommended that conception be avoided for 3 months after the last pill is taken. In those cases where the woman becomes pregnant while on the pill, a higher risk of fetal abnormality has been reported.

Source: Modified from Hellman, 1969.

containing only one active ingredient went on the market. They are manufactured by Syntex, which calls its preparation NOR-Q-D, and Ortho, calling its brand MICRONOR. Both brands contain only 0.35 mg of the synthetic progestogen (norethindrone) which is about a third of that found in the combo pills. Since synthetic estrogen is lacking, most of the side effects associated with combos and sequentials have been eliminated. The minipill works not necessarily by inhibiting ovulation but mostly by making the endometrial lining inhospitable to implantation (Guttmacher, 1973b). Women begin taking the minipill on the first day of the menstrual cycle and continue taking a pill at the same time each day for as long as they wish to prevent pregnancy. In fact, NOR-Q-D means "everyday" in Latin.

There are two problems associated with the minipills. First, they are not as effective as other types of pill. Effectiveness has been calculated at three pregnancies per 100 users, which is a higher pregnancy rate than found for the combos and sequentials. Second, a higher incidence of breakthrough bleeding and irregular cycles have been reported. However, people experiencing unpleasant complications associated with the other pills or who desire not to have ovulation inhibited may find that the minipill is an acceptable alternative.

Postcoital Pill

A great deal of controversy exists about the use of the *postcoital* or "morning after" pill. The dispute centers around its most commonly used ingredient—the synthetic estrogen DES or diethylstilbestrol. This compound has been available by prescription for many years, and has been used, among other things, in treating symptoms of menopause and cancer of the prostate gland. Women who miscarry easily have been treated with DES in order to maintain their pregnancies. Herein lies the source of the controversy. Recent studies have shown that maternal use of DES during pregnancy appears to increase the risk of a type of vaginal cancer developing several years later in the exposed offspring (Herbst et al.). It should be pointed out that a pregnancy involves treatment for an extended period of time—usually beginning with the sixth week of pregnancy and lasting at least through the first trimester; whereas the postcoital pill is given for only 5 days.

It has been shown that high doses of estrogens including DES will "intercept" a zygote and prevent implantation from taking place (Morris and Van Wagenen). Thus, on the one hand DES can maintain a pregnancy already in existence, and on the other hand it can prevent implantation. When administered early, following ovulation and within 72 h of unprotected intercourse, DES has been shown to effectively eliminate the possibility of pregnancy (Morris and Van Wagenen). In this case, 50 mg of DES are given daily for only 5 days beginning with a period not later than 72 h after intercourse. The primary side effect is nausea, which occurs in about 50 percent of patients. This necessitates the use of antinausea pills such as Compazine to be taken along with the DES. When given in the form and dosage of a postcoital pill, DES has not as yet been associated with the development of any type of cancer. Based upon this conclusion, the Food and Drug Administration on

February 22, 1973, gave its approval for the use of DES in postcoital pills, but only in emergency situations. It could be used in cases of "rape, incest, or other emergencies so deemed by the physician."

Researchers have found that other types of estrogen can be used in postcoital pills (Board and Bhatnagar). These estrogens (e.g., Premarin) have not as yet been associated with cancer production and are given as alternatives to DES in postcoital pills on some college campuses.

The mechanism of postcoital-pill action upon the endometrial lining remains unclear. One theory, explaining how a zygote normally implants, involves the availability of natural progesterone during the second half of the menstrual cycle (Board and Bhatnagar). High levels of progesterone supposedly stimulate the production of an enzyme by the endometrial cells (carbonic anhydrase) which is responsible for maintaining an alkalinity. The alkaline environment is apparently conducive to implantation, the zygote becomes "sticky" and sinks into the endometrium. It has been suggested that DES given in a postcoital regimen decreases the normal progesterone levels and this reduces carbonic anhydrase activity. The endometrial environment remains acid and therefore hostile to the implantation process.

Because of the severe nausea and vomiting, postcoital pills should never be used routinely as a contraceptive technique. If a woman is treated once or twice throughout her fertile life, this would be more than enough.

Male Pill?

A male pill is not commercially available at the present time. The major reason for its current lack of availability is that sperm production and testosterone secretions require a constant, relatively high level of pituitary stimulation. To reduce the constant pituitary control, comparatively massive dosages of inhibitor would have to be continually given—much higher than found in combo or sequential pills. Experiments have shown that many adverse side effects occur when large dosages of inhibitor are continually administered. Jackson provides a summary of research in the area of chemical methods of male contraception. These include pituitary inhibition of sperm production, direct action of chemicals on the testes, and sperm maturation in the epididymis. Currently the best hope may be in using a combination of testosterone and progestogen in low doses. By itself, testosterone can be given in large doses, which inhibit spermatogenesis but are toxic to the liver. Large amounts of progesterone also inhibit sperm production, but side effects include shrunken testicles, enlarged breasts, and decreased libido. Given together, small doses of both hormones may decrease spermatogenesis without side effects.

INTRAUTERINE DEVICE

An *intrauterine device*, or *IUD*, is an object that is placed in the uterus. "Ten years ago the IUD was considered the best hope for control of population growth" (Povey). IUDs have been used for thousands of years in one form or another. Arab camel drivers are known to have inserted small pebbles or fruit pits into the uteri of camels, thereby preventing pregnancy of the animals during a long desert trek. In 1920, the German scientist Grafenberg devised a number of IUDs made out of silkworm gut and metal to be used for women. By 1962, extensive use of a variety of plastic IUDs began under the guidance of the Population Council in America. Two years later, only 50 percent of women who had begun using IUDs remained with them. Pregnancy, irregular bleeding, abdominal cramps, and chronic expulsion were cited as the major reasons for the low rate of continuation (Tatum). All of this seriously altered the IUD's destiny as a contraceptive panacea.

"Inert" and "Active" IUDs

Today, IUDs can be classified as "inert" when the device only acts mechanically and does not exert a chemical effect on the uterine wall and "active" when they also are vehicles for antifertility agents such as copper and progestogen. The various types of IUDs are pictured in Fig. 11-1. They are manufactured

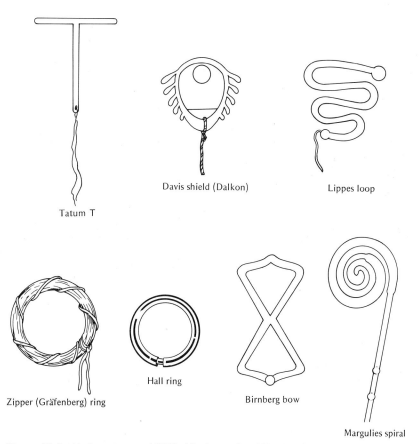

Tatum T

Davis shield (Dalkon)

Lippes loop

Zipper (Gräfenberg) ring

Hall ring

Birnberg bow

Margulies spiral

Figure 11-1 Various types of IUD's (*Redrawn from Tatum, 1972.*)

from polyethylene or polypropylene plastic and impregnated with metal salts such as barium sulfate, making them easily detectable in x-ray pictures. Occasionally, it becomes necessary in cases where the IUD perforates the uterine wall and shifts its abdominal position to locate it by x-ray analysis. In addition to the plastic, the "active" IUDs currently on the market have a fine copper wire or sleeve entwined around the central support (Fig. 11-2).

IUD Insertion Procedure

An IUD is inserted by a physician usually during the last 2 or 3 days of a woman's menses. At that time, the cervix is flexible, the woman, most likely, is not pregnant, and any additional bleeding due to insertion should be camouflaged by normal menses and therefore unalarming to the patient. Generally the smaller, more flexible IUDs are easier to insert, especially in women who have never been pregnant. An anesthetic is not used in the process of insertion. The size and shape of the uterus is carefully examined, and the IUD is positioned in the uterus using a special plastic inserter. The woman is taught to feel for the nylon threads that hang down into her vagina: when the IUD is properly in place the threads are easily detectable. Only a physician is qualified to remove the IUD upon the request of the woman (Rudel, 1973). In a 5-year clinical study of 2,300 patients, only 2.2 percent experienced severe pain immediately following insertion without an anesthetic (Portnuff et al.).

Mechanism of IUD Action

The exact mechanism by which an IUD prevents implantation of a zygote into the uterine lining is not thoroughly understood. The current theory for inert IUDs most accepted by scientists is called the *sterile inflammation reaction* (Tatum). Foreign bacteria are usually introduced into the uterine cavity whenever an IUD is inserted. The body's response is to increase the number of white blood cells in the vicinity of the uterine lining, and they remove the foreign bacteria. Within approximately 25 h, the bacteria have been destroyed but the white blood cells remain, hence the term *sterile* (no bacteria) *inflammation* (presence of white blood cells). The theory claims that some of these white

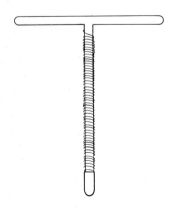

Figure 11-2 Example of an active IUD, the copper T (TCu-200.) (*Redrawn from Tatum, 1972.*)

blood cells die and disintegrate, liberating toxic chemicals that create an environment inhospitable for implantation (Tatum).

The active IUD's main contraceptive effect is due to the presence of copper ions, which when liberated into the uterine cavity influence many biochemical reactions (Orlans). One major effect suggested is that copper antagonizes the action of zinc that is needed to make the endometrial lining hospitable for implantation (Kincl and Rudel). Without zinc, implantation is resisted (Salaverry et al.).

Complications with the IUD

The most common side effects encountered with the inert IUDs are listed in Table 11-6. Generally the larger the surface area of an IUD the less the possibility of pregnancy. Unfortunately, the greater surface of an IUD is also correlated with a greater number of removals due to complaints of pain and irregular bleeding (Fortier et al.). The rate of expulsion is less when an IUD is stiff; however, rigid devices tend also to have smaller surface areas and are thus less likely to prevent pregnancies. Recently the Food and Drug Administration recalled the Majzlin Spring IUD because it has been associated with a higher number of complications than other inert forms.

In 1970, a new inert device called the "crab" or "Dalkon Shield" was designed with a relatively high surface area but small overall dimensions. Expulsion supposedly would be reduced, since the crab possessed a number of small projections extending out from its margins, tending to aid retention in the uterine cavity (Tatum). It was to be a better device for women who had never been pregnant. Since introduction of the Dalkon Shield, 2.2 million women are estimated to have used it. However, in July 1974, the Department of Health, Education, and Welfare startlingly banned the continued use of the "crab" in 3,000 federally supported birth control clinics in the United States. The Planned Parenthood Federation asked also that its doctors no longer prescribe it. A recent study made by the U.S. government's Center for Disease Control showed that women had a higher rate of pregnancy when using the shield than

Table 11-6 Complications Occurring with Inert IUD (Based on 2,547 Individuals Using IUDs)

	Lippes loop		Birnberg bow		Saf-T-coil		Total	
	No.	%	No.	%	No.	%	No.	%
Increased flow	351	23.3	45	26.6	223	25.4	619	24.3
Irregular flow	370	24.6	55	32.5	240	27.4	665	26.1
Cramping	194	12.9	22	13.0	106	12.1	322	12.6
Expulsion	269	17.9	32	18.9	18	2.1	319	12.6
Infection	16	1.1	2	1.2	9	1.0	27	1.1
Perforation	13	0.8					13	0.8
Pregnancy	60	3.9	5	2.9	24	2.9	89	3.4

Source: Portnuff et al., 1972.

when using other IUDs. In addition, women hospitalized with a disease related to their pregnancies were twice as likely to have been wearing a "crab" as not. Since 1966, 8.8 million women have used the IUD. Thirty-six deaths have occurred in association with an IUD, eleven of which involve the Dalkon Shield.

Early reports on the lack of complications arising from use of copper IUDs were encouraging in that they showed fewer removals for pain and bleeding and a lower rate of expulsion than for the "inert" Lippes loop D. However, long-range studies (taking at least 2 years) showed that "although removals for bleeding and pain were slightly lower, pregnancies and expulsions were in the same range for both 'inert' and 'active' devices" (Orlans) (see Table 11-7).

To date no evidence exists that suggests IUDs of any kind cause cancer (Orlans).

THE DIAPHRAGM AND SPERMICIDAL JELLY OR CREAM

The *diaphragm* is a thin latex dome stretched over a flexible metal ring and is designed to fit over the opening of the uterus (see Fig. 11-3). Diaphragms range in diameter from 45 to 105 mm, and if the size is correct, the diaphragm will fit snugly over the cervix. The size is determined by a physician, and a recheck normally occurs once a year or, in cases where the woman is new at experiencing intercourse, every 3 months. Also a recheck of cervical diameter would be appropriate following a pregnancy or gain in weight of 10 or more lb (Peel and Potts). The diaphragm is to be used in conjunction with spermicidal cream or jelly. The spermicide is applied to the surface of the diaphragm adjacent to the cervix and along the rim. Physicians recommend that the diaphragm and spermicide be inserted by the woman at least 2 hours before intercourse. A new application of spermicide should be used if intercourse is delayed beyond 2 hours. Insertion of a diaphragm is easiest when the woman is crouching, squatting, lying down, or standing with one foot on a chair. The diaphragm is collapsed between two fingers, inserted into the vagina, and rocked into place on the cervix. Care should be taken not to penetrate the latex with fingernails and rings. A woman can usually urinate with little worry of dislodging the diaphragm but should check the fit following defecation. Manufacturers recommend that the diaphragm be left in place at least 6 to 8 h following intercourse. After removal, the diaphragm can be washed, using a mild soap in lukewarm water, carefully dried, and examined for rips and holes by holding it up to the light. It can then be dusted with baking soda, which is generally free of harmful chemicals, and stored in its plastic case for future use.

THE CONDOM

The *condom*, or rubber, is a sheath of thin, flexible material that fits over the penis like a rubber glove; it is the most commonly used contraceptive device in the world today (Peel and Potts). The term *condom* comes from the Latin

Table 11-7 Expulsion, Pregnancy, and Removal for Bleeding and Pain in Women with a Copper IUD (TCu-200) Compared with an Inert IUD (Lippes Loop D)

Type of IUD	No. of insertions	Woman months of use	Expulsions rate	Pregnancy rate	Bleeding/ pain	Removals Other medical	Removals Planned pregnancy	Removals Other personal	Continuation rate
One-Year Rates:									
T Cu 200			9.8	3.2	8.8	N/A	N/A	N/A	N/A
Lippes loop D			12.1	3.2	13.3	N/A	N/A	N/A	N/A
Two-Year Rates:									
T Cu 200	6,801	52,133	13.0	6.1	17.1	7.5	9.8	6.7	52.7
Lippes loop D	7,419	105,199	14.3	5.5	20.5	6.3	5.4	5.6	53.9

Source: Orlans, 1973.

195

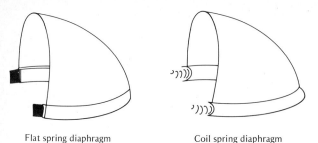

Flat spring diaphragm   Coil spring diaphragm

Figure 11-3   Types of diaphragms (*Redrawn from Peel and Potts, 1969.*)

condus, meaning receptacle. In England the device is called the French "letter" (modified from the term *envelope*); whereas the French call it *la capote anglaise.* Today, most condoms consist of a sheath of latex rubber with a dome-shaped tip or reservoir end. Some brands are lubricated and stored in a package containing a silicone fluid. A number of reusable forms, much more expensive than the latex, are made of sheep's intestine and are called "skins." The latex condoms are extremely cheap to manufacture, costing only one dollar a gross wholesale. Most condom-manufacturing companies take great care to maintain high standards of quality control. It is estimated that 99.7 percent of all condoms sold in the United States are without defects (Rudel). Tests are made before and after aging of a representative sample of the finished product. Aging is accelerated by heating rubbers to 70°C (158°F) for 7 days and allowing them to cool for 12 h before tests. The minimum thickness of a condom must be 0.05 ± 0.01 mm, and this is determined by passing an electric current through a stretched condom and calculating the electrical resistance. American companies examine for holes by filling each rubber of a test sample with about 300 ml of water, tying off the end, and rolling it on blotting paper. The British measure bursting strength by filling each condom of a test sample with about 3 q of fluid and recording whether or not it breaks under the pressure.

With so many tests for quality, any failure of a condom is usually attributed to faulty use. Manufacturers recommend that a condom be rolled over the penis leaving a little slack at the tip of the glans. Air should be pinched out of the tip in order to prevent air bubbles from traveling down the penile shaft to the vagina. When pulling the penis out following ejaculation, the condom can be kept on by holding the base with two fingers. Only a non-petroleum-base jelly should be used if a lubricant is desired. Any petroleum product tends to destroy latex.

THE FUTURE OF CONTRACEPTION

The following is a list of some of the possible contraceptive methods to be used in the future:

1   Synthetic estrogens used in the postcoital pill are effective in preventing implantation; however, they also cause nausea and cycle abnormalities. Recent clinical experiments using progestogens instead of estrogens have been successful in preventing implantation without the side effects (Kesseru et al.).

2   Some day IUDs will be impregnated with progestogen. When in the uterus, the slow release of progestogen will inhibit implantation without the current side effects of IUDs (Tatum).

3   Progestogen-impregnated rings will be available to be placed in the vagina beginning with day 5 and ending with day 26 of a given menstrual cycle. The progestogen slowly released into the blood stream will effectively inhibit ovulation (Mishell et al.).

4   Women may eventually be immunized against their husbands' sperm. Antibodies will be given that immobilize sperm.

5   A pill will be developed that will create changes in cervical mucus blocking entry of sperm into the uterus (Moghissi).

6   A method will be found that will prevent maturation of sperm in the epididymis.

7   A method will exist that will prevent capacitation of sperm once in the vagina.

8   A drug will be developed that will specifically speed up or slow down the transport of a zygote in the fallopian tubes. When the zygote reaches the uterus it will be either too early or too late for implantation (Gaddum-Rosse and Blandau).

BIBLIOGRAPHY

Adams, R. N., et al. 1973. Effect of pyridoxine hydrochloride (vitamin B_6) upon depression associated with oral contraceptives, *Lancet*, 1(7809):897–904.

Anonymous. 1970. Two brands of birth control pills are going off the market, *Chem. and Eng. News*, Nov. 2. p. 17.

Barglow, P., and D. Klass. 1972. Psychiatric aspects of contraceptive utilization, *Am J. Obstet. Gynecol.*, **114**:93–96.

Baunach, A., and M. Baunach. 1964. Erfahrungen mit ovulen, ernem neuen ovulation-shemmer, *Med. Welt.*, **41**:2207–2211.

Blake, J. 1973. The teenage birth control dilemma and public opinion, *Sci.*, **180** (4087):708–712.

Board, J. A., and A. S. Bhatnagar. 1972. Postcoital antifertility agents, *South. Med. J.*, **65**:1390–1392.

Cartwright, A. 1970. *Parents and Family Planning Services*, Routledge, London, and Atherton, New York.

Fortier, L., et al. 1973. Canadian experience with a copper-covered intrauterine contraceptive device, *Am. J. Obstet. Gynecol.*, **115**(3):291–297.

Gaddum-Rosse, P., and R. J. Blandau. 1973. In vitro studies on ciliary activity within the oviducts of the rabbit and pig, *Am. J. Anat.*, **136**:91.

Goldzieher, J. W. 1969. Oral contraceptives: which one and for whom? in Alan Rubin (ed.), *Family Planning Today*, pp. 43–57. Davis, Philadelphia.

Guttmacher, A. F. 1973a. *Planned Parenthood-World Population*, 65.

Guttmacher, A. F. 1973b. Population control at the grass roots, in R. W. Kistner (ed.), *Reproductive Endocrinology*, chap 34. Medcom Learning Systems for Wyeth Lab., Philadelphia.

Hellman, L. 1969. Oral contraceptives: safety and complications, in A. Rubin (ed.). *Family Planning Today*, pp. 29–42. Davis, Philadelphia.

Herbst, A. L., et al. 1972. Clear-cell adenocarcinoma of the genital tract in young females, *New Engl. J. Med.*, **287** (25):1260–1264.

Inman, W. H. W., and M. P. Vessey. 1968. Investigation of deaths from pulmonary, coronary, and cerebral thrombosis and embolism in women in child-bearing age, *B. Med. J.*, **2**:193–199.

Inman, W. H. W., et al. 1970. Thromboembolic disease and steroidal content of oral contraceptives. A report to the committee on safety of drugs, *Br. Med. J.*, **2**:203–209.

Jackson, H. 1973. Chemical methods of male contraception, *Am. Sci.*, **61**:188–193.

Kesseru, E., et al. 1973. Postcoital contraception with D-norgestrel, *Contraception*, **7**:367.

Kincl, F. A., and H. W. Rudel. 1971. Possible mechanism of the antifertility effect of copper, in A. Ingelman-Sundberg, and N. O. Lunell (eds.), *Current Problems in Fertility*, pp. 187–190. Plenum, New York.

Loraine, J. A:, and E. T. Bell. 1968. *Fertility and Contraception in the Human Female*. E. and S. Livingstone, Edinburgh and London.

Metzger, R. J., and J. S. Golden. 1967. Psychological factors influencing female patients in the selection of contraceptive devices, *Fertil. Steril.*, **18**(6):249.

Mishell, D. R., et al. 1972. Inhibition of ovulation with cyclic use of progestogen-impregnated intravaginal devices, *Am. J. Obstet. Gynecol.*, **113**:927–932.

Moghissi, K. S. 1972. The function of the cervix in fertility, *Fertil. Steril.*, **24**:295.

Morris, M. L., and G. Van Wagenen. 1973. Interception: the use of postovulatory estrogens to prevent implantation, *Am. J. Obstet. Gynecol.*, **115**:101–106.

Nixon, R. M. 1972. *Statement by the President on the Commission's Report*. In Commission on Population Growth and the American Future, Sup. Doc., U.S. G.P.O., Washington, D.C.

Orlans, F. B. 1973. Intrauterine devices. Copper IUDs, performance to date. *Population Report Series B, no. 1*, p. 20. Dept. of Med. and Publ. Off. Sci. Communication Div. Geo. Wash. U. Med. Cent. Washington, D.C.

Pearl, R. 1932. Contraception and fertility in 2,000 women, *Hum. Biol.*, **4**:363–407.

Peel, J., and M. Potts. 1969. *Textbook of Contraceptive Practice*. Cambridge, London.

Pincus, G., et al. 1959. Effectiveness of an oral contraceptive, *Science*, **130**:81–83.

Portnuff, J. C., et al. 1972. The intrauterine contraceptive device. A prospective 5 year clinical study, *Am J. Obstet. and Gynecol.*, **114**:934–937.

Povey, W. G. 1972. Intrauterine contraception, an overview, *Postgrad. Med.*, **51**:221–225.

Report of the Commission on Population Growth and the American Future, The. 1972. New American Library, New York.

Rudel, H. W., et al. 1965. Role of progestogens in hormonal control of fertility, *Fertil. Steril.*, **16**:158–169.

Rudel, H. W., et al. 1967. Assay of the antiestrogenic effects of progestogens in women, *J. Reprod. Fert.*, **13**:199–203.

Rudel, H. W., et al. 1973. *Birth Control, Contraception and Abortion*. Macmillan, New York.

Ryder, N. B., and C. F. Westoff. 1971. *Reproduction in the United States, 1965. National Fertility Study,* Princeton University Press, Princeton, N.J.

Salaverry, G., et al. 1973. Copper determination and localization in different morphologic components of human endometrium during the menstrual cycle in copper intrauterine contraception device wearers, *Am. J. Obstet. Gynecol.,* **115** (2):163–168.

Sartwell, P. E., et al. 1969. Thromboembolism and oral contraceptives: an epidemiological case-control study, *Am. J. Epidemiol.,* **90:**365–380.

Shettles, L. B. 1972. Predetermining children's sex, *Med. Aspects Hum. Sex.,* **6:**172.

Spellacy, W. N., and S. A. Birk. The effect of intrauterine devices, oral contraceptives, estrogens, and progestogens on blood pressure, *Am. J. Obstet. Gynecol.,* **112** (7):912–919.

Tatum, H. J. 1972. Current developments: intrauterine contraception, *Am. J. Obstet. Gynecol.,* **112:**1000–1023.

Tausk, M. 1972. General summary, in G. Peters (ed.), *Pharmacology of the Endocrine System and Related Drugs: Progesterone Progestational Drugs and Antifertility Agents,* vol. II. Pergamon, New York.

Taymor, M. L. 1964. Effect of synthetic progestins on pituitary gonadotrophin excretion, *J. Clin. Endocrinol. Metab.,* **24:**803–807.

Tietze, C., et al. 1950. Time required for conception in 1,727 planned pregnancies, *Fertil. Steril.,* **1:**338–346.

Tyler, E. T. 1973. Conception control: the pill is best for most, in R. W. Kistner (ed.), *Reproductive Endocrinology,* pp. 37–39. Medcom Learning Systems for Wyeth Lab., Philadelphia.

Vessey, M. P., and R. Dall. 1969. Investigation of relation between use of oral contraceptives and thromboembolic disease. A further report, *Br. Med. J.,* **2:**651–657.

Vorys, N., et al. 1965. The effects of sex steroids on gonadotropins, *Am. J. Obstet. Gynecol.,* **93:**641–658.

Westoff, C. F., et al. 1961. *Family Growth in Metropolitan America.* Princeton University Press, Princeton, N.J.

Sterilization, Abortion, and Artificial Insemination

Who shall be responsible for transmitting genes to the next generation? Who shall reproduce and who shall not? To what extent can society infringe upon individual freedom in order to have a better supply of genes for the future? To what extent is abortion murder? To what extent does giving birth to an "unwanted" child negatively influence that child as well as the parents? These and others like them are the primary social questions of our time and are reflected in the current controversies around the right of a woman to control her own body versus the right to life of a conceptus. No other questions of sexuality so obviously combine aspects of law, biology, and ethics. The medical procedures involved in these questions currently are sterilization and abortion.

STERILIZATION

All surgery specifically performed to prevent conception, whether on women or men, is termed *sterilization.* Close to 4 million persons have been sterilized in the United States, about 75 percent of whom are men. Throughout most of the United States, voluntary sterilization is legal provided informed consent is given by the patient. Although the consent of the spouse is not required, most physicians will obtain it in order to protect themselves from future malpractice suits. Voluntary sterilization generally occurs either for purposes of birth control or for therapeutic reasons where the person has a medical condition that would be exacerbated by pregnancy.

In addition, 25 states have laws that allow for compulsory sterilization of various grades of mental retardation or mental disease that may be inherited. However, as of February 1974, new guidelines on compulsory sterilizations were announced by the Department of Health, Education, and Welfare. The issuance of new rules followed news reports that two young black girls underwent compulsory sterilizations as a condition for remaining on the welfare rolls in Montgomery, Alabama. The new rules state "in no case may sterilization be performed unless the procedure is initiated on the basis of a voluntary request by the patient or his or her representative" (Weinberger). Requests must be made in writing and are to be reviewed in every case by a committee of at least five members. The review committee's approval must be referred to a court in order to get a final determination of the patient's best interests, and at least 72 h must elapse between final consent and the actual sterilization.

Vasectomy

A *vasectomy* involves the blocking or cutting of both sperm ducts or vas deferens. The procedure prevents the passage of sperm during an ejaculation (Wortman and Piotrow). Vasectomies can be performed quickly (from 10 to 20 minutes), inexpensively (as compared to female sterilization), and with almost no mortality.

Today, there are as many specific techniques of vasectomy as physicians performing them. Most doctors use only a local anesthetic (usually a few milliliters of 1 to 2 percent lidocaine) injected into a thin portion of skin that is devoid of blood vessels and located high in the scrotum. A general anesthetic, one in which the person would be put to sleep, is avoided except in cases of an unusually thick scrotal skin or where isolation of the vas deferens will be difficult (Blandy).

The two sperm ducts can be identified through the scrotal skin before an incision is even made. Each sperm duct is actually part of a spermatic cord containing small arteries, veins, some fine nerves, and lymphatic channels. With the thumb and index finger, a physician can feel the spermatic cord on each side and gradually locate the sperm ducts which feel rather hard like whipcords and do not pulsate like blood vessels. After the sperm ducts are identified and anchored, a single incision is usually made in the skin between them. Some physicians, however, prefer two incisions, one over each duct. Whatever the preference, the sperm duct must be clearly and carefully separated from the other structures in the spermatic cord. Severing a testicular artery, vein, or nerve could lead to atrophy of the testes. When both sperm ducts are cut, a small portion from each is removed, and the ends are sealed by clipping, tying, or coagulating with a needle electrode (Wortman and Piotrow).

The sealed ends are turned away from each other and often buried in the surrounding connective tissue. There is some disagreement as to the amount of each duct that must be removed, but the majority of physicians take out from 1 to 3 cm (Davis). After the ducts have been cut and sealed and all bleeding has stopped, the scrotal skin is sutured.

Following the vasectomy, the patient is asked by his physician to avoid unprotected intercourse until he has had 12 ejaculations and two consecutive sperm counts that are found negative (Wortman and Piotrow). Since intact sperm ducts help support the testes, a vasectomy may cause a temporary feeling of heaviness in the scrotal sacs. Wearing a special pair of "y"-fronted underpants is recommended to reduce the uncomfortable feeling.

According to most evidence, a vasectomy performed on a psychologically well-adjusted and healthy individual does not drastically affect sexual motivation, ability to maintain an erection, testosterone production, or ejaculation of semen. One study showed that the strongest reason for not having a vasectomy was disagreement of husband and wife over its advisability (Ferber et al.). Any disagreement seemed to favor development of future psychological problems on the part of the man. Other studies suggest that only couples with certain identifiable characteristics are best suited for sterilization, whereas others may be better off using oral contraceptives or IUDs. If a couple desires a permanent form of birth control and the husband is not particularly hypochondriacal or overly concerned about his masculinity, then a vasectomy may be the best technique available for them (Ziegler et al.). The couple and their physician should thoroughly discuss all ramifications and consequences before deciding on a vasectomy.

Cross-culturally, a relationship between type of male-role identity and acceptance of a vasectomy seems to exist. Vasectomies are very popular in India and Pakistan, but extremely unpopular in countries such as Yugoslavia, Greece, and Latin America where feelings of machismo or masculine prowess dominate the culture.

Scientists have become increasingly concerned about a major complication of vasectomy. In some cases, antibodies against a man's own sperm have been found in the blood due to a vasectomy (Rumke). Recall that only a few substances can cross the walls of the seminiferous tubules, so that the interiors of the tubules are chemically isolated from the rest of the body. As a result, if sperm products get into the bloodstream, the body considers them to be foreign substances, that is, antigens, and forms antibodies against them. Apparently antibody formation after a vasectomy is brought about in the following way: Sperm production generally continues at a normal rate after the sperm ducts are blocked. The sperm will accumulate in the epididymis and are engulfed and digested by certain kinds of cells called phagocytes. If for any reason this digestive process is faulty, then incompletely digested sperm can escape to the blood from the phagocytes and cause antibody formation against them. Once antibodies are formed in the blood, they may leak back into the testes. Sperm that are developing normally in the testes will be caused to abnormally clump together. The problem is quite severe if the man wishes to reverse the vasectomy in an attempt to have children, as once antibodies are formed their presence may be permanent and clumped sperm will not fertilize an egg. Currently, the success of reversibility itself is not good. Claims of 90 percent success are based upon finding a normal number of sperm in samples of semen following reversal. However, the key point is pregnancy, and experts in the field who have performed reversals say that only 30 percent of the patients are successful in impregnating their wives (Schmidt). The low rate of impregnation may more readily reflect the effects of antibodies on normal sperm rather than faulty techniques in reversing the operation.

Experimental attempts to improve on current vasectomy techniques and its possible reversal are being made. Plastic plugs inserted in each sperm duct are being tried but so far without success. "On-off" valves made of gold and stainless steel have been designed to be inserted into each vas deferens, but so far they have worked only in guinea pigs. Research in the area is voluminous, and new breakthroughs will undoubtedly occur soon.

Female Sterilization

Although removal of the ovaries, uterus, or fallopian tubes will render a woman sterile, these operations are rarely performed strictly for birth control purposes. The most common sterilization technique is the *Pomeroy tubal ligation.* This technique, done through an incision of either the abdominal or the vaginal wall, involves tying off the middle third of each fallopian tube and then excising it (see Fig.12-1). A general anesthetic is used with the abdominal incision, but a local is all that is required with the vaginal route. Alternative techniques include the Madlener, where a section of each tube is crushed, then tied but not cut, and Irving's method, which involves removing a section of each tube and then burying all cut ends into the surrounding tissue. The specific technique selected depends primarily on the operating physician's experience.

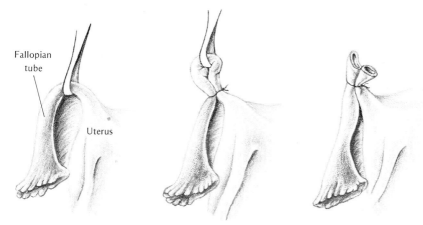

Fallopian tube

Uterus

Figure 12-1   Pomeroy sterilization procedure. (*Redrawn from Reid, 1972.*)

Evidence indicates that the safest time for performing a sterilization is at or immediately following delivery (Phatak). The tubes are less susceptible to infection at this time, and the patient will not have to receive a second anesthetic.

Whereas the above methods can involve at least 2 days' hospital recovery time, the following new methods are outpatient procedures, using a local anesthetic and an occasional sedative. In *culdoscopy sterilization,* an instrument called a culdoscope is inserted through the vagina into the abdominal cavity for purposes of observing the fallopian tubes. Once the tubes can be seen via the culdoscope, they are tied and cut, or a section of each is fused shut with an electric current. In the culdoscopy method, the patient is positioned so that the knees touch the chest, whereas in other techniques the legs are extended. The advantages of the culdoscopy technique include clear visualization of operative technique, rapidity of procedure, and lack of a visible scar on the exterior of the body (Clyman).

Another technique, *laparoscopy sterilization* (Steptoe), is one that has been used successfully at times other than immediately following childbirth. The operation takes only 20 min and involves a minimum of surgical trauma; the patient usually leaves the hospital in 24 h and returns to her normal activities within a week. It is relatively easy to train personnel in this technique, but the equipment involved is costly, at least $1,500, so that in poor countries where large numbers of sterilizations are performed, the method would have limited value. The patient is admitted on the same day as the surgery following about 12 h of fasting. A local anesthetic is given, and the abdomen is distended with an inert gas that will give the physician a clear view of the fallopian tubes. A small incision is then made in the abdominal wall beneath the umbilicus and a telescopelike device with a "cold" light source called a laparoscope is inserted through this opening. Looking through the laparoscope, the surgeon now has a clear view of the fallopian tubes. A second incision is made about 8 cm from the umbilicus and a special type of forceps is then inserted. Each tube is seized, cauterized, cut, and cauterized again using the special forceps. Afterward the instruments are removed, surgical clips are placed on the small abdominal incisions and covered with adhesive bandages (Neuwirth). A modification of the method is to make only one small abdominal incision, inserting a type of laparoscope which has the cauterizing forceps attached to it. The entire operation can be performed through the single opening (Johnson).

An even newer and faster procedure still in the experimental stage is called *hysteroscopic sterilization* (Guerror et al.). Under local anesthesia another type of telescopelike device with built-in "cold" light source and cautery device is inserted into the uterus through the cervix. The scope is called a *hysteroscope,* from the Greek word *hystera,* meaning "womb." The fallopian tubes are visualized and cauterized with an electric current at the site of entry into the uterus. Scar tissue forms and eventually blocks the tubes. The technique is relatively painless, does not involve abdominal incisions, takes about 15 minutes, and requires only 2 to 4 h recovery time for the patient. So far the primary disadvantage has been a comparatively high failure rate. In up to 25 percent of cases, the fallopian tubes fail to remain blocked. However, the failure rate is less when the operation is performed early in the proliferative phase of menstruation. At this time, the endometrial lining has not thickened, and the surgeon can maneuver far more easily with the hysteroscope.

Although all sterilization techiques are currently considered irreversible, some studies have reported about a 17.2 percent pregnancy rate following attempts to reconnect the fallopian tubes (Garcia). Some workers have recently been experimenting with the use of chemicals and plastics that when injected into a fallopian tube causes scar tissue to develop that ultimately blocks the tubes' cavity (Corfman et al.). If this procedure is successful, it may have great potential for reversibility where the present techniques of cutting, tying, and cauterizing make sterilization practically irreversible. The necessity that sterilization be reversible has, however, been somewhat exaggerated. Estimates are that 1 in 2,000 cases of female sterilization and 1 case in 400 vasectomies ever request the operation for reversal (Johnson).

The risk of mortality due to female sterilization has been estimated at 25 per 100,000 operations (Johnson). This tends to be lower than the mortality rate due to pregnancy but higher than the rate due to therapeutic abortion.

ABORTION

What Is Abortion?

The Manual of Standards in Obstetrics and Gynecology defines *abortion* as termination of pregnancy prior to 20 weeks of gestation counting from the first day of the last menstrual cycle. At 20 weeks the fetus weighs about 500 g, is approximately 16.5 cm in length, and rarely can survive outside the uterus even if the best medical treatment is available. As medical technology advances, it may eventually be possible to routinely save the life of a fetus even younger than 20 weeks. This will necessitate, of course, a change in definition of abortion. For now, the definition stands and includes the categories of spontaneous abortion, which is the medical term for miscarriage, and induced abortion, which is purposeful termination of pregnancy.

Spontaneous Abortion

A pregnancy that terminates on its own for any reason is termed a *spontaneous abortion,* or miscarriage. Since a miscarriage does not take place by induction or force, it cannot be considered a form of birth control. Twenty-seven percent of all pregnancies have been estimated to terminate in spontaneous abortions (Stickle). The actual incidence may be much higher but cannot be measured accurately because of the difficulty in identifying the number of fertilized zygotes that slough off without ever implanting. The possibility of spontaneous abortion decreases as a pregnancy progresses. Estimates of incidence show close correlation with the woman's age, the maximum rate occurring in women over 35 having their fourth or more pregnancy (Peel and Potts). Miscarriages generally occur, on the average, 2 weeks after the embryo has died. Chromosomal abnormalities are found in about 25 percent of spontaneous abortions (Carr). Of these the most common problem is either lack of one of the sex chromosomes or one too many of a chromosome pair other than X or Y. Some suggested causes of spontaneous abortion of normal-chromosome fetuses are an abnormal placenta, poor implantation, premature rupturing of the membranes, congenital malformations due to a poor fetal blood supply, and problems with an abnormal umbilical cord. A commonly held misconception is that orgasm at any time during pregnancy can lead to spontaneous abortion. All current evidence indicates that this is doubtful. Masters and Johnson (1966) have suggested that coitus leading to orgasm can be allowed at any time during a pregnancy up to about 18 days of the due date. Exceptions would be if the woman shows any sign of vaginal discharge or abdominal pain.

Induced Abortion

An abortion is called *induced* if it results from a procedure that was done for the purpose of terminating the pregnancy. Whether an induced abortion is legal or illegal depends on the interpretation of the law.

The Legal Status   Prior to 1973, the legal status of abortion was determined mostly by state and local legislatures (Sarvis and Rodman). Often abortion procedures within individual hospitals in a given area were determined by the political attitudes of resident physicians and administrators. Then on March 27, 1972, the President's Commission on Population Growth and the American Future, chaired by John D. Rockefeller III, published its report. The majority of the commission concluded: "Therefore with the admonition that abortion not be considered a primary means of fertility control, the Commission recommends that present state laws restricting abortion be liberalized along the lines of the New York state statute, such abortions to be performed on request by duly licensed physicians under conditions of medical safety. In carrying out this policy, the Commission recommends: That federal, state, and local governments make funds available to support abortion services in states with liberalized statutes; That abortion be specifically included in comprehensive health insurance benefits, both public and private" (Commission).

Five out of the twenty-four commissioners did not concur with the majority opinion and wrote minority statements. Senator Alan Cranston from California wrote: "I am unable to join in this recommendation because I hesitate to endorse governmental sanction of the destruction of what many people consider to be human life. I am particularly concerned by the social and ethical implications of such action now, given the general atmosphere of violence and callousness toward life in our society and in our world. Ours has become an incredibly violent time" (Cranston). Other dissenting commissioners were concerned that "Impulsive, irresponsible sexual involvement can be rationalized without fear of pregnancy if abortion is open, legal, and free"

(Chandler), and that "this section of the report does not even make an attempt to provide a legal accounting for the unborn developing child" (Cornely). The President of the United States, although finding many parts of the report "of great value in assisting governments at all levels of public policy," specifically found the recommendation on abortion written by the majority as "unacceptable." However, despite this lack of support from the Executive Branch, the Supreme Court of the United States was strongly influenced by the report's conclusions. In a seven-to-two decision, the Supreme Court on January 22, 1973, declared unconstitutional two state laws regulating when abortions can be performed (*Roe v Wade,* Texas, and *Doe v Bolton,* Georgia). The court indicated that states had no compelling reason to interfere with the rights of a woman if she should decide to have an abortion for any reason during the first 3 months of a pregnancy: "The attending physician in consultation with his patient is free to determine without regulation by the state, that in his medical judgement the patient's pregnancy should be terminated." The court spelled out clearly that states may require that only qualified physicians perform abortions, but can no longer enforce that abortions during the first 3 months of pregnancy take place only in accredited hospitals. Early abortions may now be performed in such places as a doctor's office or clinic not associated with any hospital. Between the third and seventh month of pregnancy, the court concluded, states may enact only those laws that protect the health of the mother, including stipulations as to where an abortion can take place. During the last 3 months of pregnancy, the court maintained that states may prohibit all abortions except when the physical and mental health of the mother is at stake.

Almost immediately after the court's decision, the antiabortion forces, initially caught off guard by the ruling, regrouped, and by July 1973, seventeen federal constitutional amendments prohibiting abortion in all situations except to save the life of the mother were sent to the Congress of the United States. The proposed amendments included one written by United States Senators Mark O. Hatfield of Oregon and James L. Buckley of New York. Hatfield said to a news conference, "Abortion is a form of violence that cheapens human life, and as an alternative there should be broad-ranging sex education and more access to contraceptives" (*San Francisco Chronicle,* June 1, 1973). Buckley was quoted as saying he "would prefer abstinence for people out of wedlock and if not abstinence then, I would prefer contraception to killing" (*San Francisco Chronicle*). The Senators' amendment as well as many others have been criticized by various constitutional lawyers on the grounds of being ambiguous and poorly written. The amendment of Hatfield and Buckley proposes, for example, that American embryos and fetuses be given United States citizenship and thus be protected under the law as any other citizen. If this amendment should pass, the legal problems of tax exemption for unborn children, obtaining extra passports for the fetus when a mother travels abroad, and so on, would necessitate broad and far-ranging changes in many other laws of the land.

Medical Procedures   The technique used in a legal abortion depends primarily on the duration of the pregnancy (Altchek). Although not safer than contraception, a legal abortion performed by a well-trained physician before the twelfth week of pregnancy is said to be one of the safest of surgical procedures. However, the risk of death is almost nine times greater when the abortion is performed from the thirteenth to twenty-seventh week of gestation. The traditional method usually used up to the twelfth week of gestation is *dilatation* and *curettage* or D and C. A local or general anesthetic is given, and the cervix is dilated using graduated instruments. A long handled device with a spoon-shaped end called a curette is used to scrape away the inside of the uterus. The products of conception usually are broken into small pieces and removed with ovum forceps.

A newer technique called *suction curettage* or *uterine aspiration* is claimed to be faster, easier, and relatively bloodless (Peel and Potts). A local anesthetic is given and dilation of the cervix takes place using a special vibrator. The suction apparatus consists of a long tube called a vacurette attached to a glass container via a piece of rubber tubing (See Fig. 12-2). The vacurette is placed inside the uterus, and a suction pump also attached to the glass container is turned on with about 300 mmHg pressure for 20 to 40 s. The products of conception are sucked out and can be seen in the glass container. With this technique the uterus easily contracts, reducing blood loss considerably. Occasionally, ovum forceps must be used to remove persistent material. Suction curettage is recommended only up to 11 weeks gestation because in abortions beyond this period, the vacurette and rubber tubing tend to become clogged by large pieces of tissue (Altchek).

In keeping with the evidence that earlier abortions show fewer complications, a new method coming into vogue called *menstrual extraction* is being used during the 2 weeks immediately following the first missed menstruation. It is still experimental in many states but promises to be the most economical and possibly the safest method of abortion available. It is basically similar to suction curettage but utilizes narrower gauge tubing in conjunction with a manual or foot suction pump.

Problems to be solved with the menstrual extraction technique include the possibility that many women having it done may not even be pregnant. Standard pregnancy tests sometimes do not give an accurate reading at such an early stage. Other women may utilize this technique every month as a form of contraception. However, long-term effects of regular use have not been studied. Some groups have suggested that paraprofessionals and nurses, instead of physicians, could administer the technique because of its simplicity. Most physicians disagree with this concept, believing that complications of bleeding and infection can occur with any technique of abortion and only personnel trained to handle such emergencies should be involved.

The size of a fetus between the thirteenth and fifteenth week of gestation is generally too large for suction curettage and too small for techniques of late abortion to be discussed in the next paragraph. If the patient's pregnancy has reached the twelfth week of gestation, many physicians will wait until the

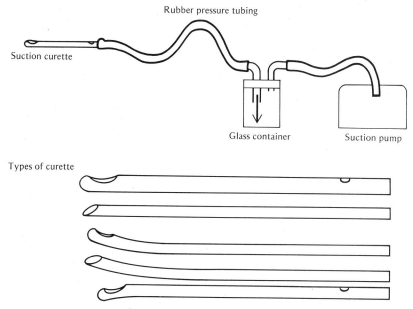

Figure 12-2 Apparatus for uterine aspiration. (*Redrawn from Peel and Potts, 1969.*)

sixteenth week before attempting abortion. A few gynecologists will extend the 12-week limit and use the method of dilation and curettage.

Current methods for termination of pregnancy between the sixteenth and twenty-fourth week of gestation are not fully satisfactory in terms of rapidity and safety. *Hysterotomy* resembles a minor cesarean section. A small abdominal or vaginal incision is made and the products of conception are removed via this opening. However, the most common method used throughout the United States is the *salting-out* technique involving saline injection. Under local anesthesia, a small quantity, about 200 cc, of amniotic fluid is removed from the uterus. (Amniotic fluid is the liquid that bathes the fetus and acts as a shock absorber.) An equivalent quantity of a salt solution (2 percent of NaCl, which is saltier than amniotic fluid) along with an antibiotic is introduced into the uterus. Within 24 h, the fetus is expelled as in a spontaneous abortion. In about 10 percent of cases, only the fetus is expelled and the placenta has to be removed in a special operation. Many patients have experienced nausea, abdominal pain, and vomiting. The most severe complication is that sodium derived from the salt may appear in the patient's blood in excessive amounts.

Prostaglandins are potent drugs that cause uterine contraction. They have been recently isolated and synthesized and currently are being routinely used in Great Britain to terminate pregnancies beyond the twelfth week of gestation. They can be administered via the patient's blood, through her vagina, or directly into the amniotic fluid (Toppozada et al.). Some side effects occur with use of prostaglandins, but these are not as severe as with salting-out techniques. Use of prostaglandin may well be the method of the future for late abortions.

The Prevalence of Induced Abortion   "Abortion is obvious evidence of social failure. Ideally, conception should have been prevented" (Guttmacher). This statement made by the President of Planned Parenthood comes at a time when the population division of the United Nations reports that even in the face of recent advances in contraception, induced abortion is probably the most common birth control method in the world. As of the early part of 1974, Russia had close to two and one-half times as many abortions as babies born—an incredible 2,355 abortions per 1,000 live births. This rate compared with 271 abortions both legal and illegal per 1,000 live births in the United States indicates that contraception instead of abortion is generally an American option. Nevertheless, in the wake of the recent ruling made by the United States Supreme Court, estimates have been made that 1.6 million American women will seek legal abortions each year.

The Controversies on Abortion   The subject of abortion has evoked more statement, opinion, and emotional outcry than any other area of sexuality. According to most recent polls, the American public is almost evenly divided, with those in favor of allowing a woman to obtain an early abortion slightly ahead. The difficulty in resolving the issue is that both sides present a number of valid viewpoints which when analyzed essentially boil down to a matter of rights. The American Civil Liberties Union has stated that women have the right to decide when and whether their bodies are to be used for procreation without control of the state or due process of law. The Commission on Population Growth and the American Future concluded that legal restrictions against abortion "stand as obstacles to the exercise of individual freedom: The freedom of women to make difficult moral choices based on their personal values, the freedom of women to control their fertility, and finally, freedom from the burdens of unwanted childbearing." The Commission also recognized the problems of "bringing into the world an unwanted child particularly when the child's prospects for a life of dignity and self-fulfillment are limited."

On the other hand, Pro-Life viewpoints hold that at the moment of conception a new human life is formed and that no qualitative or essential difference exists between the zygote and the adult human being. "Voluntary abortion is, therefore, an assault upon the life of an innocent human person that is not essentially different from any other willful destruction of an innocent human life" (Shenan et al.). Dissident members of the Commission on Population Growth and the American Future have asked, "How is abortion distinguished from infanticide?" (Erlenborn), and have challenged the majority's opinion in that "for all its language about moral sensitivities, the text seems completely oblivious of the fact, much less the implications of defining a segment of humanity as unwanted. The Commission does not face the question: What does it mean as public policy to legitimate the destruction of unwanted children?" (Cornely).

Each and every citizen regardless of final decision must face these problems and only by keeping thoroughly informed and up to date about all aspects of abortion can the process of analysis be made with wisdom.

ARTIFICIAL INSEMINATION AND SEMEN PRESERVATION

Some scientists recommend that prior to a vasectomy a man study the possibility of storing samples of his sperm for later efforts at fathering children via artifical insemination. Semen introduced into the cervix by mechanical devices instead of intercourse constitutes *artificial insemination.* The storage and preservation of semen samples for purposes of artificial insemination have a number of advantages and disadvantages:

1 A man's semen could be available even after a vasectomy should he change his mind about having children in the future. However, Planned Parenthood feels it is vitally important that men contemplating vasectomies be made fully aware of the fact that semen-preservation techniques have not yet been thoroughly studied or regulated legally.

2 Men with low sperm counts could accumulate semen reserves over a period of time in a sperm bank. Eventually they would have enough to successfully inseminate their wives.

3 Semen samples of different men could be available for possible artificial insemination of a woman with an infertile husband. Herein lies a number of legal, moral, and ethical problems (Francoeur). Let us assume a woman is married to a chronically impotent man. The couple strongly desire to raise a family, and the man verbally consents to artificial insemination of his wife using another man's thawed semen. In this case, who is the legal father? If a divorce ensues, would the husband be responsible for child support? Could adultery be charged? If the child is born with a physical or mental defect, could the donor or the physician be sued in a malpractice suit? The law has not kept up with these questions, and only in California and Oklahoma is artificial insemination legal. The California Civil Code 216, for example, written in 1969, states: "A child born to a woman as a result of conception through artificial insemination to which her husband has consented in writing, is legitimate if the birth occurs during the marriage or within 300 days after the marriage has been dissolved." This code assumes that the husband must support the child even after a divorce.

4 Semen could be stored for purposes of selective breeding. This raises the specter of eugenics as well as such serious concerns as what human characteristics are desirable for propagation. Who is to make the decisions of selection? Do we even wish to pursue a course of eugenics in humans? Some say that the government should control our selective-breeding procedures. Others say that people themselves should exert their individual rights in these decisions. Currently, some physicians have taken it upon themselves to identify what they call "superior" individuals, obtaining samples of their sperm for artificial insemination in situations where a donor other than the husband is requested. One gynecologist in California beset with requests for artificial inseminations, sent an open appeal for semen samples to a top university. One hundred students responded to his appeal. Besides giving samples of semen, each student was required to take the Stanford-Binet IQ test and complete questionnaires designed to reveal stability of personality. The IQ test, of course, measures only abstract reasoning and omits aspects of creativity, the ability to memorize, and adaptability. In addition, many social scientists have been critical of the cultural bias inherent in most verbal IQ tests. Furthermore, the correlation between high scores of IQ tests and emotional stability versus physiological characters of semen deemed superior have never been measured. Does high IQ always correlate with top-quality semen in terms of sperm count and motility?

Because selective breeding has been successful in producing high-quality cattle and other domestic animals, some scientists feel that it should work as easily for humans. True, more than 100 million calves and about 400 humans have been conceived with thawed semen. The human children as well as the calves have appeared normal; however, careful biochemical tests for enzyme deficiencies which would reflect genetic abnormalities have never been made. I. Michael Lerner has suggested reasons why conditions for success with selection in animal breeding may not necessarily be met for human populations. First, characteristics worthy of selection in humans are almost impossible to determine; we need writers, artists, scientists, people with manual dexterity, physically strong people, individuals with social responsiveness, ad infinitum. Even with domesticated animals, what is desirable one time may not be later on. Lerner cites that prior to World War I pigs with heavy back fat were desired. After the war, and the discovery that heart disease was correlated with fat in the diet, lean pigs were desired. "It is difficult to believe that very many specific aspects of human behavior are predictable with respect to their desirability 1,000 years, or let us say 30 to 35 generations ahead, when we do not even know what we want in a pig." The second reason that Lerner cites is closely related to the first. Breeding leads ultimately to a homogeneous population. For instance, when all or most of the pigs in a population possess a uniformly low quantity of back fat, then the direction of selection is considered successful. However, one of the principles of evolution is that species who have the most genetic heterogeneity are the ones that are most likely to adapt to environment changes and survive. This principle applies to the human species as well. The physical, mental, and behavioral qualities that make a human being most successful today may be a handicap tomorrow. We certainly would not want to breed out all the genetic potential for slightly different humans. Third, much experimentation takes place in animal breeding where matings are frequently made between parents and siblings; however, from all indications, humans are not ready yet for incest. Fourth, animal breeding takes place rapidly and continuously with very little time between pregnancies. Humans have entered the age of birth control. Time between pregnancies is prolonged and results of selection would take an inordinate amount of time to analyze. Last, when a particular characteristic is selected for, the "harmonious whole" usually is disrupted. An organism exists in relationship to the environment, and each of its characteristics has evolved as a compromise between the demands of its habitat and functional capacity. Each individual characteristic works harmoniously with all others in the survival of the organism. If we artificially select for one, it will develop out of proportion to the others. So when breast meat was selected for in turkeys, huge-chested turkeys resulted that have lost all capability of copulation and can only be propagated by artificial insemination.

Some eugenists insist that they are "not seeking some kind of superior man, but are interested in the survival and increase of men with diverse genetic potentials, each appropriate to particular environments" (Osborn). Whether these and other lofty goals can be accomplished remains to be seen.

Currently, the technology of human sperm storage and preservation is still in the experimental stage. Operators of commercial sperm banks in the United States confess that only about 1,000 men have deposited samples of their sperm. Legal requirements for labeling, disposing of unused sperm, proper processing of samples, and handling of freezing equipment have not been spelled out (Gatov). The major technical concerns are with rate of cooling of semen samples, the temperature they should be stored at, the type of storage vial used, and the kind of medium mixed with semen that would allow for maximum sperm survival (Carlborg).

The temperature of a semen sample must be cooled below its freezing point without the formation of ice crystals. This process is called supercooling. The formation of ice crystals inside sperm cells would cause permanent damage, and this must be prevented. Supercooling is a gradual process, the slower the better (Behrman). Before freezing, semen is mixed in a protective medium usually containing glycerol only or more rarely a glycerol–egg-yolk–citrate combination. The protective medium provides a stable environment for sperm, usually preventing loss of critical salts, fats, and proteins. Samples of medium and semen are placed inside small plastic straws called "pailletes" for storage. Glass ampoules were formerly used but would frequently burst during the thawing process (Carlborg). Pailletes usually are filled with $1/2$ ml of fluid containing about 20 million sperm each. The long-term storage temperature for semen samples is about $-321°C$ in liquid nitrogen. Controversy exists concerning how long sperm may survive at such low temperatures. Most samples used in human inseminations have been frozen for not longer than $2^{1}/_{2}$ years. However, Tyler reports that sperm have been frozen and brought to full function as long as 15 years later. Some workers believe that the longer sperm are stored, the poorer their ability to fertilize, and this is based upon the observation that sperm motility, or ability to swim, is reduced after freezing. However, recent evidence suggests that the amount of motility is not correlated with fertility. Many pregnancies have resulted from artificial inseminations using thawed sperm with reduced swimming ability (Behrman). According to one study, the pregnancy rate using thawed sperm in donor inseminations is 48.2 percent as compared to 68 percent using fresh sperm (Behrman). In order to obtain this pregnancy rate, an average of seven inseminations over a period of about four months was necessary. Ninety-three percent of the patients got pregnant in the first 6 months using the thawed sperm.

BIBLIOGRAPHY

Altchek, A. 1973. The art of abortion, *Emergency Medicine*, Sept. Issue:145–180.

Behrman, J. J. 1971. Preservation of human sperm by liquid nitrogen vapor freezing, in A. Ingelman-Sundberg and N. C. Lunell (eds.), *Current Problems in Fertility*, chap. 2. Plenum, New York.

Blandy, J. 1971. Male sterilization. in A. J. Smith (ed.), *Contraception Today*, Family Planning Association. pp. 101–107. London.

Carlborg, L. 1971. Some problems involved in freezing and insemination with human sperm, in A. Ingelman-Sundberg and N. O. Lunell (eds.), *Current Problems in Fertility*, chap. 4. Plenum, New York.

Carr, D. H. 1965. Chromosome studies in spontaneous abortions, *Obstet. Gynecol.*, **26**:308.

Chandler, M. B. 1972. *Separate Statement of Marilyn B. Chandler in Commission on Population Growth and the American Future, Population and the American Future.* Sup. Doc., GPO, Washington.

Clyman, M. J. 1968. Operative culdoscopy, *Obstet. Gynecol.* **38**:840.

Commission on Population Growth and the American Future. 1972. *Population and the American Future.* Sup. Doc., GPO, Washington.

Corfman, P. A., et al. 1965. Response of the rabbit oviduct to a tissue adhesive, *Science*, **148**:1348.

Cornely, P. B. 1972. *Separate Statements of Paul B. Cornely, M. D., in Commission on Population Growth and the American Future, Population and the American Future.* Sup. Doc., GPO, Washington.

Cranston, A. 1972. *Separate Statements of Alan Cranston in Commission on Population Growth and the American Future, Population and the American Future.* Sup. Doc., GPO, Washington.

Davis, J. E. 1972. Vasectomy, *Am. J. Nurs.*, **72**(3):509–513.

Doe v. Bolton. 1970. 319 F. Supp. 1048 (N. D. Ga).

Erlenborn, J. N. 1972. *Separate Statements of John N. Erlenborn in Commission on Population Growth and the American Future, Population and the American Future.* Sup. Doc., GPO, Washington.

Ferber, A. S., et al. 1967. Men with vasectomies: a study of medical, sexual, and psychosocial changes, *Psychosom. Med.*, **29**:354–366.

Francoeur, R. T. 1973. *Utopian Mother-Hood.* Perpetua, So. Brunswick and New York.

Garcia, C. R. 1969. Oviduct anastomosis procedures, *Paper Presented at the Conference on Human Sterilization*, Cherry Hill, N.J., Oct. 28–31.

Gatov, E. (ed). 1973. *Sex Code of California.* Graphic Arts of Marin, Inc., Sausalito, Calif.

Guerror, R. Q., et al. 1973. Tubal electrocauterization under hysteroscopic control, *Contraception*, **7**:195.

Guttmacher, A. 1973. Quoted from *San Francisco Examiner*, Sunday, Feb. 4.

Johnson, D. S. 1972. Female sterilization: prognosis for simplified outpatient procedures, *Contraception*, **5**:155–163.

Lerner, I. M. 1972. Polygenic inheritance and human intelligence, in T. Dobzhansky et al. (eds.), *Evolutionary Biology,* vol. 6, chap. 15. Appleton-Century-Crofts, New York.

Manual of Standards in Obstetrics and Gynecology, 2d ed. 1965. American College of Obstetricians and Gynecologists.

Neuwirth, R. S. 1972. Nonpuerperal sterilization by laparoscopy, in R. M. Richart and D. J. Prager (eds.), *Human Sterilization,* chap. 11. Charles C Thomas, Springfield, Ill.

Osborn, F. 1973. The emergence of a valid eugenics, *Am. Sci.,* **61**(4):425–429.

Peel, J., and M. Potts. 1969. *Textbook of Contraceptive Practice.* Cambridge University Press, Cambridge.

Phatak, L. V. 1972. Evaluation of the optimal time for tubal ligation, in R. M. Richart and D. J. Prager (eds.), *Human Sterilization,* chap. 9. Charles C Thomas, Springfield, Ill.

Roe v. Wade. 1970. 314 F. Supp. 1217 (N. D. Texas).

Rumke, P. 1968. Sperm-agglutinating autoantibodies in relation to male infertility, *Proc. R. Soc. Med.,* **61**:275–277.

Sarvis, B. and H. Rodman. 1973. *The Abortion Controversy.* Columbia, New York.

Schmidt, S. 1968. Vasectomy: indications, technique and reversibility, *Fertil. Steril.,* **19**:192.

Sharp, H. C. 1909. Vasectomy as a means of preventing procreation in defectives, *J. A. M. A.,* **53**:1897–1902.

Shenan, Cardinal L., et al. 1968. The right to life. Relaxation of Maryland's abortion law opposed by bishops, *Catholic Mind,* March Issue.

Steptoe, P. C. 1968. Sterilization by laparoscopic techniques, *Sixth World Congress on Fertility and Sterility.*

Stickle, G. 1968. Defective development and reproductive wastage in the United States, *Am. J. Obstet. Gynecol.,* **100**:442.

Toppozada, M., et al. 1971. Induction of midtrimester abortion by intra-amniotic administration of prostaglandin F2α, *Contraception,* **4**:292–303.

Tyler, E. T. 1972. Frozen semen banks, *Medical Tribune,* March 22 Issue.

Weinberger C. W. 1974. *Statement Made by Secretary of Dept. of HEW,* Tuesday, February 5.

Wortman, J. and P. T. Piotrow. 1973. Sterilization-vasectomy: Old and new techniques. Population Report, Dept. Med. Public Affairs. Geo. Wash. U. Med. Cent. Series D(1):1–19.

Ziegler, F. J., et al. 1969. Psychosocial response to vasectomy, *Arch. Gen. Psychiatry,* **21**:46–54.

Chapter 13

Common Infections of the Genital Tract

During any week, the communicable disease record of any big city hospital might look like this:

Disease	Number of Cases
Smallpox	0
Chickenpox	0
Influenza	0
Measles	0
Mumps	2
Hepatitis	25
Syphilis	13
Gonorrhea	300

The fact that syphilis and gonorrhea have reached epidemic proportions in the United States is becoming painfully apparent. Some people with full knowledge of what they are doing may even spread genital infections around. One female student related how, following an act of intercourse, her male partner, a comparative stranger, offered this sage advice, "Better get checked; I have gonorrhea." Even more prevalent are the so-called minor infections such as trichomoniasis, "crabs", and thrush. These latter infections induce discharges and/or irritations that are more of a nuisance than a hazard to health. Unfortunately, the organisms that cause these minor infections can be highly resistant to currently available drugs, and treatment may require a good deal of perseverance on the part of patient and physician. Many people simply adjust to the infection and resign themselves to a life of "drip," "itch," and sometimes painful intercourse.

When an infection is transmitted primarily by sexual intercourse it is called a *venereal disease.* The venereal diseases include gonorrhea and syphilis as well as several other disorders that are less well known to the public. The less serious vaginal infections can also be transmitted venereally. However, many of these organisms are found in the air, on the body, or in the vagina itself, and very often they cause no trouble unless the vaginal environment is upset. The reason stems from the fact that the vagina is normally inhabited by certain forms of bacteria (Döderlein's bacilli) that are very important in maintaining the vaginal fluids at an acid pH of 3.8 to 4.2. This highly acid environment is usually hostile enough toward the less harmful foreign organisms to prevent symptomatic infections. However, the vaginal environment is altered toward alkalinity with menstruation, ovulation, pregnancy, use of contraceptive pills, douching, increasing age, and just plain getting run down. Antibiotic therapy can destroy the Döderlein's bacilli and thereby cause a shift toward alkalinity. Many of the more common organisms causing vaginal discharge can then invade the vagina while others, which are already present in a dormant state, become activated by the newly provided alkaline environment.

TRICHOMONIASIS

Incidence

The most common cause of vaginal discharge and irritation is a flagellated one-celled organism called *Trichomonas vaginalis.* (A flagellum is a hairlike structure functioning in swimming. The tail of a sperm is a flagellum.) About 25 percent of gynecological patients in the United States are infected by this organism. It is estimated that trichomoniasis also infects 4 percent of the males living in the United States. In these cases, the parasite lives in the urethra, but symptoms are often absent in the male, thereby making incidence of infection difficult to ascertain.

Symptoms

The first noticeable symptom is a greenish yellow vaginal discharge that is usually accompanied by varying degrees of irritation, swelling, and reddening of labial structures. A vulvar examination commonly reveals a frothy or bubbly ooze that smells bad and can irritate the adjacent skin of legs, crotch, and thighs upon contact. The infection is most often confined to the vagina; however, the urethra, bladder, and Bartholin's glands may also be affected, and intercourse, at the time of infection, can be painful. The organism can inhabit the urethra of the male but causes little or no discharge or discomfort.

Transmission

Sexual intercourse is the primary method of transmission; however, bath water, swimming pools (with low chlorination), towels, and douche nozzles have all been implicated. Other species of *Trichomonas* live in the mouth and rectum, but these cannot survive in the acid vaginal environment and are not considered a source of vaginal infection. The wide discrepancy between the incidence in females and males may be due to a relatively high rate of nonvenereal transmission and/or the possibility that the disease is transient in males but longer lasting in females.

Diagnosis

A small quantity of vaginal discharge is placed on a slide, mixed with a drop of saline solution, and examined under a dark field or phase contrast microscope (see Fig. 13-1).

Treatment

Trichomonas vaginalis thrives in a relatively alkaline environment, and treatment is effected by returning the vaginal fluids to normal acidity thereby killing the organism. Tablets of 200 mg metronidazole (Flagyl) are taken orally three times a day for about one week. This compound is 80 percent to 90 percent successful in eliminating infection.

VAGINAL THRUSH

Incidence

Vaginal thrush (monilia) is caused by a fungus, *Candida albicans,* and occurs in 36 percent of pregnant women and 16 percent of nonpregnant women. The organism thrives in the presence of sugar and is very common among women

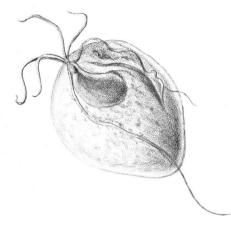

Figure 13-1 *Trichomonas vaginalis* in vaginal smear.

who are diabetic, but will also flourish in women who have recently completed antibiotic therapy for other infections and in pregnant women. (Recall that the Döderlein's bacilli change sugar to an acid; the sugar content of the vagina increases during pregnancy.)

Symptoms

White patches may be seen on the vulva, vaginal wall, and cervix and when removed leave a raw, bleeding surface. The discharge may be cheesy-white in appearance or watery in consistency and results in a vulva that itches severely.

Transmission

Vaginal thrush probably is venereal, although a fungus infection of the male urethra is not common. It may also be acquired in a hundred other ways, since the fungus is present everywhere—mouth, anus, skin, and even the air. If the vaginal environment is not conducive to growth, the fungus will lie dormant, becoming symptomatic when conditions are right—diabetes, pregnancy, menstruation, and so on.

Diagnosis

The fungus is yeastlike, single cells budding off each other, but may also develop whitish, threadlike structures called *hyphae.* A small sample is specially stained and examined under a microscope (see Fig. 13-2).

Treatment

Candida albicans is a hardy fungus and often persists even under adverse conditions. Treatment should be continued for the prescribed length of time and not curtailed when symptoms disappear. Nystatin or Candicidin supposi-

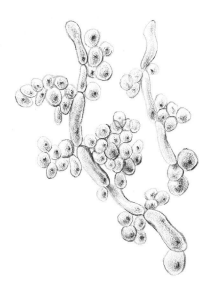

Figure 13-2 Moniliasis (*Candida albicans*) in vaginal smear.

tories are usually prescribed to be used twice daily for two weeks. Immediate relief from a stubborn itch may be secured by painting the vulva and vagina with a 1 percent Gentian Violet solution. This can be messy, but ah the relief!

THE "CRABS"

Incidence

The "crab" is really a louse (an insect belonging to a group called "biting lice") and causes an annoying condition of the skin called pediculosis pubis (see Fig. 13-3). No accurate information on incidence is available; however, reports from various communes in the San Francisco Bay area indicate that it may be the most prevalent infection associated with the genitalia among these groups. T. Rosebury reports sharp increases of this condition in England and Wales.

Transmission

Although sexual intercourse is a primary method of conveyance, clothing, bedding, and towels are excellent additional sources of "crabs."

Symptoms

Crab lice usually congregate in and around hair, particularly pubic and anal, although occasionally they are found in the arm pits and rarely in eyebrows and among beards. The distance between the coarse hairs in these areas is equivalent to the width of the louse's body, from claw to claw of the extended legs. This allows the lice to cling tenaciously between two adjacent hairs (Nuttall). The louse buries its head under the skin and feeds on blood. Tiny bluish gray spots are formed at these feeding grounds, and the louse's feeding and incessant movements cause severe itching and irritation. The eggs, called nits, can be observed as tiny, black periods attached to the base of a single hair creating the appearance of a forest of exclamation points!

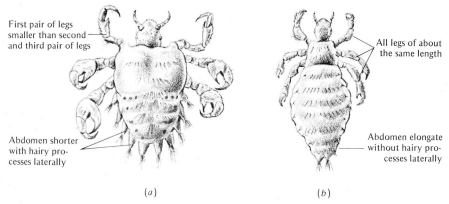

First pair of legs smaller than second and third pair of legs

All legs of about the same length

Abdomen shorter with hairy processes laterally

Abdomen elongate without hairy processes laterally

(a)   (b)

Figure 13-3 Lice commonly found on man: (a) the crab louse, (b) generalized structure of the body and head lice. (*Public Health Service, 1953.*)

Treatment

The old way involved shaving off all the hair and applying a 10 percent DDT powder which was to be left on for 24 h. A more recent and less obnoxious treatment involves applying a 2 percent solution of Dicophan BPC to be left on for 24 h. Today patients use Kwell by prescription.

HERPES SIMPLEX VIRUS TYPE 2

Incidence

The exact incidence of type 2 *herpes simplex* virus (HSV-2) is unknown but extimates indicate that about 350,000 cases occur each year and that it ranks behind gonorrhea as the second most common venereal disease in the United States.

Symptoms

Usually a group of tiny blisters form on the glans penis, prepuce, and scrotal skin in males. The blisters are filled with fluid and are painful to the touch. Often the blisters rupture and form tiny ulcers on the surface of the skin. In females, the blisters form on the inside of the vagina, on the cervix, and more rarely on the vulva, thighs, and buttocks. They also can ulcerate and are painful. Some people experience flulike symptoms such as enlarged lymph nodes, fever, and headache along with the blisters on the genitalia. Symptoms may last from 1 to 4 weeks. Then the ulcers and blisters dry up and disappear. However, immunity to the virus does not develop, and symptoms can reappear periodically, especially if the person is under some form of psychological or physical stress. Pregnant women infected with HSV-2 should seek advice as to the possibility of the virus seriously damaging the fetus. Some physicians estimate that there is a 25 percent chance of congenital malformation occurring in a fetus carried by an infected mother. Cancer of the cervix is several times more likely to occur in women who have had the virus than in women who have not.

Transmission

Sexual intercourse is the primary mode of transmission from person to person.

Diagnosis

The *herpes simplex virus-2* can be detected by microscopic examination of material from a pap smear or can be cultured and grown in a special medium. Also a blood test for antibodies against the virus can be given. Many physicians can simply diagnose the infection by direct examination of the blisters.

Treatment

Currently no treatment is 100 percent effective in curing the disease. Analgesics are given to reduce the pain and frequent saline baths for hygiene purposes are recommended by some physicians. Recent use of an inexpensive dye painted over the blisters with the whole area exposed to the light from an ordinary lamp has proven successful and at the same time controversial. Using the light-dye technique clears the infection up in a few days and reduces by one-half the possibility of a recurrence. However, one researcher is claiming that the technique itself may stimulate cancer production in some people. Research is currently going on with the possibility of developing a vaccine against the disease.

PROSTATITIS

Incidence

Prostatitis is an inflammation of the prostate gland and is caused by various bacterial agents—*Neisseria gonorrhoeae,* the organism that causes gonorrhea, staphylococcus, and streptococcus—and the flagellated organism *Trichomonas vaginalis.* Prostatitis occurs in many young men but usually the infection is slight and does not show obvious symptoms. About one man in every 2,000 will show the severe symptoms of prostatitis including urethral discharge, fever, and painful groin.

Symptoms

The man with prostatitis usually suffers from pain in the groin and lower back. His sexual motivation is reduced, and urination and ejaculation may be painful. Severe infections are often accompanied by a loss of appetite, fever, chills, and vomiting.

Transmission

Some organisms that cause prostatitis are passed on via sexual intercourse (*Neisseria, trichomonas*). Others can invade the prostate via the blood and lymphatic channels from other parts of the body (staphylococcus, streptococcus). Men who drive heavy construction equipment or frequently ride bicycles or horses are particularly susceptible to prostatitis. The constant vibration or pounding of the groin area can weaken the prostate and seminal vesicles making them more susceptible to infection.

Diagnosis

Prostatitis is determined through examination of urethral fluids and by rectal examination.

Treatment

Formerly heat therapy was applied to the groin area in order to help reduce the formation of pus in the inflamed prostate. Current methods of treatment for prostatitis include the giving of antibiotics—e.g., tetracycline. Prostatic massage is performed only when the infective organism has been destroyed and pain in the groin has been reduced.

GONORRHEA

Incidence

Many times more common than syphilis, *gonorrhea* is a disease of the mucous membranes in the genital tract and is caused by a coffee-bean-shaped bacterium, *Neisseria gonorrhoeae.*

According to the World Health Organization, the 1971 ranking of most prevalent communicable diseases places gonorrhea second only to the common cold. Evidence that the rate in the United States is still rising is derived from the fact that from April to June of 1971, 299 cases of gonorrhea were reported for every 100,000 people as compared with statistics for all of 1970 of 285.2 cases per 100,000. Atlanta, Georgia, and the San Francisco Bay area ranked first and second, respectively, in cases reported and were unprecedented in leading the nation. The high incidence does not necessarily reflect widespread promiscuity but rather a more efficient system of reporting and a larger number of medical units capable of coping with the problem. It is disconcerting, however, to note that seven out of eight cases of syphilis and eight out of nine of gonorrhea (Anonymous) go unreported. Contrary to popular opinion, increases in the rate of gonorrhea during the years from 1956 to 1970 are not confined to the teenagers or the twenty- to twenty-four-year-olds but are occuring similarly in all age groups (VD Statistical Letter, November 1971).

Gonorrhea essentially involves the genital lining but can also be present in the rectum. Rectal infection is fairly common, especially among male homosexuals who frequently perform anal intercourse. Gonorrhea of the mouth and throat is rare and involves infection localized in the adenoids and tonsils.

Symptoms

From 2 to 5 days (up to 3 weeks) after exposure males notice a burning sensation when urinating. By squeezing the penis, an infected male will observe a yellowish discharge (watery at first but thicker in a day or so) oozing from the urethra. If left untreated, the disease will infiltrate deeper portions of the genital tract such as the posterior urethra, prostate gland, seminal vesicles, and epididymis. After several weeks or months, scar tissue in these areas may obstruct passageways, thereby restricting the movements of sperm and urine. Urethral obstruction, at least, will have to be cleared by insertion of a metal rod or catheter. Fortunately this degree of infection is relatively rare, as treatment is usually obtained when symptoms first appear.

In a female, the problem becomes relatively acute because early symptoms, if any, are not easily detectable. If present, symptoms usually include a mild irritation and discharge resembling the drip caused by a fungus or other minor infection, which fools the person into thinking it is not important. At first, the disease affects the urethra and Bartholin's glands, but if left untreated, it travels to the cervix, uterus, and fallopian tubes. After a few months, a female develops abdominal pains sometimes resembling an appendicitis attack. Eventually scar tissue that has formed in the tubes blocks the movement of egg and sperm, and the infected person is rendered sterile.

Rarely, in both sexes, the organism will enter the blood and travel to other parts of the body causing heart valve trouble and acute arthritis of wrist and knee.

Gonorrheal infection of the rectum usually shows up as a slight discharge or wetness in the anus, pus in the stools, and pain when the person passes gas.

The conjunctiva (thin outer covering of the eyeball) of newborn babies is very susceptible to gonococcal infection. Babies pick up the disease at birth while passing through the mother's infected cervix. Symptoms show up in 48 h and include swollen eyelids, red conjunctiva, and discharge of pus. In all states except three (New Jersey, Maryland, and Nebraska) physicians are required to put silver nitrate, penicillin, or another antibiotic in the eyes immediately following birth. This procedure is 100 percent effective in eliminating the problem.

Scientists believe that many strains of *Neisseria gonorrhoeae* exist. When a person contracts one particular strain, the body produces antibodies against it, and sometimes antibody production is sufficient to cure the disease. Immunity to this strain then occurs; however, the immune individual is not protected against other strains, and infections may occur several times, each by a new strain of gonococcus.

Transmission and Diagnosis

The primary method of transmission is sexual intercourse. When a male is being examined for gonorrhea, it is recommended by the Department of Health, Education, and Welfare that a smear of the urethral discharge be taken with a cotton swab, rolled on a slide, fixed and stained (gram-negative), and examined microscopically (see Fig. 13-4).

If the organism cannot be identified in the smear, a culture specimen should be obtained and inoculated into a special chocolate agar medium (broth base with heated blood or hemoglobin plus antibiotics to retard growth of other bacteria).

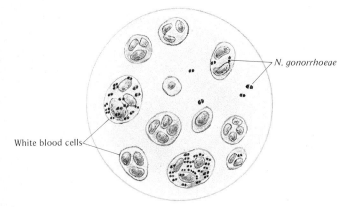

N. gonorrhoeae

White blood cells

Figure 13-4 Smear showing *Neisseria gonorrhoeae*, the organism that causes gonorrhea.

Neisseria gonorrhoeae does not survive well outside of the body's mucous membranes and must be maintained at an optimum temperature of 35 to 36°C (95 to 96.8°F), optimum pH of 7.2 to 7.6, and with a moist atmosphere containing 8 to 10 percent CO_2. A special oxidase reaction will cause the organism to change color from pink to black, indicating its presence. In homosexuals, culture specimens should also be obtained from the rectum and mouth.

In females, *Neisseria* are rarely revealed by microscopic examination of stained slides, and a culture specimen should be obtained from the cervix and rectum and inoculated into the special medium as explained above.

Treatment

As of April 1971, the Department of Health, Education, and Welfare recommended penicillin, in large doses, as the antibiotic of choice. Some strains of gonorrhea, which may be traced to Vietnam, have shown increased resistance to penicillin. Vietnamese prostitutes have been known to receive low doses of penicillin over a long period of time in an effort to reduce venereal diseases. However, because of variations in resistance already present, low doses kill only some of the organisms while allowing others to survive. Those that survive reproduce new populations with an even greater resistance to penicillin than the original population, and these hardy strains are carried home by returning GIs.

Uncomplicated gonorrhea in males and females requires 4.8 million units of aqueous procaine penicillin divided into two injections given at the same visit. Follow-up tests and therapy should take place 5 to 7 days after the initial injections. Severe and advanced cases are treated on an individualized basis. The large doses of penicillin will usually eliminate syphilis as well as gonorrhea, but treatment with other antibiotics requires a follow-up serologic test for syphilis. Oral doses of tetracycline may be given as an alternative for patients who are sensitive to penicillin (although this is not recommended for pregnant women).

Several states (Alaska, Arkansas, California, Colorado, Connecticut, Hawaii, Maryland, Nebraska, North Carolina, New Jersey, Oregon, Rhode Island, South Carolina, South Dakota, and the District of Columbia) allow minors over 12 years of age to receive treatment for gonorrhea and syphilis without parental consent, although parental communication is encouraged.

At the present time, there is no known blood test for gonorrhea; however, one may soon be available which will cut down the time involved in diagnosis (Norins).

SYPHILIS

Although a controversy rages as to the origin of *syphilis* (Rosebury), most evidence points to a long and close association between man and the causative agent—a corkscrew-shaped (spirochaetes) bacterium called *Treponema pallid-*

ium (see Fig. 13-5). The infective organism can be grown experimentally in rabbits and other animals, and its presence does not produce a disease as it does in man. Syphilis is specifically a disease of man.

Incidence

For the first time since 1943, an increase in the incidence of syphilis, including all stages, has occurred. There were 46.9 cases per 100,000 nonmilitary persons reported from April to June in 1971 compared to a rate of 43.8 cases in all of 1970. True, the length of time involved is not equivalent; but barring the discovery of a miraculous vaccine, all indications point to an upward trend. It is encouraging to note, however, that the largest increase seems to be in the early stages of the disease, indicating perhaps that more people are reporting it sooner, receiving treatment, and thereby never experiencing the later stages. Curiously, it is the thirty- to forty-nine-year-olds who show the greatest rate increases since 1956 rather than the teenagers or twenty- to twenty-four-year-olds. The total number of deaths due to syphilis in the United States has drastically declined from 14,064 in 1940 to 510 in 1969. Syphilis in newborn infants shows a one-tenth increase in rate per 100,000 population from April to June of 1971 compared to all of 1970.

Transmission

The spirochaetes are transferred from open lesions of infected persons to mucous membranes or skin abrasions of the second person during sexual intercourse (vaginal, anal, or oral) and kissing. The organism cannot survive a transfer without moisture and will die in seconds on dry toilet seats, towels, and so on. Since *Treponema* enters the blood, blood transfusions once were a method of transmission—fortunately this is no longer true. Blood is now kept under refrigeration, and the spirochaetes cannot survive cold temperatures. Some rare cases have been reported where transmission took place from freshly used condoms mistaken for balloons, shared lipsticks, and tattooing needles. Physicians, nurses, and police officers have been known to pick up syphilis through skin abrasions on their hands from the secretions of syphilitic babies.

Congenital syphilis (syphilis in the newborn) occurs because *Treponema pallidum* is one of the rare forms of bacteria capable of passing through the placenta. Infection generally takes place after the eighteenth week of fetal life because a special protective layer of the placenta normally atrophies and disappears during the sixteenth week (Rasmussen).

Symptoms

Clinical manifestations are divided into six stages (Willcox): The first four, incubation, primary, early latent, and secondary, are collectively called early syphilis; the last two, latent and tertiary, may be observed years after the initial infection. It is only during early syphilis that the disease is contagious, particularly during the primary and secondary stages.

The *incubation period* for any disease is the time between initial exposure

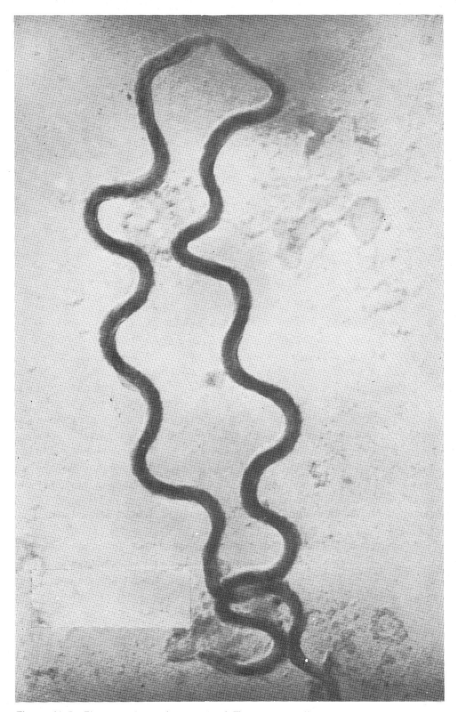

Figure 13-5 Electron photomicrograph of *Treponema pallidum*, the organism that causes syphilis. The organism has been magnified 36,000× and is shown dividing. (*Public Health Service, 1968.*)

and the appearance of the first disease symptoms. In syphilis, this ranges between $1^1/_2$ and 8 weeks, with an average of 21 days. The length of time depends primarily on the number of spirochaetes transferred, their rate of reproduction, and the number needed at the spot to cause a primary chancre sore (Rosebury). Spirochaetes are single cells that reproduce by division into two equivalent cells every 30 to 33 h. It has been estimated that during sexual contact a few hundred spirochaetes are transmitted to a given spot on the mucous membrane or crack in the skin. When the count reaches 100 million, a chancre sore develops (usually 3 weeks later).

The *primary stage* begins with the development of a tiny, painless pimplelike chancre sore often with a hard, outer ring present at the site of initial spirochaete penetration (usually on the penis or cervix). A swelling of lymph nodes in the groin area is frequently associated with the sore. Symptoms last 2 weeks on the average, with a range from 1 to 5 weeks and up to 3 months in rare cases. They then disappear, signaling the beginning of the *early latent stage,* a period during which the person is symptomless.

One to six months following initial appearance of the primary chancre sore, syphilis enters the *secondary stage.* A variable amount of rash appears over the body with concentration in moist areas. The sores of the rash swarm with spirochaetes and are highly contagious, especially if they ulcerate. The rash may be accompanied by a sore throat, headache, mild fever, falling hair, tender lymph nodes, mucous patches on the lips, and inflammation of the iris.

After several weeks, the secondary symptoms vanish and the latent stage begins. During the *latent stage* the person generally has no outward symptoms and may think he is cured. The rash, however, may reappear periodically for up to a period of 5 years. If untreated, the progress of syphilis during the latent stage is highly variable. Evidence for this comes from an incredible study of 1,404 untreated syphilitics in Oslo, Norway (Clark and Denholt). The study began in 1891, and follow-up reports were made in 1929 and 1959. One-third of the patients showed a spontaneous cure, another third exhibited positive blood tests but did not develop tertiary or late symptoms, and the final one-third developed symptoms of the *tertiary stage* 10 to 20 years later. The symptoms of tertiary syphilis include large ulcerlike sores called gummata, brain and spinal cord damage, heart disease, and aneurism (swollen blood vessels).

Diagnosis

Although many tests are available, the United States Department of Health, Education, and Welfare, in a pamphlet dated May 1971 and entitled *The Laboratory Aspects of Syphilis,* specifies the three laboratory procedures most often employed to be: (1) the Venereal Disease Research Lab Test (VDRL)—the routine serological test; (2) looking for spirochaetes under the microscope providing the only *absolute* diagnosis for early (infectious) syphilis; (3) a fluorescent antibody test (FTA)—a serological test primarily reserved as a verification procedure.

Serological tests are based on antibody-antigen reactions, and for syphilis they are performed on samples of blood and spinal fluid. Usually an antibody will react with only one type of antigen. But in some cases an antigen causes formation of not only specific antibodies but also more general antibodies that can react with several different types of antigens. These general antibodies are called "nonspecific." The VDRL test is used to detect a "nonspecific" antibody called reagin which is produced by the body as a result of the interaction between the spirochaetes and the body tissue. The VDRL test does not use spirochaetes for the antigen but rather a substance called cardiolipidlecithin derived from beef hearts. A small sample of antigen and blood serum is mixed, and if reagin antibodies are present, a distinct clumping will be observed. Since a number of other infections can cause a positive VDRL test, this method is used only for screening. Positive VDRLs should be followed up with the FTA procedure. The FTA test utilizes dead *Treponema pallidum* obtained from rabbits as the antigen. When this antigen is mixed with blood serum from a person with syphilis, specific antibodies that are present (not reagin) will coat the dead spirochaetes. The reaction is not visible but is made so under a fluorescence microscope by adding a fluorescent dye capable of combining with the coated spirochaetes.

Treatment

For early syphilis, the long-acting benzathine penicillin G is given during a single visit by injecting 1.2 million units into each buttock. Short-acting forms of penicillin can be given in larger quantities over longer intervals of time. Persons having sexual contact with syphilitic patients should be notified and treated immediately. Latent and tertiary stages of syphilis require even heavier doses of penicillin (6 to 9 million units) given over a period of weeks. In 1969, the United States Department of Health, Education, and Welfare reported that 6.2 reactions to penicillin occurred out of 1,000 patients receiving treatment; however, due to better history taking and more highly purified forms of penicillin, this rate of reaction is less than in former years. Erythromycin and tetracycline (not recommended for pregnant women with syphilis) are alternate antibiotics that may be used for people that react to penicillin.

SOME COMMON QUESTIONS

Two basic questions about venereal disease are asked so frequently by students that they merit some comment. Where did VD come from in the first place, and what can we do to send it back? The answer to the first question is, we don't know, and in some specific cases we may never know. However, based on our knowledge of parasitism and evolution, we can generalize. The consensus among parasitologists is that each parasite (an organism living in or on a host and producing some degree of harm varying from slight to severe) must have evolved from a free-living (nonparasitic) ancestor sometime in the past. For example, C. J. Hackett has shown that the types of bacteria causing syphilis are identical in a number of characteristics and are closely related to the forms of bacteria causing yaws and pinta (skin infections, primarily of children living in the tropics). He hypothesizes that the common ancestor of these bacteria must have been a free-living species feeding on dead, decomposing material that accidentally entered man or an ancestor of man via some route (e.g., food) and ultimately became parasitic. The ancestor had to possess characteristics that would allow it to survive in the new environment provided by the innards of humans.

How can we rid ourselves of these venereal diseases? Again, no easy answer is available. Some (Rosebury) say we could eliminate at least syphilis and gonorrhea by a government-sponsored and -financed program utilizing technology already available. Others say increase the amount of information and educate people about VD from grammar school on up to the physicians themselves. It would help to expand our ability to locate the sexual contacts of people with VD By increasing the number of paramedicals trained for this function (Horn). The availability of free condoms would help if more men would use them. Some men claim penile desensitization when using a condom; however, no experimental evidence is available that shows the penis to be physiologically less sensitive with a condom than without one. Cases of syphilis and gonorrhea should perhaps be quarantined for the time it takes to effect a complete cure. Control of VD among prostitutes and seamen would help reduce the rate of spread. The best method may still be in the immediate future—immunological techniques that detect the disease very early before symptoms show up and before it becomes contagious (Norins).

BIBLIOGRAPHY

Anonymous. 1969. Lack of reporting masks VD climb, *J. Am. Med. Assoc.*, **207**:21–22.

Clark, E. G. and N. Denholt. 1964. The Oslo study of the natural course of untreated syphilis, *The Medical Clinics of North America,* **48** (3).

Hackett, C. J. 1963. On the origin of the human treponematoses, *Bulletin of the World Health Organization,* **29**:7–41.

Horn, J. S. 1969. *Away All Pests: An English Surgeon in People's China.* Paul Hamlyn, London.

Norins, L. C. 1967. Selected aspects of syphilis and gonorrhea research in the United States, *Br. J. Ven. Dis.,* **44**:103–108.

Nuttall, G. H. F. 1918. The pubic louse, *Parasitology,* **10** (3):383–405.

Public Health Service. 1971. *The Laboratory Aspects of Syphilis.* U.S. Department of Health, Education, and Welfare. Issue No. 111.

Rasmussen, D. M. 1968. *Syphilis and the Fetus in Intra-uterine Development,* A. C. Barnes (ed.), Lea & Febiger, Philadelphia.

Rosebury, T. 1971. *Microbes and Morals.* Viking, New York.

Wenrich, D. H. 1947. The species of *Trichomonas* in man, *J. Parasitol.,* **33**:177–88.

Willcox, R. R. 1964. *Textbook of Venereal Diseases and Treponematoses.* Heinemann, London.

Chapter 14

An Alternative Sexual Orientation: Homosexuality

"We are allowed to watch our lovers being killed in Viet Nam but not allowed to love them at home." This statement expresses the feeling of frustration experienced by many homosexually oriented women and men in our society who feel themselves denounced and outcast. A Louis Harris poll taken in 1969, at the birth of the gay movement, showed that 63 percent of the nation considered homosexuality harmful to the American way of life. Although it is not illegal to be a homosexual, some states have statutes that forbid homosexual acts. In addition, most states forbid certain forms of coitus, such as anal and oral-genital intercourse, that are used by both heterosexuals and homosexuals. Because of the general population's prejudice against homosexuality, this latter group of laws, although applicable to all people, is used most often to prosecute members of the gay community.

Our long history of being taught to despise and suppress homosexual feelings has led us to the concept that homosexuality is a crime, a sickness, or sin to be punished severely by the state—after all, people who do nasty things with their genitals must be punished. Recently, and coupled with the increased communication and education about sexuality, gay organizations throughout the country are requesting and in some cases demanding equal treatment under the law, freedom to choose social contacts, and fair employment practices. The media and gay rights organizations have been central in the dissemination of information, helping to dispel stereotyped views of gay men and women. Panel discussions on television, newspaper articles, even rap sessions with the clergy on Sunday morning radio have involved homosexually oriented individuals and topics.

Some understanding has indeed been created by this educational process. As of April 1973, police surveillance of "gays" in San Francisco's bars and public toilets has markedly decreased. The New York Police Department has ended "entrapment" of homosexuals and issued a statement on August 20, 1973, requiring that all derogatory or inflammatory names for the homosexually oriented person be eliminated from crime reports, radio messages, and communications, and the term "gay" used instead. On August 27, 1973, a "New Humanist Manifesto" signed by 120 scientists, writers, and philosophers called for the right to sexual freedom and privacy: "While we do not approve of exploitive, denigrating forms of sexual expression neither do we wish to prohibit by law or social sanction sexual behavior between consenting adults." A new federally sponsored gay rights bill has the word "affection" added to it in order to offset the myth that gays are "oversexed" and constantly on the make. The gay life style involves as much love and affection between individuals as is found in any other group. The bill, sponsored by 24 members of Congress would make it illegal to discriminate against a person's affectional or sexual orientation in areas such as employment, housing, and public accommodation. Much recent evidence indicates that a dramatic shift in public opinion toward a more positive view of gays has occurred in the last 3 to 4 years, and some members of Congress are becoming aware of this shift.

Along with these shifts in attitude about homosexuality, the long controversy as to whether nonheterosexual orientations constitute illness of the body or mind, or distortion of social development, is subsiding. Indeed, many persons, particularly social scientists, have accepted the "normality" of homosexuality and wish only to describe the social structure of homosexual life without trying to look for cause. "One might as well try to trace the etiology [cause] of 'committee-chairmanship' or 'Seventh Day Adventism' as of 'homosexuality'" (McIntosh). Others believe that a thorough analysis of the cause of alternative sexual orientations will enlighten us about all aspects of sex, including heterosexuality.

This chapter will serve to acquaint or remind the reader of the current definitions of homosexuality, its incidence, characteristics, language, and social structure, the theories about cause, and the attitudes about homosexuality prevalent in American society. The material will be presented, hopefully, with a minimum of value judgment and in a way that will illustrate the enormous variation in all aspects of the subject.

DEFINITION

Definitions of homosexuality depend mostly on the background and beliefs of the person doing the defining—nowhere does professional chauvinism become so obvious. Social scientists emphasize that homosexuality is a "way of life" involving a ". . . community of understanding wherein members of one's own sex are defined as the most desirable sexual objects" (Goffman). Some psychiatrists (a minority) believe homosexuality to be a mental derangement or a deviation from what is "normal," "right," and "correct." "When a member of one sex is mainly or exclusively attracted to those of his own sex, he becomes a homosexual and is then perverted" (Allen). Some educators follow this concept of "perversion" and their textbooks classify homosexuality as a sexual *aberration.* In keeping with the idea of an aberration, some psychiatrists concerned with therapy and cure diagnose a patient as homosexual when that person has a history of repetitive erotic arousal with members of the same sex—"whether sporadic or continuous" (Bieber, 1965). Kinsey et al. (1953) believe homosexuality to be not an illness or a perversion but one of the many possible types of sexual orientation found among humans as well as other species. They defined it as sexual "responses or contacts between individuals of the same sex." The majority of psychiatrists agree with Kinsey but, like most gay women and men, believe that a definition should include concepts of "attraction," "desire," and "permanency" rather than emphasizing only specific acts or behavior patterns. Thus, Martin Hoffman uses the term *homosexual* "to refer to those individuals who have a sexual attraction toward partners of the same sex over at least a few years of their lives." Others disagree that a definition should necessarily include concepts of drive or motivation. These parameters are difficult to measure, whereas some form of actual behavior can be more easily identified. Thus, Mark Freedman simply defines homosexuality "as sexual relations between members of the same sex." Freedman further qualifies this statement when he says that homosexuality "is more often involved with needs central to the individual's personality such as the need for companionship, love, dependency" rather than a mere satisfaction of physical urges for sexual contact. Thus, homosexuality is an affectional and sexual orientation toward persons of the same sex. Many experts argue that use of the terms "heterosexual" and "homosexual" as nouns should be abandoned altogether because they imply that a person absolutely fits a category without variation. Indeed, Kinsey et al. (1953) showed that more than a third of American men, for example, have been homoerotically aroused to orgasm even though many of them are predominantly heterosexual. The term "homosexual" has associated with it so much negativism that it tends to release more emotion than rational thinking. Thus, "homosexual orientation," "homophile," or just plain "gay person" are more acceptable terminology. Most homosexual men prefer to be called gay, and most homosexual women gay or lesbian.

Some confusion exists about the meaning of transvestism, transsexuality, and bisexuality as they relate to homosexuality. A *transvestite* is a person, generally male, who derives pleasure and/or increased sexual arousal from wearing clothes of the opposite sex. The vast majority of gay people are not transvestites. Transvestites can be found among all sexual orientations, but most often they are heterosexual. The term transvestite has become somewhat more difficult to interpret because of the return to unisexual characteristics of clothing in the current fashions. Many people appear to cross-dress, yet would not fit the category of transvestite as "illness or psychological problem." Perhaps the person who best fits the definition of a transvestite would be one who is so concerned about cross-dressing that he seeks out help in some form of therapy. H. Benjamin has proposed that transvestism is just one end of a "sex orientation scale" with the other end consisting of the transsexual. A *transsexual* is a person who psychologically is one sex but physically is the opposite sex. The person despises his or her own genitals and wants to be rid of them. Transsexuality is a total psychosexual reversal of identity. The person involved has an intense belief that he or she is trapped in the wrong body and wishes conversion by means of hormone treatments and special surgery.

A *bisexual* is a person who enjoys sexual contacts with individuals of both sexes, whereas a *homosexual* has sexual contacts and forms sexual relationships primarily or exclusively with members of his or her own sex. Neither of these terms says anything about the sexual self-identity of the person. Most male homosexuals consider themselves males; and most lesbians feel female. Few gay people have much interest in dressing like the opposite sex or in undergoing sex-conversion treatment.

INCIDENCE

Because sexual orientations, other than heterosexual, are often not admitted by people being interviewed, incidences are difficult to ascertain. The best evidence for incidence of homosexuality comes from Kinsey et al. (1948; 1953), followed up approximately 20 years later by a survey published in *Psychology Today*. According to these sources, 4 percent of adult white males and 2 percent of adult white females in the United States are homosexual. This means that approximately 500 homosexually oriented persons per 10,000 individuals in the population (6 million) exist in the United States. San Francisco appears to be a center of homosexual activity with an estimated 1 in 10 individuals being gay, 106 gay bars, and several bath houses catering particularly to individuals of this group. It is probable that most big cities have a relatively large gay population composed of natives plus others who have immigrated from small urban and rural areas. Many people argue that the incidences quoted above fall far short of reality. Lyon and Martin write that gay women are as numerous as gay men and "may run as high as ten million women." Jess Stearn's main theme in *The Sixth Man* is that one out of every six males is gay. Statistical discrepancies arise from different methods of analysis, bias as to the nature of the sample, and the fact that many people simply do not fit into any single category. Those who do admit to a category of sexual orientation sometimes change after a variable amount of time. Indeed, Kinsey et al. (1948; 1953) believed that any large population sample taken in the United States could be arranged along a continuum as to sexual preference and behavior. He called it a heterosexual-homosexual rating scale. The scale is based on a balance between heterosexual and homosexual experience of any one person during a particular period of time. Heterosexuality and homosexuality are seen as opposite extremes, and gradations of bisexuality lie along the scale between extremes. The midpoint of the scale refers to women or men who have had equal amounts of heterosexual and homosexual experience. Mary McIntosh has rearranged Kinsey's data into a table (Table 14-1) that compares males and females at selected ages. It is apparent that a sizable group believes itself to be bisexual, for example, 22.5 percent males and 10 percent females at 20 years of age. The data also show a reduction with age in this percentage for males but a slight increase for females. McIntosh has thus hypothesized that men become more "specialized" and "narrow" in sexual orientation, whereas women "broaden their sexual experiences" as they get older.

LANGUAGE

Subgroups within any general population tend to develop and maintain a special language or jargon peculiar to that group. If the subgroup is highly ostracized, that language becomes of extreme survival value—not only must individuals communicate and understand each other but they cannot afford to reveal their identities to the general populace. Theoretically the language contains phrases and words that convey meaning only to individuals within the subgroup; however, the media's frequent and extensive use of the language has made it easy to decipher and readily discernible to all elements of society. Thus, the dialect will have to change constantly, and nonverbal elements of communication will serve when words are no longer useful.

E. Sagarin has summarized some of the language of the homosexual subculture (see Table 14-2) and states that in addition to the need for secrecy,

Table 14-1 Comparison of Male and Female Heterosexual-Homosexual Ratings: Active Incidence at Selected Ages

Sex	Age	Percentage of each age group having each rating								
		(No interest in either sex) X	(Hetero-sexual) 0	1	2	3	4	5	(Homo-sexual) 6	Totals of 1–6
Male	20	3.3	69.3	4.4	7.4	4.4	2.9	3.4	4.9	27.4
Female		15	74	5	2	1	1	1	1	11
Male	35	0.4	86.7	2.4	3.4	1.9	1.7	0.9	2.6	12.9
Female		7	80	7	2	1	1	1	1	13

Source: McIntosh, 1968. Based on Kinsey (1948), p. 652, Table 148; and Kinsey (1953), p. 499, Table 142.

Table 14-2   Some Terms Used by Gay Women and Men

Term	Meaning(s)
λ	The Greek letter lambda, a scientific symbol for activism, has been chosen by the Gay Activist Alliance to represent gay pride
AC-DC	Bisexual orientation—"A person who can function no matter what the source of energy"
Basket	A person's genitals
Butch	Masculine appearing
Cruising	The search for homosexual contacts
Dyke	A very masculine appearing lesbian
Femme	Feminine appearing
Front marriage	Homosexually oriented male marries a homosexually oriented female—have or adopt children of their own, all done for the purposes of convenience
Gay	A person whose affectional and sexual orientation is toward members of the same sex
Homophile	A homosexually oriented person—stress on love; used as an adjective to describe gay organizations
Humphreys	Homosexual contacts in public restrooms (T-rooms)
Lesbian	A gay woman
Lesbian feminist	A gay woman in the feminist movement
Nellie	Feminine or feminine appearing—usually male
Poppers	Isoamyl nitrite, a drug which, when inhaled prior to climax, can heighten and lengthen the event
Queen	General term used to describe a gay person—usually male or depending on context; one who is a "Nellie"
Closet queen	One who does not publicly admit to being homosexually oriented or one who does not like to be associated with other gays and spends much time in the straight world
Screaming queen	A gay person who purposely exaggerates characteristics of being feminine
Size queen	Gay male who desires a big penis on his partner
Straight	Heterosexual orientation
T-rooms	Public restrooms
To bring out (bringing out)	To initiate another person in homosexual activity or the first homosexual contact that an individual found enjoyable and which ended in orgasm; sometimes used synonomously with "to come out"
To come out	(a) Self-recognition; usually after some struggle with self-identity that he or she is homosexually oriented. This may include simultaneous public announcement or appearance in the gay community (b) To be openly gay to nongays as well as to gays

Source: Modified from Sagarin, 1970; and Dank, 1971.

gay language is a reflection and reinforcement of a particular way of life. Thus the term *gay*, coined in 1949 (DeForrest) to refer to homosexual, comes from the description of "a gay blade" as a person who lives with joy and pleasure and is supposed to reflect the fact that homosexually oriented individuals are happy, healthy, and well adjusted.

No other term better describes the struggle for self-identity than "to come out." Barry Dank describes the feeling of relief expressed by many gay individuals when they come to accept their homosexuality: "A person's identification of himself as being homosexual is often accompanied by a sense of relief, of freedom from tension. . . . Coming out, in essence, often signifies to the subject the end of a search for identity."

Nonverbal communication is extensively used when words no longer fit a situation. Often gay-oriented women and men will visit a specific bar, discotheque, or other gay place, their mere presence signifying desire for contact. In sexual courting, lengthy stares, looking a person up and down, and a glance at a person's "basket" (genitals) will operate to communicate desire for contact. Sometimes an inquiry as to the "time," a statement about the "weather," a comment concerning the current "political climate" serve to confirm the gay person's intentions much as they act as openers in heterosexual interactions.

CHARACTERISTICS

The gay population consists of as many different types of body build and personality as exist in the nongay community. The limp-wristed, effeminate male and broad-shouldered "butch" female are but a small minority within the gay population. Evidence from a variety of sources indicates that body build and personality or whether one is effeminate or butch bears little relationship to one's affectional and sexual orientation. "Screaming queens" and "dykes" get most of the publicity, and this tends to create false stereotypes. As in any group of people, concern does exist regarding age, attractiveness, and good grooming. But what constitutes sex appeal among gays is as highly variable and dependent upon conditioning as in any other subculture.

Contrary to popular belief, homosexuality is *not* synonymous with promiscuity and amorality. Although homosexuality is becoming more acceptable to the general population, many gays and bisexuals still run the risk of losing friends and jobs if their sexual orientations are generally known. Some of these people feel that public exposure is most easily prevented if their activities take the form of brief encounters with strangers. Consequently, some males cruise for contacts in parks, T-rooms (public restrooms), and, more frequently, in gay bars. Lesbian cruising in bars is not at all uncommon, but searching for contacts in parks and T-rooms seems to be an almost exclusively male activity. However, at this time, no one knows exactly how common cruising in general is among gay men or women. Obviously, gays who have not "come out" and who must meet in bars, in the park, or at the beach cannot afford to spend much time in cultivating interpersonal relationships. However, even during brief encounters, respect is shown for the other's person's wish to remain anonymous, and force or coercion in sexual behavior is not tolerated (Freedman).

Most people, gay or straight, need and seek out sexual relationships that will, in addition, fulfill needs for emotional support and companionship. Despite the need for discretion, long-term affairs have always been common among gay men, marriages without certificate coupled with a great deal of fidelity are known to last for 30 years or a lifetime. Long-term emotional attachments involving love may be even more common among homosexually oriented women. Gay marriages may also involve caring for children.

Sexual behavior among homosexually oriented men and women involves much of the same kind of activity as that found among heterosexuals. Simple kissing, tongue kissing, hugging, caressing are all common. Additionally, among American men, fellatio and anal intercourse are common methods of sexual arousal. English men also appear to enjoy the "rub off," which involves simply rubbing the penis against the partner's body until orgasm and not necessarily inserting it into any oriface (Hoffman). Some American men experience sexual activity in twos, threes, or in larger groups depending upon the size of the place where the activity occurs. Bath houses usually have small rooms for pairs of individuals and larger ones with tumbling mats for group sex. Activity in groups sometimes involves a central core of fellating individuals, but as one moves to the periphery, anal intercourse, mutual masturbation, hugging, and kissing may predominate. A few individuals on the outer rims simply masturbate while looking on. Those men who enjoy cruising T-rooms often find large holes between stalls for insertion of the penis, where fellatio can take place anonymously. How common this type of behavior may be is not known. Men experience and enjoy homosexual behavior long before "coming out" and acknowledging a homosexual identity.

This contrasts with females where "homosexual identification precedes actual sexual behavior" (Freedman). Active sexual involvement among lesbians usually is preceded by extensive romantic involvement (Simon and Gagnon). Lesbians enjoy much the same methods of foreplay as any other group. Kissing, hugging, tonguing, and breast stimulation all precede cunnilingus and manual manipulation of the mons, clitoris, and labia. Occasionally, a face-to-face coital posture will be assumed, and orgasm will be achieved by rubbing the vulva on each other's body. A dildo or fake penis is hardly ever inserted into the vagina. Activity shows as much variation as the people themselves. Women, however, rarely get involved with large-group sexual activities.

It is commonly believed that gay couples, whether men or women, are always composed of a butch and a "femme" partner. No evidence exists to support this contention, and gay couples may show as many types of interactions as are found among heterosexuals.

SOCIAL STRUCTURE

As in the lives of all people, sexual behavior is but a part of the overall striving for happiness and success in interpersonal relationships. When viewed in the context of how individuals relate to one another, sex per se is only one of the possible means of communication that has been emphasized in much of the current popular literature. In actuality, the gay individual living in a large city is usually part of a complex "community of understanding," consisting of service organizations such as SIR (Society for Individual Rights), Daughters of Bilitis, and the Gay Activist Alliance, which provide places for social interaction and facilitation of contacts. In addition, gay bars, which function much like bars for swinging singles, baths, restaurants, and other businesses cater directly to the gay community. Relationship to these institutions depends on a given person's set of needs and values but also on whether he or she has "come out" and accepted the gay life. In 1956 Leznoff and Westley found that the homosexual population in a large city consists of at least two groups: a minority of "overt" individuals who have "come out," and the larger "secret" group of people who "fear recognition as a status threat." Although a certain amount of mobility between groups does exist, a "reciprocal hostility" has developed which maintains a social distance between them. A change in orientation from "overt" to "secret" appears to occur among individuals showing "upward mobility." The "secret" group consists of a number of small cliques frequently interacting but maintaining only a partial relationship to the gay life. They demand total concealment and discretion concerning love affairs and sexual contacts. "Overt" individuals form tightly knit associations where activity is openly homosexual and involves considerable interaction with the heterosexual society. In Leznoff's and Westley's intensive study of 60 homosexually oriented men based in a large Canadian city, occupations of the overt individuals were of lower economic and professional status where concealment was unnecessary.

In the 1970s, some of the behavior described by Leznoff and Westley seems to be changing. For example, the gay rights movement has led to the emergence of many professional and civil rights groups consisting of overt gay women and men with middle and upper economic status. The National Gay Task Force, the country's largest gay civil rights organization, is headed by a former university professor; Lambda Legal Defense and Education Fund is a corporation of gay lawyers in New York City; the Gay Nurses Alliance is headquartered in Philadelphia; the Gay Academic Union has an annual Thanksgiving weekend symposium, which is attended by over a thousand lesbians and gay men from universities. Currently, there also exists a greater openness and social integration of overt gays with the heterosexual world.

Individuals who acknowledge their gayness come to accept their self-identification only after considerable struggle. Indeed, having homosexual experiences and accepting one's homosexuality do not coincide. One statistical analysis of the process of "coming out" showed that the average age, among 182 males, of identifying oneself as homosexually oriented was 19.3, but the time interval between "age of first sexual desire toward same sex" and age of self-identification was 6 years (Dank).

Differences between the sexes exist as to age of first sexual experience. Thus sexual desire and behavior in males occur on the average at 13.5 years of age. In contrast, initial sexual experiences among homosexually oriented women occur much later at an average of 19 or 20 (Kaye). The social context in which "coming out" occurs is quite variable but usually takes place in a situation where information about homosexuality is freely available. The most common context for both men and women appears to be during a love affair with another gay person. The affair usually takes place between two people of similar age and rarely involves seduction by an older individual, as is commonly thought.

Although friendships and social contact between groups and cliques are minimal, interaction for sexual purposes is a major reason for mobility between groups. Evidence indicates that at least among gay men, individuals who serve sexual needs are kept distant from those who serve social needs (Sonenschein). Except for marriages and cohabitations, first-order friends considered to be the "really close" associations within a clique were the least desirable for sexual contacts. On the other hand, one night stands and the slightly longer sexual relations of "being kept" and "affairs" were made with complete or relative strangers from other groups or cliques.

The recent research on social structure has revealed something about the makeup of a gay community as it relates, primarily, to the male. It is hoped that more work will be forthcoming that will not only extend our knowledge of the social relationship among gay males but similarly help in our understanding of the community of gay females. Practically no thorough research has been done on the social structure of the lesbian community, but a number of recently published books do report the attitudes and life styles of a sampling of lesbians (for example, see Wysor).

CAUSE

To some experts, any discussion of causes is suspect; to others, it is a necessity. If homosexuality is an illness, and some believe it is, then the revelation of causes could lead to appropriate treatment and cure. In this case, cure could mean a reversal toward heterosexuality or better adjustment within the homosexual orientation. Others believe homosexuality to be not a "condition" but one of the many possibilities found in a species that is predisposed to variation. It becomes an illness only if some label it as such. Still other psychologists believe that homosexuality does not represent either an abnormal *or* normal entity. A person identified as homosexual does not necessarily demonstrate any characteristics in common with other homosexuals. In the same way, saying that two persons are heterosexual does not allow one to predict any other traits they have in common.

Experts who view homosexuality as an alternative orientation instead of a "condition" sometimes feel that discussions of causes are meaningless and even harmful. They fear that looking for causes will only perpetuate the label "homosexual" and thereby the stigma. However, we must not fail to consider the possibility that each and every topic of human concern should be subjected to as thorough an analysis as possible, limited only by the sophistication of the investigator and availability of techniques. This can be done solely for the purpose of enlightenment. But several points should be kept in mind throughout such an investigation. First, current research indicates that homosexuality has multiple causes. This conclusion is hardly surprising, because homosexuals, like heterosexuals, have many different character traits, personalities, and family histories. Second, one cause or a particular group of causes may apply to one person, but a different set of causes may apply to another individual. Third, if a person has experienced an event that is known to be one of the causes of homosexuality, he or she may not necessarily develop a homosexual orientation. And, finally, causes interact. Researchers in the areas of biology, psychology, and social science must always struggle to investigate fully within their own specialties and still remain aware of the greater picture.

Genetic Factors

Although various experts believe that genetic theories accounting for homosexuality should be rejected (Miller et al.), the problem of genetic causes needs further research. To date, specific genetic or chromosomal differences have not been found among individuals with a homosexual orientation when compared with those with other orientations. A sample of male homosexuals was found to possess the normal complement of X and Y chromosomes in every cell examined (Pritchard). Similar studies on females and examination of the other 22 pairs of chromosomes have not been made. Genetic differences can exist in many forms that would not necessarily show up in observations of chromosomal structure or numbers.

Other genetic evidence is indirect. Recent statistics have shown that homosexually oriented men tend to be born late in order of siblings and to relatively older mothers (Slater). Genetic irregularities can accumulate and be more prevalent among older mothers, be more often transmitted to the last offspring, and thus provide a genetic propensity for unusual or rarer forms of sexual development such as homosexuality. This concept has been criticized on the grounds that genetic propensity is unnecessary to explain the fact that many youngest children tend to identify more with their mothers and interact with them in such a way that a psychological propensity for homosexuality could occur (Karlen). However, no one has explained why many youngest children never become homosexually oriented or why many oldest children do become homosexually oriented despite all the "propensities."

The most often criticized work on genetic causes is Franz Kallman's study on the incidence of homosexuality among identical twins versus fraternal twins. Of 40 identical twins, when one individual was exclusively homosexual the other twin was also found to be exclusively homosexual or nearly so. The author reports that even though both twins in the sample were raised together, their sexual orientation was developed independently and often far apart from each other. All of the identical twins denied any "mutuality" of sexual orientation and knowledge of the other twin's sex practices. This high concordance of sexual orientation was not observed among a sample of 45 fraternal twins, each pair also having been raised together. That is, when one member of a set of fraternal twins was exclusively homosexual, the other member was not necessarily so and could be exclusively heterosexual. The fact that all twins were raised together casts some doubt on theories which propose a type of family interaction as a primary cause of homosexuality. If family influence was important, a greater concordance should have been found among the sexual orientations of fraternal twins.

Many people criticize Kallman on grounds that are not based on the data actually presented by him. For example, Kallman has never suggested that a specific gene, or even a specific group of genes, is responsible for homosexuality. Yet he is criticized for having said this. Instead, he proposes only that an interaction must exist between certain genetic combinations and the development of personality. He recognized the importance of environmental triggers acting on genetic potentials and had difficulty in separating hereditary from environmental factors. On the other hand, reports from psychiatrists and doctors actually working with patients have shown that even identical twins may have divergent sexual orientations, so that the genetic problem continues to remain unresolved. Indeed this last evidence does not rule out genetic influences, but only suggests that other factors are probably involved. Identical twins are often treated by parents, siblings, friends, and teachers as if they were one person; whereas fraternal twins are often treated as separate individuals. This tendency accounts for the greater concordance among Kallman's identical twins. Research is needed that would compare identical twins reared apart from birth.

We should keep in mind that, if genetic differences between homosexuals and heterosexuals are discovered, this will not necessarily imply an abnormality in one group or the other—only a difference.

Hormonal Theories

These theories like the genetic are generally rejected by most psychologists. Injections of testosterone given to homosexually oriented males do not cause a switch in orientation but may increase sexual motivation. Recent evidence from two areas of research is causing a resurgence of interest in hormonal mechanisms. The organizing effect of hormones on the developing brain and the blood levels of testosterone and estrogen in a variety of adult individuals is being extensively studied.

Organizing Effect   Evidence from work with rats, hamsters, guinea pigs, and Rhesus monkeys has shown that absence of androgens during early differentiation of the brain favors the development of female control centers for feminine behavior and estrus cycles occurring in postpuberty (Money and Ehrhardt). When androgen is present, it influences the differentiating brain by disorganizing prospective female control centers by potentiating a prospective male circuitry (Whalen and Edwards). Experiments that disrupt the usual process of brain development—such as injections of testosterone into female rats at birth or castration of newborn male rats—will modify sexual behavior in these individuals as adults, and orientations become homosexual. Newborn female rats given large amounts of testosterone propionate (100 to 500 mg) will not only show reduced feminine behavior as adults but will fail to ovulate. In addition, in the presence of a normal estrus female, they will display components of masculine behavior and will mount the presenting female (Money and Ehrhardt).

Adult male rats, castrated at birth and thus lacking in the organizational properties of testosterone, will show a relatively high proportion of femalelike responses such as lordosis toward normal males and a relatively low incidence of mounting responses toward normal females in estrus (Dorner). In all Dorner's experiments, males castrated as newborns were given injections of testosterone propionate when sexually mature and still showed a preponderance of female responses toward normal males. Control groups of male rats castrated as adults and given testosterone injections failed to show lordosis responses to normal males.

Extrapolation of such evidence to the human situation can be dangerous and must be viewed with caution. Nevertheless Feldman and MacCulloch utilizing the above information have come up with a theory that homosexually oriented men are of two types: primary and secondary. The authors believe this is also true for women although the evidence is less clear. Persons with homosexuality of a primary sort have never experienced a pleasurable sexual contact with the opposite sex. The authors theorize that "primary homosexuals differ from secondary homosexuals in that their developing brains have been preconditioned, prior to birth, by an imbalance of sex steroid." For example, the authors imply that a lack of testosterone at the "critical" time of brain development in the male or too much of the hormone in the female can lead to a homosexual orientation later in life. The effect is not necessarily on the orientation per se, but on a whole constellation of behaviors conducive to the influence of environmental factors that can trigger homosexuality. Behavior patterns are not considered "all female or all male" but lie along a continuum between extremes. A small proportion of primary homosexuals are considered by the authors to be transsexuals in that they desire a total sex change. Therapeutic techniques fail to switch orientations in primary homosexuals. Secondary types of homosexuals are those individuals who through conditioning *learn* to avoid heterosexual contacts. By aversion techniques of reconditioning they can learn to become heterosexually oriented.

It must be made clear that the effects of the presence or absence of androgen on the developing brain can also influence brain centers that control nonspecific behaviors such as aggressiveness, level of muscular activity, and sensitivity of sense organs to stimuli. These factors could influence the way parents interact with a child. For example, a passive versus an aggressive child would be treated differently by parents, other relatives, and peers.

Blood Levels of Sex Hormones in Adults   For reasons that will be shortly given, caution must be used in interpreting the following results: Thirty homosexually oriented men had blood levels of testosterone approximately one half of that found in fifty heterosexually oriented men (Kalodny et al). In another study, a small sample of exclusively homosexual females was found to possess higher levels of testosterone and lower levels of estrogen in their urine when compared to heterosexually oriented women (Loraine et al.). In still another study, the urinary levels of two breakdown products of testosterone were found to differ. The ratio of the two products found in urine was reversed in men with the homosexual orientation when compared to men with the heterosexual orientation (Margolese). Other reports have failed to confirm Margolese's results.

Before we accept the results of the above studies, we have to ask ourselves the following question: Does the behavior result from hormonal differences or do hormonal differences reflect the behavior? Also, other factors such as stress can influence hormonal levels—for example, stress is known to lower testosterone levels. It is possible that society's stigma and ostracism could create a continual level of stress in homosexually oriented persons leading to hormonal differences (Green).

Learning and Psychodynamic Theories

There are numerous theories that try to describe the psychological basis of behavior. They can primarily be divided into learning theories and psychodynamic theories.

The learning theorist approaches homosexuality as he does any other form of behavior, always looking for ways in which the individual was conditioned for this behavior. The theorist assumes the presence of both homosexual and heterosexual interests in all people, and, working from this assumption, he takes one of two approaches: Some theorists show how homosexual interest is selectively cultivated by the individual's family and by other close social-environmental forces. For example, they look for factors in family dynamics that positively reinforce the homosexual interest through reward and punishment. Other learning theorists take the opposite approach and search for ways in which heterosexual interest may have been selectively eliminated from the person's repertoire of behavior.

The psychodynamic theories (psychoanalysis and its updated and related schools) again begin with the assumption that all persons have homosexual interests. These theories include the concept that homosexual interest is fostered to the exclusion of the heterosexual interest by unsuccessful completion of a phase of development. This lack of development is caused by some limiting circumstances in the family relationship.

Basically most of the theories involve the concept that conditioning during childhood in association with an indifferent father and overpowering mother in the case of males and "the close-binding, overly intimate father in the case of females" can lead to homosexuality (Bieber, Kaye). The development of fear of the opposite sex, a flight from the strain of living up to a specific role whether feminine or masculine, and actual hatred for the opposite sex are all considered results of pathological home life.

The learning and psychodynamic theories have been heavily criticized on the ground that the data have been obtained mostly from psychiatric patients. These theories assume that all homosexuals had a disturbed family relationships because those who seek treatment did. This assumption is as invalid as saying that all heterosexuals had a pathological home life because some heterosexuals need mental health care. Actually, the majority of gay women and men have no background of psychiatric need or care. If homosexuality were indeed a result of a "crippling inhibition" of development in the heterosexual direction, we would at least expect to find evidence of neuroticism and widespread lack of adaptation on the part of homosexually oriented persons. Evidence tends to refute this expectation (Miller et al., Freedman). For example, E. Hooker gave the Rorschach test to 30 heterosexually and 30 homosexually oriented men. Three psychologists examined the results of the tests and found that the majority of men with homosexual orientations showed superior to average adjustment and were not characterized by any form of mental illness. Similar results were found for women (Armon). The methods used by these authors have been challenged. A. Karlen has criticized the methods used by Hooker stating that ". . . all her subjects were carefully selected for their good adjustment." This criticism still does not distort the fact that many homosexually oriented persons are well adjusted; otherwise there would be no such sample to choose from. Karlen also denies the importance of the Rorschach tests beyond that as an "adjunct to diagnosis."

There is widespread feeling among psychiatrists that therapeutic techniques should be available to those who want help. A variety of therapeutic techniques from shock therapy to Freudian analysis have been used to treat those in need. Treatment has not proved very successful in causing changes of orientation but has helped persons adjust within the context of their current sex-role identities. Apparently those persons most receptive to treatment are also those most receptive to change—for example, they tended to be bisexual or secondary homosexuals and acted positively toward therapeutic techniques.

Recently the American Psychiatric Association and the American Psychological Association have excluded homosexuality from the list of mental disorders and illnesses. This action reflects the growing scholarly evidence that homosexuality per se does not involve any impairment of general social and vocational capabilities, reliability, judgment, or stability.

Social Theories

Social scientists are sensitive to violation of the person in his or her attempt to live within the social environment. They deal harshly with the role demands of such social institutions as femininity, masculinity, sexual normality, and marriage. They point out that these roles demand types and standards of behavior that do not suit everyone's character traits, personality, or interests. Thus some people reject these roles in order to preserve their own mental health. Some forms of homosexuality represent such a rejection plus a search for affectional sexual relationships that better fit the person's needs. Modern society with its advanced technology and increased urbanization has been identified as a possible factor leading toward the genesis of homosexuality (Hoffman). Within our society everyone is expected to be heterosexually oriented and thus, according to some, without a unique identity. By being a variant, one gains comradeship with a few others who share the difference. The hatred of authority on the part of some and the search for a self-concept unique in a world of peas in a pod can contribute to acceptance of variant orientations. The exhilaration of experiencing something considered against the law contains the elements of danger and once again brings to light the idea that many people seek out sexual behavior in direct proportion to how illegal it is. It seems possible that the homophile and heterophile organizations available to strengthen identity for their respective orientations leave the large middle ground of bisexuality with the least support for identity and thus the most guilt and clandestine behavior.

Recent evidence casts light on the controversy about homosexuals and their social and mental health status. Myrick studied attitudinal differences between heterosexually and homosexually oriented males. The homosexually oriented males in the study were "characterized by lower self-esteem, personal competence, and self-acceptance; less power; and fewer norms" than the heterosexually oriented males. The author concluded that these results support the concept that the gay person suffers primarily from social condemnation and "needs to adjust to himself as a homophile because of his inability to cope with life and to determine the results of his behavior" (Myrick). The same study also concluded that "overt gay people" possessed even less self-acceptance and suffered more social isolation than "covert gay people." Myrick rejected the concept that homosexuality is a sickness caused by factors other than social attitudes.

HOMOSEXUALITY AND THE LAW

In most of the United States, legal sexual activity is confined to heterosexual intercourse within the context of marriage. There are a number of views as to what the relationship should be between homosexuality and the law (*The Challenge and Progress of Homosexual Law Reform*). These can be summarized as follows:

1 Homosexual acts performed in private by consenting adults without force or coercion should not be the concern of the law or law enforcement agencies. This is the essence of the Wolfenden Report in Great Britain (Schur).

2 Homosexual acts must be punished severely by strong laws.

3 Laws must be available but should not prosecute severely. In a society where religious and political integrity is weakened, laws are the only way society can express its frustration about behavior it deems unnatural.

4 Homosexuality is not a crime but a sickness, and individuals performing such behavior should be hospitalized or incarcerated in mental institutions instead of in jails.

Laws are designed to control behavior that would be offensive and injurious to ourselves and others. Some lawyers and judges believe that a society has every right to decide which forms of behavior are unacceptable and to punish what it considers to be wrong (Wallheim). Others believe that laws governing sexual behavior are justified only if the sex acts are performed in public, are violent, or involve minors (Slovenko). Still others in the legal profession ask: "Are we moral to create laws that govern our morals?" (Rostow and Hart). Most of the sex acts performed by adult homophiles involve mutual consent and occur in private. Many of these sex acts are considered by some lawyers as "crimes without victims." This legal category is defined by Schur as the consensual interaction between adults of strongly demanded but illegal behavior.

In the last few years, an impressive array of major national groups has urged an end to legal restrictions on consensual adult sexual behavior, whether heterosexual or homosexual. These include the American Bar Association, the American Psychiatric Association, the American Psychological Association, and several national church bodies. Interestingly, the United States is virtually the only nation in the Western Hemisphere with laws forbidding homosexual acts and it is also virtually the only one in the entire Western world.

BIBLIOGRAPHY

Allen, C. 1967. Sexual perversions, in A. Ellis and A. Abarbanel (eds.), *Modern Sex Practices, The Encyclopedia of Sexual Behavior,* vol. I. Ace, New York.

Armon, V. 1960. Some personality variables in overt female homosexuality, *J. Project. Tech.,* **24**:292–309.

Benjamin, J. 1966. *The Transsexual Phenomenon.* Ace, New York.

Bieber, I. 1962. *Homosexuality: A Psychoanalytic Study.* Basic Books, New York.

Bieber, I. 1965. Clinical aspects of male homosexuality, in J. Marmor (ed.), *Sexual Inversion.* Basic Books, New York.

Council on Religion and the Homosexual, Daughters of Bilitis, Society for Individual Rights, and Tavern Guild of San Francisco. 1968. *The Challenge and Progress of Homosexual Law Reform.*

Dank, B. 1971. Coming out in the gay world, *Psychiatry J. for the Study of Interpersonal Processes,* **34**:180–197.

DeForrest, M. 1949. *The Gay Year.* Woodford Press, New York.

Dorner, G. 1969. Zur frage finfe neuroendokrinen pathogenese, prophylaxe und therapie angeborener sexualdeviationen, *Dtsch. Med. Wochenschr.,* **94**:390–396.

Feldman, M. P. and M. J. MacCulloch. 1971. *Homosexual Behavior: Therapy and Assessment.* Pergamon, New York.

Freedman, M. 1971. *Homosexuality and Psychological Functioning.* Brooks Cole Pub., Belmont, Calif.

Freedman, M. 1975. Homosexuals may be healthier than straights, *Psych. Today,* March Issue, p. 28.

Goffman, I. 1963. *Stigma: Notes on the Management of Spoiled Identity.* pp. 143–144. Prentice Hall, Englewood Cliffs, N.J.

Green, R. 1972. Neuroendocrine and anatomical correlates of atypical sexuality, in J. L.

McGaugh (ed.), *The Chemistry of Mood, Motivation, and Memory.* Plenum, New York.

Hoffman, M. 1968. The roots of homosexuality, Chapter 8 in *The Gay World.* Basic Books, New York.

Hooker, E. 1959. Symposium on current aspects of the problems of validity: What is a criterion? *J. Project. Tech.,* **23**:278–286.

Jones, K. L., e al. 1969. *Sex.* Harper & Row, New York.

Kallman, F. 1952. Twin and sibship study of overt male homosexuality, *Am. J. Hum. Genet.,* **4**:136–146.

Kalodny, R., et al. 1971. Plasma testosterone and semen analysis in male homosexuals, *New Engl. J. Med.,* **285**:1170–1174.

Karlen, A. 1971. *Sexuality and Homosexuality, A New View.* Norton, New York.

Kaye, H. E. 1972. Lesbian relationships, *Sexual Behavior,* Apr. Issue.

Kinsey, A. C., et al. 1948. *Sexual Behavior in the Human Male.* Saunders, Philadelphia.

Kinsey, A. C., et al. 1953. *Sexual Behavior in the Human Female.* Saunders, Philadelphia.

Leznoff, M., and W. A. Westley. 1956. The homosexual community, *Social Problems,* **3**:257–263.

Loraine, J. A., et al. 1971. Patterns of hormone excretion in male and female homosexuals, *Nature,* **234**:552–555.

Lyon, P., and Del Martin. 1972. *Lesbian Woman.* Bantam, New York.

Margolese. 1970. Homosexuality: a new endocrine correlate, *Horm. Beha.,* **1**:151–155.

McIntosh, M. 1968. The homosexual role, *Social Problems,* **16**(2):182–192.

Miller, P., et al. 1968. Review of homosexuality research (1960–1966) and some implications for treatment, *Psychotherapy: Theory, Research, and Practice,* **5**(1):3–6.

Money, J., and A. A. Ehrhardt. 1971. Fetal hormones and the brain: Effect on sexual dimorphism of behavior—a review, *Arch. Sex. Beha.,* **1**(3):241–262.

Myrick, F. L. 1974. Attitudinal differences between heterosexually and homosexually oriented males and between covert and overt male homosexuals. *J. Abnorm. Psychol.,* **83**(1):81–86.

Pritchard, M. 1962. Homosexuality and genetic sex, *J. Ment. Sci.,* **108**:616–623.

Rostow, E. V., and H. L. A. Hart. 1961. The use and abuse of criminal law, *Oxford Lawyer,* **4**:7–12.

Sagarin, E. 1970. Language of the homosexual subculture, *Med. Aspects Hum. Sex.,* **4**(4):37.

Schur, E. 1965. The Wolfenden report, *Am. Sociological Review,* **28**:1055.

Simon, W., and J. H. Gagnon. 1967. The lesbians: A preliminary overview, in J. H. Gagnon et al. (eds.), *Sexual Deviance,* pp. 247–282. Harper & Row, New York.

Slater, E. 1962. Birth order and maternal age of homosexuals, *Lancet* **1**:69–71.

Slovenko, R. 1971. Sex laws: are they necessary? in A. M. Barclay et al. (eds.), *Sexuality: A Search for Perspective.* Van Nostrand, New York.

Sonenschein, D. 1968. The ethnography of male homosexual relationships, *J. of Sex Research,* **4**(2).

Stearn, J. 1962. *The Sixth Man.* MacFadden Books, New York.

Wallheim, M. 1959. Crime, sin and Mr. Justice Devlin, *Encounter.* Nov. Issue, pp. 34–40.

Whalen, R. E., and D. A. Edwards. 1967. Hormonal determinants of the development of masculine and feminine behavior in male and female rats, *Anat. Rec.,* **157**:173–180.

Wysor, B. 1974. *The Lesbian Myth.* Random House, New York.

Chapter 15

Problematic Sexual Behavior

Understanding the difference between "normal" and "abnormal" sexual behavior has been and will always be a central focus of human concern. The basic problem is that all of us may show variant forms of behavior but "a sharp line of distinction cannot always be drawn between healthy and neurotic sexuality" (Marmor, 1971). Definitions of abnormal sexual behavior vary culturally—an abnormality being "anything and everything" the particular society declares it to be (Ellis). Concepts of normalcy vary also with time. Formerly, the term "perversion" was used to describe abnormal sexual conduct. Today, softened labels such as "deviations" or "variations" are used to describe the same behavior, thereby reflecting shifts in attitude toward greater understanding and objectivity with respect to sex.

Some authors claim the possible existence of an optimal level of sexual adjustment that transcends culture (Marmor, 1971). The ability to control one's emotions and drives, self-acceptance, and confidence certainly are desirable cross-culturally. Nevertheless, any definition of "optimal" behavior generally depends upon its cultural context and specifically upon the one doing the defining. Thus, a physician in our society would define abnormal behavior as unhealthy; whereas, a social scientist would assert that "abnormal" sexual behavior is unacceptable socially and results from distortion of the learning process. Law-enforcement agencies consider any behavior that breaks the law as abnormal. In this sense, the only legal sexual activity in most of the United States is voluntary face-to-face intercourse between married persons or others who could legally get married (Gatov).

Biologists have stressed that many types of sexual activity such as oral-genital contact and anal stimulations are "normal" adaptations having a long evolutionary history (Kinsey). For example, nonhuman mammals utilize a variety of oral-genital and anal techniques in their courtship behavior. Because many people in this society wish to remove the weight of criminality from such behavior, they claim that any sexual act between adults that is consensual, lacks force, and is performed in privacy away from unwilling observers should be considered normal and out of reach of the law. The key words are *adult, privacy, consent,* and *lack of force.* "The issue here is really not sex but rather protection of the helpless from indecent behavior or attack" (Slovenko). Since minors according to law are "helpless," they are incapable of giving their consent even if willing.

The necessity for privacy during sexual acts appears to be one of the most common concepts found in virtually all cultures studied. The function of privacy is not clearly understood. Humans are very sensitive to external stimuli during sexual intercourse. A door slamming, a telephone ringing, a child screaming can interrupt coitus, causing a reduction in vaginal lubrication and a lessened erection. One suggestion is that privacy helps to reduce these distracting stimuli (Jensen). Of interest, seclusion during coitus is also well developed in chimpanzees and other nonhuman primates. Another theory states that primitive humans have learned that seclusion during sexual acts reduces social tensions arising from viewing the genitalia of other individuals (MacLean). Some species of nonhuman primates, for example, use the genital display in territorial behavior and this, according to the theory, has been retained in humans (MacLean). Whatever the function, cultural influence seems to reinforce positively sexual behavior performed in private. Seemingly a difficult legal question is the meaning of the "in private" or its antithesis "in public." Can intercourse performed in the relative seclusion of a stall in a public toilet be considered private?

The concepts of consent and lack of force reflect the view of many psychologists that problematic sexual acts arise as conflict between social constraints and sexual motivation. Evidence from one study, in a college setting, indicated that when sexual intimacy between male and female proceeded with initial consent, the male reacted with physical force if consent was withdrawn just prior to intercourse (Kanin). A majority of the females involved responded by "screaming, fighting, crying, and pleading," which usually deterred the male from further assault. Less than 1 percent of the victims, however, were willing to report their partner's aggressions. Kanin indicated that the women did not wish to identify their degree of sexual activity or get the male partner in trouble. The most significant point of the study was the apparent lack of communication between the sexes about the meaning of erotic involvement. "The young female generally perceives of sex activity in terms of partial gratification and stabilization; whereas, the male is prone to interpret progressive sexual compromise as signifying potential intercourse" (Kanin).

This evidence does not mean that assaults are always due to overwhelming sex drives suddenly released. More often sexual assaults are motivated by the presence of hostility on the part of the attacker. In heterosexual assault, this is usually a general hostility toward the opposite sex. Frequently the perpetrator also views sex as filthy and dirty and is essentially paying the victim back for being unfaithful, untrustworthy, and imperfect. Sexual assaults are thus seen as an extreme case where the functions of intercourse include not only the expression of love but may "also be a vehicle for establishing one's sense of power" by controlling the behavior of the partner (Halleck). The husband who feels by giving his wife an orgasm he will "own" her and the wife who refuses intercourse so as not to be "owned" are examples of power plays which simply lack the violence. The problem is how do we classify this last form of behavior—as deviant along with the aforementioned sexual assaults?

In a pluralistic society where a large number of choices can be made between a variety of alternatives, variations in sexual behavior will also exist. Under our current social system, behavior that deprives others of their rights of personal choice, causes serious injury, and takes advantage of a victim who does not or cannot give his or her consent is considered deviant (Wolfgang). Additionally, "habitual and preferential" use of outlets of sexual release not involving mature adults are considered deviant. Examples are sexual acts with children, animals, dead people, and inanimate objects.

Many sexual offenses, such as most rapes, occur opportunistically. A man sees a woman alone on a dark street, and the scene is set. Other offenses occur as a response to stress or in the "heat of passion." Thus the sexual offender does not always possess a psychological disorder or persistent personality problem. The person who does have such a problem resulting in habitual deviant acts is rare (Mohr). The chronic sexual offender is an individual who has great difficulty developing and maintaining mature interpersonal relations with other adults. "Easier" outlets are chosen which eventually become major alternatives to "mature" relationships. The individual often has a history of family problems where one parent is overwhelmingly dominant and the other indifferent. "Disturbances in core family relationships, impairment in gender identity development, poor ego development, and specific conditioning experiences are all involved" (Marmor, 1971).

Evidence is also accumulating that indicates some chronic sexual deviation may have its roots in disorders of brain function. Epstein studied 13 cases of fetishism where sexual arousal and gratification was usually achieved with an inanimate object. Nine of these individuals showed abnormal electroencephalograms (brain waves) and five exhibited chemical evidence of brain disease. Brain wave abnormalities have also been found in cases of transvestism (Walinder). Since this is preliminary data, one should proceed with caution in attributing all or even most cases of deviation to errors in brain function (Stoller). Nevertheless, whereas psychoanalysis fails to reverse most deviant behavior, preliminary data do indicate that removal of damaged brain areas and treatment with drugs acting on brain circuitry can reduce certain forms of deviation. Particularly important has been the use of cyproterone acetate, the most powerful antiandrogen currently known. Physiologically, the level of androgen in both sexes and the capacity of certain brain areas (limbic system, hypothalamus) to respond to androgen are major determinants of sexual behavior. Cyproterone acetate competes with androgen for receptor sites in these brain locations and thus essentially blocks pickup of male hormone by the sexual control centers. The effect in males is to reduce libido, erection, and orgasm in that order (Lasche). The results of therapy with the drug are most clearly seen in the syndrome of exhibitionism. An exhibitionist is defined as one who preferentially and habitually gets sexual gratification from exhibiting his genitals to unwilling observers, usually women or children. An exhibitionist, usually male, reacts to the shocked expression of a surprised victim with an erection. In one study, cyproterone acetate accomplished a rapid and impressive cure in 27 cases of exhibitionism, reducing libido and the ability to obtain an erection (Lasche). All cases remained rehabilitated even when the drug was withdrawn.

It would appear that drugs used to control deviation may be the therapy of the future. However, care must be taken to ensure that consenting patients are fully informed about the nature and possible side effects of drug treatment and that evidence of success is significantly different from placebo effects (Stoller).

FORCIBLE RAPE

Forcible rape is defined as an act of intercourse or penile-vaginal contact, however slight, that is forced upon a woman against her consent (Gatov). Forcible rape involves actual physical violence or threat of violence; however, a rape conviction may also be reached if the victim was simply constrained against her will. A male, regardless of age, must generally show sufficient physical strength to be accused of rape. The victim's age makes no difference in an act of forcible rape. Rape is the nation's number one crime against women—close to 32,000 forcible rapes were reported in 1973 by the Federal Bureau of Investigation; many more go unreported.

In some states, a charge of rape can be made if a man knowingly has intercourse with a woman who is intoxicated, high on drugs, or is mentally retarded. In California, if a woman is led to believe that a man is her husband and thus consents to intercourse with him, he can be charged with forcible rape (Gatov). Laws governing rape make no provisions for sexual assaults on a wife by her husband; however, he can be prosecuted under "wife beating" or assault and battery statutes. Similarly, rape laws do not protect one from homosexual assaults. Again, other statutes which prosecute persons for oral-genital and anal intercourse are used in this case. In addition, women are rarely accused and prosecuted under rape statutes. One woman, however, in 1971 was convicted of rape because she held a weapon on her husband forcing him to have intercourse with another female.

The penalty for forcible rape varies with the state but generally involves a sentence of not less than 3 years to a maximum of life imprisonment or death. The extent of physical harm sustained by the victim and whether a weapon was used in committing the assault are factors that determine individual sentencing (Kling). Recently, attempts have been made by some state legislatures to reduce these sentences. In California, for example, a measure pending in the state assembly would lower the penalty for rape from the 3 years to life to 2 to 10 years for the first offense.

Evidence of Rape (Graves and Francisco)

Evidence for rape is very difficult to obtain. Generally a physician is called in to examine the garments and physical state of the victim and the accused, the alleged location of rape, and to act as an "expert witness" for the court. Blood and semen stains, hair, fibers, and any other material that can identify the rapist and rape site are searched for on all garments. Dried semen on nylon appears shiny, on cotton has a stiff feel, and can be positively identified by acid phosphatase tests. Blood type can be identified either from blood or semen stains. The victim's face and body will be examined for signs of struggle. Samples of vaginal secretions will be checked for sperm. However, absence of sperm may simply mean that during the rape the man did not ejaculate, did ejaculate but outside the vagina, or ejaculated but had no sperm. Also, the possibility that the victim may have douched immediately afterward cannot be discounted. A torn hymen may constitute evidence only if it can be proved that it was previously intact. The presence of gonorrhea will be determined.

The accused will be examined only if he gives his permission, and lack of it does not prove guilt. His fingernails will be studied for debris, genitals examined for trauma, and skin observed for scratches, bruises, and blood stains. A smear will be taken from the urethra and the presence or absence of gonorrhea will be determined.

If rape took place within 72 h, the postcoital pill will be given to prevent possible implantation. Evidence suggests the possibility that rape could cause ovulation reflexively. It is well known that cats and rabbits ovulate only following coitus. Humans are generally spontaneous ovulators; however, victims of rape show a higher rate of pregnancy compared to a control group (Goldsmith). This may mean that the physical trauma of a rape triggers ovulation under some situations. The crime of rape can be so traumatic as to leave permanent physical and mental scars for the rest of a victim's life. Psychotherapy will be given the woman, with an attempt to emphasize any and all positive relationships she has had with men. She and her family will be assured that a full recovery from the experience is probable. Often the family's hysterics can prolong the victim's agony, and they will receive counseling to reduce this possibility.

Nature of the Rapist (Schiff, 1972)

The majority of forcible rapes are committed by men who find themselves in a situation conducive to the act; these men rarely repeat the offense. In contrast, the rarer chronic rapist goes looking for opportunities and repeatedly rapes until caught. The personality of the chronic rapist includes hostility and fear of women. Sex, in this case, is considered filthy and demeaning, and intercourse is a method of performing a "despicable act" with one whom the rapist despises. Tracing the family history of a chronic rapist shows once again a cool, indifferent father and an overdominant mother especially restrictive of the son's sexual behavior. The rapist often feels a lack of control over his own destiny, and the act of rape is an attempt to direct the future. Evidence shows chronic rapists to have a relatively low association with pornography as compared to other sex offenders.

Nature of the Victim

Schiff cites two studies where the age of the victim most often raped was fourteen (range from one to eighty-eight). The author speculates that fourteen-year-old girls are more susceptible to rape since older women would have learned to shy away from potentially dangerous situations. Additionally, fourteen-year-olds can be more easily frightened into submission and immobilized by threats of violence. They are also just beginning to mature physically and would be more attractive to a rapist than someone younger.

The majority of victims are single and conspicuously alone more frequently than married women. In most reported rapes the rapist and victim are strangers, but in about one-third of the cases, the victim is known to the perpetrator in a casual manner. Schiff states that about 16 percent of rapes in his study could have been precipitated by seductive behavior on the part of the victim at a party or bar.

How to Avoid Rape

Most preventative measures for avoiding a rape involve common sense. Here are some suggestions:

1   Always hitchhike with a partner and carefully study the driver for unusual mannerisms and nervousness.

2   Avoid lonely streets at night.

3   Before getting into your car, check that no one is hiding in the back seat.

4   Wear long hair up when walking alone at night so it won't be so easy to pull.

5   If followed, never head the suspect to your home but rather to a police station.

6   Avoid panic—keep your cool.

7   Sometimes carrying a readily available "weapon" that is legal may deter an assailant; for example: hat or hair pin, letter opener, hair brush with stiff bristles, a lighter, a purse with weights in it, knitting needle, a police whistle, hair spray, sharp pencil, and so on.

8   Learn karate, kung fu, or another form of self-defense, but be sure to practice against men as well as women.

9   Help in developing legislation that would reduce the social stigma and

rough treatment of the victim on the part of law-enforcement personnel, lawyers, and judges.

10 Of course, if rape is inevitable, submitting to the rapist is far better than getting killed or maimed for life.

UNLAWFUL INTERCOURSE

Unlawful intercourse, synonomous with *statutory rape,* is an act of coitus with a female under the age of consent. In this case the female gives her consent, but this is not acceptable under the law. The term statutory is a journalistic term and should be abandoned in the specific sense of rape, since all laws are statutes. The crime is a felony in most states, punishment ranging from 1 year to life imprisonment (Kling).

SEDUCTION

Seduction is voluntary sexual intercourse based on an unconditional promise of marriage to an unmarried woman. If the man places conditions upon the promise such as "I will marry you only if I get a divorce from my present wife" or "if you get pregnant," the charge of seduction cannot be made (Gatov). The penalty tends to be rather severe. For example, the California Penal Code 268, written in 1889, states that seduction is punishable by not more than 5 years and/or by a fine of not more than $5,000.

SADISM

Receiving sexual pleasure and gratification by physically or mentally hurting someone is defined as *sadism.* The true sadist is one who primarily achieves orgasm via sadistic acts even though regular intercourse as a sexual outlet is also available. Sadism differs from rape in that usually the victim volunteers and is often a person with masochistic tendencies. The physical violence per se may not be the primary requirement for the sadist, but the desire to dominate the partner usually is. The sadist generally is male, unmarried, and possesses deep feelings of inadequacy. By sexually assaulting someone, the sadist is unconsciously reassuring himself of his worth and denying the existence of an inferiority complex. Occasionally, a person who is able to inhibit his sadistic tendencies loses this ability when under the influence of stress, alcohol, drugs, or jealousy (Rothman).

The conditioning for sadism probably begins early in childhood punishments. "It may be related to the system of corporal punishment of children, especially in schools, since any overwhelming and big emotional experience can flood over into the sexual system, especially in early childhood, and leave its imprint for a lifetime" (Money). The suggestion that sadism may thus occur more often in countries such as England and Germany where corporal punishment is common has been made but not proven.

The term sadism was coined by Krafft-Ebing, a noted German psychologist, who wrote *Psychopathia Sexualis* in 1886. The term was derived from the name of a French nobleman living during the French Revolution who made some notorious sexual assaults on women. He was the Marquis de Sade. Lewinsohn records that the celebrated exploits of the Marquis actually included only two acts that could be termed "sadistic." Once in Paris, as a young officer, he enticed a girl (although she apparently encouraged it) into his home and then proceeded to bind her arms and legs as well as threaten her with a knife. Somehow she was able to free herself and hastily made an exit through a window. The only other act of sadism occurred when he visited a house of prostitution in Marseilles. There he treated the prostitutes to wines and liqueurs and gave them each some bonbons containing the alleged aphrodisiac Spanish Fly. Spanish Fly is neither a fly nor is it exclusively Spanish; it actually is a powder obtained from crushed beetles belonging to the blister beetle family. There are over 2,000 species of the beetle containing Spanish Fly, with over 200 of them found in the United States (Presto and Muecke). The most active ingredient of Spanish Fly is cantharidin, a type of acid that forms biologically active salts when mixed with alkali in the body. It is a potent irritant of the genito-urinary and gastro-intestinal tracts. It can cause erections and increase vaginal lubrication but the amount needed to do this is often lethal—about 10 mg (Goodman). Apparently the prostitutes given the Spanish Fly by the Marquis suffered extreme nausea, abdominal pain, and excessive salivation. One prostitute could not stand the pain and jumped out of a window and two others suffered heart and lung collapse and eventually died.

The Marquis spent 17 years in prison for his crime with Spanish Fly. Following his release from prison he became a professional writer, authoring such perverse novels as *Justine* and *Juliette,* which were full of violence and sex. No longer did the Marquis perform sadistic acts in real life. Now, as Lewinsohn has pointed out, he was simply a "pervert of the pen."

Amazingly, the terms sadism or sadist are rarely mentioned in the various legal statutes. However, sadistic acts are punishable under other laws depending on the degree of violence involved. Simple assault, child beating, and murder have all been charged in cases of sadism.

MASOCHISM

Masochism is defined as obtaining sexual pleasure and gratification by experiencing physical or mental pain and humiliation. The masochist desires to be dominated in a sexual relationship, abrogating all responsibility for involvement in an act he deems filthy and morally wrong. According to one psychiatrist, the masochist as a child experienced family attention only when being punished and consequently became conditioned to believe that love is obtainable only by submitting to domination (Marmor, 1969). Generally masochists as defined above are more likely to be single and about equally common among men and women.

Masochism as a term was coined also by Krafft-Ebing and named after the

Austrian writer Ritter Leopold Von Sacher-Masoch. Von Sacher-Masoch wrote many novels and short stories "each depicting in some fresh variant a type of man who satisfied his sexual needs by making a woman inflict pain on him" (Lewinsohn).

Masochism per se is not mentioned in any state law, but the act can be charged under indecent exposure, disorderly conduct, or assault and battery statutes (Kling).

PEDOPHILIA

One of the most hated of the sex offenders is the *pedophiliac*—a person who obtains pleasure by sexually molesting a child. About one-third of all sex offenses are acts of child molestation. The criminal classification of pedophilia depends upon the degree and nature of the offense. Thus, an offender can be prosecuted under rape, sodomy, corruption of the morals of a minor, or assault and battery statutes (Resnik and Peters). In addition, some states have laws that prohibit loitering in places where children gather—near schools and playgrounds, for example. The age limits of the victim in charging pedophilia depends upon geographic location. In Canada, the upper limit for the victim is fifteen, whereas in the United States it is twelve years of age.

Peters and Sadoff have described the psychodynamics of the child molester as an individual who is most often male, in his late thirties or early forties, and who lacks the feelings of emotional security and self-confidence observed in mature adults. Over half of the pedophiles in this study were alcoholics, a condition which apparently contributed to a reduction of their behavioral controls. "Not infrequently, the individual who presents himself sexually to a young female is a man who recently has felt rejected by his wife or girlfriend and approaches a less threatening sexual object" (Peters and Sadoff). Of course, child molestation may also include homosexual acts. Rarely is the pedophile a complete stranger to the victim. More often the offender and the victim may be blood relatives, friends, or acquaintances, the act occurring at either person's home.

The long-range effects on the victim tend not to be deleterious, and follow-up studies of the victim, show no evidence of psychological upset "unless the child was already mentally ill, continued to be neglected, or had an experience with a mentally disturbed adult" (Bender). Again, counseling of the family as well as the victim is of prime importance to prevent the hysterics more often damaging to the child than the actual act itself. Often the victim reacts to the offense with more calm and assurance than the parents.

Recently, a controversy has surfaced as to the effectiveness of electric shock therapy to cure pedophilia. Advocates say that it is quick, inexpensive, and most importantly it works. The pedophiliac is shown a slide of a naked child and simultaneously given an electric shock to the inner surface of his thigh. No shock is given when a picture of an adult is shown. In conjunction with the shock treatments, the pedophiliac is hypnotized and taught to associate objects he fears such as a snake or spider with thoughts and pictures of children. They are also given the opportunity to associate positive things such as ice cream and Disneyland with thoughts and pictures of an adult. Members of the Civil Liberties Union, however, claim that the treatment is "inherently coercive" and express doubts concerning its effectiveness. Pedophiliacs who are treated are usually inmates in prison. In a sense, they are forced to volunteer for treatment in order to be cured and subsequently released from prison.

GERONTOPHILIA AND NECROPHILIA

Other acts similar in dynamics to pedophilia include *gerontophilia,* which is deriving sexual pleasure and gratification by assaulting elderly persons, and *necrophilia*—attempting to have sexual contact with a corpse. In these cases, the possibility of rejection is reduced to a minimum or absent.

"INDIRECT" SEXUAL OFFENSES

We have been discussing sexual acts which involve direct person-to-person contact and a relative amount of violence. Another category of sex offenses is called "indirect" and does not include acts of force. These offenses are presented here beginning with the most indirect and include voyeurism, obscene telephone calling, exhibitionism, and frottage (Sadoff). The offender in the "indirect" category remains at some distance from the victim and is often completely obscure and anonymous. Rarely will he or she switch to some of the more violent acts such as rape or sadism.

    Voyeurism is defined as being sexually turned on by viewing someone in the nude or persons having sexual intercourse. To some extent most people possess voyeuristic tendencies and it only becomes problematic if the major sexual outlet is via this means and if the person takes great risks in being a voyeur. The offender is usually single, male, and on the average relatively young—about twenty-four years of age. He obtains full sexual satisfaction primarily by viewing the behavior of his victims and does not desire any physical contact with them (Sadoff). The family history of the voyeur often involves an incident of viewing his parents in sexual intercourse. So traumatic was the experience that the voyeur as an adult appears to be trying in vain to recreate the scene so as to learn to cope with it.

    Only five states have specific laws against voyeurism, whereas all others resort to various miscellaneous "catch all" and disorderly conduct statutes. In most cases, the penalty is a misdemeanor—not more than $1,000 in fine and/or 1 year in prison.

    Some variant forms of voyeurism include *scoptophilia*—sexual pleasure derived from viewing other people's genitalia, *urophilia*—sexual gratification by being urinated on or by viewing others urinating, and *coprophilia*—viewing someone defecating.

    Chronic obscene phone callers (almost always male) are said to be incapable of forming lasting positive relationships and only rarely are married or living in a family-type structure (Sadoff). They tend to be withdrawn in personality but are also relatively nonaggressive. They get sexually turned on from a distance by the frightened or shocked reaction of the victim. Arguing with him or begging him to stop only encourages the caller to continue. Although the victim gains little solace in it, evidence does indicate that the caller almost never performs any of the acts he promises over the phone. Often the caller will disguise himself as a census taker or salesperson. He will start by asking questions concerning the nature of your clothing and when he gets to the brand of your underpants it should be obvious as to his motives. Suggestions to the victim are to keep calm and if the situation is chronic, have a tape recorder that records the call. Blowing a police whistle into the receiver can deter the caller by breaking his ear drum.

Exhibitionism is defined as obtaining erotic pleasure from briefly exhibiting one's genitals to a surprised stranger, usually a child or woman. This is done most often in a public place such as the beach or park. The exhibitionist feels a compulsion to act this way and frequently returns to the same location over and over again until caught. The offender derives most of his pleasure by viewing the shocked reaction of a victim and may masturbate to orgasm following such an incident or ejaculate on the spot. If the victim reacts coolly and pays little attention, the offender is disappointed and gains little gratification. Many exhibitionists appear to have relatively normal sexual relations with their spouses but desire the variant form of activity, claiming that it gives maximum amounts of pleasure (Sadoff). On the average, exhibitionists do not show psychoses or a history of drugs and alcoholism but rather have a weak sex-role identity and need constantly to confirm their masculinity. Some psychiatrists believe that by revealing his penis the exhibitionist is demanding that everyone recognize he has one (Fenichel). Others suggest that the offender is shy and has an overpowering and aggressive spouse or mother and thus seeks release from domination (Allen). Fortunately, group psychotherapy has proven of some help in alleviating the problem.

Frottage comes from the French, meaning "to rub." As a sexual deviation, it is defined as obtaining sexual pleasure by rubbing one's genitals, usually when fully clothed, against the body of a female in a crowded place. Most acts go unnoticed and rarely do offenders seek treatment. Therefore little information exists about the psychodynamics of the frotteur. What evidence does exist indicates that the offender is a young male and the act takes place wherever people congregate—in subways, at festivals, on buses, trains, and in elevators. Apparently the frotteur is quite gratified simply to touch the legs or buttocks of his victim and rarely desires further contact.

PROSTITUTION

The only sex offense more often charged against women than men is *prostitution*. The word comes from the Latin *prostituere*, meaning to "offer for sale, set forth in public." The definition includes the factors of indiscriminate sexual relations for hire, usually without affection. "Prostitutes are those individuals who engage in sex with a variety of individuals as a paid vocation" (Bell and Gordon). In many states, such as California, prostitution per se is not against the law; however, if a person is caught soliciting, she may be prosecuted as a vagrant under the statute governing disorderly conduct. This usually is a misdemeanor, the penalty in California, for example, being a period in county jail of not less than 90 days. Other laws against operating a house of prostitution, pimping, pandering, or inducting a minor into the profession are felonies, which means that a possible penalty of more than 1 year in jail and/or $1,000 fine can be served. Only in New York, Illinois, Wisconsin, and Washington, D.C., are there laws against the customer (Basel). The penalty for patronizing a prostitute generally is that for a misdemeanor.

There are several classes of prostitute, which include the streetwalker, house prostitute and madam, call girl, mistress, and male prostitute. In all classes, a special vocabulary has evolved that reflects the prostitutes' and pimps' thinking and way of life (Table 15-1).

Streetwalker

The streetwalker is often considered the "queen" of prostitutes since she must learn to handle the rigors of the street (Hirschi). She must somehow attract customers but at the same time avoid being busted. The most important factor contributing to the financial success of a streetwalker is not so much how attractive she is but rather how capable she is in flattering and pleasing the potential trick. If she can convince him that their act together will reach heights of erotic pleasure never before experienced, she will be successful, at least initially (Hirschi).

Contrary to popular belief, interviews with many streetwalkers indicate a widespread satisfaction with their jobs. Not only can it be lucrative but they can meet a variety of people and obtain sexual satisfaction besides. There has been considerable disagreement among psychiatrists as to the ability of prostitutes to experience orgasm with their customers. Some have denied this ability, but others claim that prostitutes are "quite free of neurotic involvements and experience orgasm frequently" (Esselstyn). Interviews with prostitutes tend to support the latter contention.

The duration of a streetwalker's career is short, averaging about 7 years. Only rarely does a streetwalker continue her profession beyond the age of thirty-five. Perhaps the record for age among streetwalkers was seventy-three, held by "Baby Doll" Cowan, who was recently found dead at her home in Peoria, Illinois. She began work as a prostitute at nineteen and had 51 arrests, the last one only a few days before her death.

The pimp occupies a most significant position in the life of the prostitute. He is a "functional necessity" and may be her lover, protector, teacher, employment agent, and investor all rolled into one. The most commonly heard claim from streetwalkers is that their pimps are saving and investing their money so that some day soon they can retire.

The question most often asked by a customer is, "How did a nice girl like

Table 15-1 A Glossary of Terminology Used by Prostitutes and Pimps

Trick	A customer
John	A male customer
Jane	A lesbian customer
In the life	Being a prostitute
Hooker	Female prostitute
Pimp	"Any person who obtains support from earnings of the prostitute or who receives compensation for soliciting customers" (Gatov)
Outlaw broads	Prostitutes who do not have any connection with organized crime and must pay their own protection
Panderer	"Any person who procures a female for the purpose of prostitution or to reside in a house of prostitution" (Gatov). To procure, in this case, means to assist, induce, persuade, or otherwise encourage the female
To turn a trick	To perform sexual intercourse
Around the world	Licking of the body from head to toe followed by coitus, fellatio, and anilingus
Halfway around the world	Everything as above except the licking
Peg house	Male house of prostitution
To get burned or stiffed	To give service without getting paid
Freak	A trick with unusual sexual tastes
Turned out	Being subjected to the unusual sexual acts by a freak
Stable	A number of prostitutes controlled by one pimp. Highly chauvinistic, the term reflects the belief of some pimps that prostitutes are like "herds of domestic cattle"
Book	Used by a call girl, the book contains a list of the names and addresses of tricks
The book	Rules and regulations concerning the business of a pimp. Passed on orally
To break luck	A prostitute's first trick of any given working day
Flat-backer	A prostitute who makes her living by turning over as many tricks as possible instead of conniving to steal the money
Cookies	The payment for turning a trick
Git-down time	The time of day a streetwalker is supposed to begin her work
Sugar pimp or sweet Mack	A pimp who uses little violence and instead "sweet talks" or charms his prostitute(s) into submission
Hard Mack or gorilla pimp	A pimp who uses violence in bringing his prostitutes into submission
HO	A black pimp's term for prostitute

you get into this business?" The streetwalker will answer with a clever but fake hard-luck story designed to stimulate sympathy on the part of the "trick," hopefully resulting in additional payment. The customer also tends to counter with a yarn of his own justifying his visit to the prostitute. The people, places, and specifics of these yarns are often false, but enlightening in a general sense reflecting the functions of prostitution in our society. For example, some stories by customers reveal difficulty in developing normal adult relationships, a shy or timid personality, an individual's feelings of unattractiveness or ineptness as a lover, and a high desire for sexual variety. Many men, of course, visit prostitutes because they simply enjoy sex; whereas others do so because of the thrill of doing something illicit and illegal. There appears, however, to be a general decline in prostitution, especially the "houses," and this is due, in part, to the changing status of women and the increased use of contraceptives (Bullough).

Houses of Prostitution

These establishments, also called "brothels," "whorehouses," "disorderly houses," or "houses of ill repute," are not necessarily mansions or even large houses. They may be a one- or two-bedroom apartment occupied by only a few prostitutes plying their trade. Most often a "house" is supervised by a madam who pays the bills, including protection, and may also provide for classes in "sex education," emphasizing variety of sexual techniques on how to please the customers. In some cases, the madam has become a folk hero, and as John Steinbeck once said, "There is something very attractive to men about a madam. She combines the brains of a businessman, the toughness of a prize fighter, the warmth of a companion, the humor of a tragedian. Myths collect about her" (Gentry). The classic brothel run by an older madam has greatly declined since the end of World War II. On the rise has been the call-girl system of operation and massage parlors where services range from "discussions only" to fellatio and anilingus. Evidence indicates that prostitution, rather than increasing, is shifting from the centralized big-city market to suburbs, small towns, and cities where salesmen and other male travelers congregate. In some cases, even mobile homes are used to carry a masseuse with special lotions for "local" massages almost to your very doorstep. In places such as Des Moines, Wichita, and Colorado Springs, one can find massage parlors, nude photo labs, counseling, and escort services as easily as the "deliver-a-pizza" shop. Apparently, the massage-prostitution business is lucrative. One parlor in Minneapolis with only two masseuses is said to have grossed $50,000 in 1974.

Call Girls

Call girls typically obtain clients primarily by telephone, as individual referrals, and perform the sex act in either their own or the customers' residences. Bryan studied 33 call girls working in the Los Angeles area and found they go through a variable-length apprenticeship before becoming full members of the profession. The novice is introduced into the apprenticeship by another call girl or pimp. She will share an apartment with a more experienced call girl and there learns how to use the telephone and is given some philosophical advice which includes the concept that tricks are exploitive persons not to be trusted. She will be allowed to share a few of the older call girl's customers but eventually must develop her own clientele. Of interest, when steady customers discover the presence of an apprentice they often switch over to her permanently. The basis of the change is the customer's desire for variety and sexual experience with a younger woman.

An apprenticeship may last up to 8 months, but, on the average, they usually end abruptly in 2 to 3 months. The terminating factor depends upon the size of the apprentice's accumulated clientele and not on any degree of professional understanding or competence. Occasionally the abrupt ending may be due to a misunderstanding between apprentice and trainer, often pertaining to thievery of clients.

Mistress

Perhaps the category of mistress or "kept" woman should not be considered under the topic of prostitution as it no longer conforms to the classic view of a young woman set up in an apartment paid for by an older man and readily available to him primarily for sexual purposes. To be sure, the mistress occasionally is wealthier than the man and who "keeps" whom becomes a rhetorical question. The mistress is often married herself to a man of relative accomplishment and success. This marriage, however, usually does not possess the same sexual satisfaction and interpersonal meaning developed in her mistress association. The importance of sex in the totality of the mistress-man relationship is highly variable. In some situations, the mistress may share intellectual or political pursuits with her man, sex playing only a minor role. Certainly a relative amount of affection exists, sometimes greater than in the man's relationship with his wife. John Cuber has studied the "mistress in American society" and defines her as "a woman who has formed and maintained a lasting, intimate relationship with a man to whom she is not legally married and has no expectations of marriage to him." Some mistress relationships can be quite durable with longevities of 15 to 20 years.

Male Prostitutes

Male prostitutes have a clientele that is almost exclusively male, only rarely do they engage in sexual relations with females. T. C. Esselstyn has characterized the white male prostitute working in a city such as New York or San Francisco as between the ages of fifteen to twenty-five, rarely older, and not effeminate in demeanor, but instead going to great lengths to appear supermasculine in posture, physique, and clothing. They possess average or better IQs, generally have a high school diploma, but rarely attend a university. Most do not admit to being homosexually oriented unless as an excuse to keep out of the draft. They hang around streetcorners and in doorways as well as in lobbies of hotels and theaters or coffee shops located in certain areas of the city. They will stand in a provocative pose and solicit quietly by staring down at the trick's pants or into his eyes. Each prostitute has his own sexual ritual and these tend to be restrictive—fellatio and anal intercourse will be performed on the prostitute or on the customer, but rarely both. Prices tend to average $5 to $10, but older tricks are charged more. Some male prostitutes work out of organized "peg" houses or sauna baths and massage parlors. A few good-looking prostitutes become "kept boys" by an older wealthy man with primary or occasional homosexual desires. Often the "kept boy" is given an assumed title such as "auto mechanic," "private secretary," "plumber," "chauffeur," or "gardener."

BIBLIOGRAPHY

Allen, C. 1961. Sexual perversions, in A. Ellis and A. Abarbanel (eds.), *Modern Sex Practices*, vol. 1, *The Encyclopedia of Sexual Behavior*. Ace, New York.

Basel, A. S. 1970. Why do married men visit prostitutes? in *Viewpoints, Med. Aspects of Hum. Sex.,* **4**(7):84.

Bell, R. R., and M. Gordon. 1972. *The Social Dimension of Human Sexuality.* Little, Brown, Boston.

Bender, L. 1969. Childhood sexual abuse, in *Answers to Questions, Med. Aspects Hum. Sex.,* **3**(8):87.

Bryan, J. H. 1965. Apprenticeships in prostitution, *Social Problems,* **12**:278–297.

Bullough, V. L. 1970. Why do married men visit prostitutes? in *Viewpoints, Med. Aspects Hum. Sex.,* **4**(7):93.

Cuber, J. F. 1969. The mistress in American society, *Med. Aspects of Hum. Sex.,* **3**(9):81–91.

Ellis, A. 1952. What is normal sex behavior? Complex No. 8: 41–51.

Epstein, A. W. 1973. The relationship of altered brain states to sexual psychopathology, chap. 14 in J. Zubin and J. Money (eds.), *Contemporary Sexual Behavior: Critical Issues in the 1970's,* Johns Hopkins, Baltimore.

Esselstyn, T. C. 1968. Prostitution in the United States, *Ann. Am. Acad. Pol. and Soc. Sci.,* **376**:124–135.

Fenichel, O. 1945. *Psychoanalytic Theory of Neurosis.* Norton, New York.

Gatov, E. R. 1973. *Sex Code of California. A Compendium.* Graphic Arts of Marin, Inc., Sausalito, Calif.

Gentry, C. 1964. *The Madams of San Francisco.* Doubleday, Garden City, N.Y.

Goldsmith, S. 1974. *Personal Communication.* Planned Parenthood, San Francisco.

Goodman, G. 1955. *The Pharmacological Basis of Therapeutics,* pp. 1022–1023. Macmillan, New York.

Graves, L. R., and J. T. Francisco. 1970. Medicolegal aspects of rape, *Med. Aspects Hum. Sex.,* **4**(4):109–120.

Halleck, S. L. 1969. Sex and power, *Med. Aspects Hum. Sex.,* **3**(10):8–24.

Hirschi, T. 1962. The professional prostitute, *Berk. J. Sociology,* **7**(1):33–39.

Jensen, G. D. 1973. Human sexual behavior in primate perspective, in J. Zubin and J. Money (eds.), *Contemporary Sexual Behavior: Critical Issues in the 1970's.* Johns Hopkins, Baltimore.

Kanin, E. J. 1970. Sex aggression by college men, *Med. Aspects Hum. Sex.,* **4**(9):25–40.

Kinsey, A. C., et al. 1948. *Sexual Behavior in the Human Male.* Saunders, Philadelphia.

Kling, S. G. 1965. *Sexual Behavior and the Law.* Pocket Books, New York. Originally by Bernard Geis Associates.

Lasche, U. 1973. Antiandrogen in the treatment of sex offenders: mode of action and therapeutic outcome, in J. Zubin and J. Money (eds.) *Contemporary Sexual Behavior: Critical Issues in the 1970's.* Johns Hopkins, Baltimore.

Lewinsohn, R. 1958. *A History of Sexual Customs.* Bell Publishing Co., Inc., New York.

MacLean, P. D. 1973. Special award lecture: New findings on brain function and sociosexual behavior, in J. Zubin and J. Money (eds.), *Contemporary Sexual Behavior: Critical Issues of the 1970's.* Johns Hopkins, Baltimore.

Marmor, J. 1969. Sadomasochism in answers to questions, *Med. Aspects Hum. Sex.,* **3**(9):45.

Marmor, J. 1971. "Normal" and "deviant" sexual behavior, *J. Am. Med. Assoc.,* vol. 217.

Mohr, J. W. 1969. Assessment of treatment needs, in *The Treatment of Sexual Offenders.* H. L. P. Resnik, Moderator Symposium. *Med. Aspects Hum. Sex.,* **3**(8):35–49.

Money, J. 1973. Pornography in the home: A topic in medical education, in J. Zubin and J. Money (eds.), *Contemporary Sexual Behavior: Critical Issues in the 1970's.* Johns Hopkins, Baltimore.

Peters, J. J., and R. L. Sadoff. 1970. Clinical observations on child molesters, *Med. Aspects Hum. Sex.,* **4**(11):20–32.

Presto, A. J. III, and E. C. Muecke. 1970. A dose of Spanish Fly, *J. Am. Med. Assoc.,* **214**(3):591–592.

Resnik, H. L. P. and J. J. Peters. 1967. Outpatient group therapy with convicted pedophiles, *Int. J. Group Psychother.* **17**:151.

Rothman, G. 1971. *The Riddle of Cruelty.* Philosophical Library, New York.

Sadoff, R. L. 1972. Anonymous sexual offenders, *Med. Aspects Hum. Sex.,* **6**(3):118–123.

Schiff, A. F. 1972. Rape, *Med. Aspects Hum. Sex.,* **6**(5):76–84.

Slovenko, R. 1971. Sex laws: Are they necessary? in D. L. Grummon and A. M. Barclay (eds.), *Sexuality: A Search for Perspective,* pp. 142–158. Van Nostrand, New York.

Stoller, R. J. 1973. Psychoanalysis and physical intervention in the brain: the mind-body problem again, in J. Zubin and J. Money (eds.), *Contemporary Sexual Behavior: Critical Issues in the 1970's.* Johns Hopkins, Baltimore.

Walinder, J. 1965. Transvestism, definition and evidence in favor of occasional derivation from cerebral dysfunction, *Int. J. Neuropsychiatry,* **1**:567–573.

Wolfenden Report, The. 1963. *Report of the Committee on Homosexual Offenses and Prostitution.* Stein and Day, New York.

Wolfgang, M. F. 1969. General sociological comments on sexual deviance, in *The Treatment of Sexual Offenders.* H. L. P. Resnik, Moderator Symposium. *Med. Aspects Hum. Sex.,* **3**(8):35–49.

Appendix

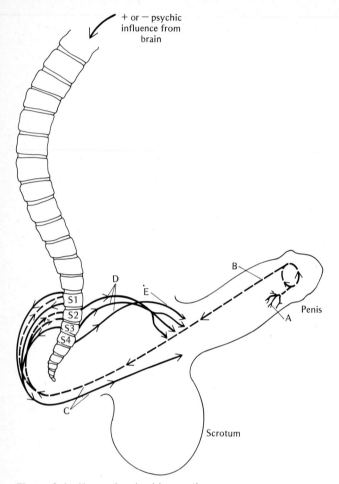

Figure A-1 Nerves involved in erection:
A = receptors
B = dorsal nerve of penis
C = pudendal nerve carrying information from dorsal nerve of penis to erection center and from erection center to muscles of penis causing contraction
S1–S4 = erection center (sacral segments 1 to 4)
D = nervi erigentes
E = pelvic plexus sending information to arteries of penis causing dilation and engorgement of cavernous bodies

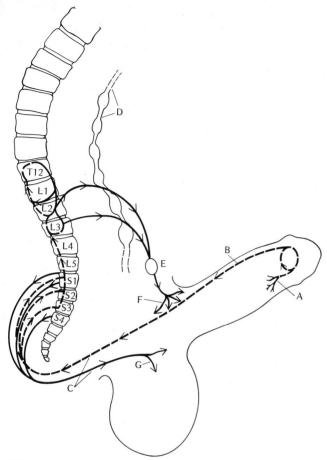

Figure A-2   Nerves involved in ejaculation:
A = receptors
B = dorsal nerve of penis
C = pudendal nerve
T12–L5 = ejaculatory center (Thoracic segment 12 to lumbar 3)
S1–S4 = erection center (sacral segments 1 to 4)
D = sympathetic chain of ganglia
E = hypogastric ganglia
F = nerves communicating with smooth muscles of vas deferens, epididymis, and internal sphincter of bladder causing emission
G = nerves communicating with striated muscle of penis causing expulsion

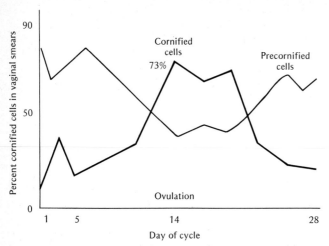

Figure A-3 Summary of changes in vaginal smears during the normal menstrual cycle. *Preovulatory smear* (ninth day of 28-day cycle): (1) Moderate amount Döderlein's bacilli and leukocytes. (2) Approximately 12 percent cornified vaginal cells which stain red; each possessing a tiny dark nucleus resembling a period. Remaining precornified cells stain blue and possess large nuclei. (3) Fewer total number of cells. *Ovulation smear* (fourteenth day of 28-day cycle): (1) 73 percent cornified vaginal cells. (2) Low bacilli and leukocytes. *Postovulatory smear* (twenty fifth day of 28-day cycle): (1) Eighteen percent cornified vaginal cells, remainder precornified. (2) Cells in clumps; many with folded edges and wrinkled cytoplasm. (3) Moderate bacilli and leukocytes. (*Based on De Allende and Orias, 1950.*)

Glossary

Abortion   Spontaneous or induced expulsion from the uterus of the products of conception.

Abstinence (sexual)   (1) Celibacy: refraining from all forms of sexual contact at all times. (2) Method of birth control: (*a*) total abstinence: refraining from coitus at all times; (*b*) rhythm: avoiding coitus during woman's time of maximum fertility.

Adolescence   Culturally defined stage in human life; begins around time of average puberty and terminates at socially and legally defined age of adulthood.

Adrenocorticotropin (ACTH)   Hormone secreted by pituitary gland; acts on adrenal cortex.

Adultery   Voluntary coitus between two people, at least one of whom is married to a third party.

Amenorrhea   Absence of menstrual flow.

Anaphrodisiac   Any food, drug, or beverage that when ingested decreases one's sexual motivation.

Androgens   Male sex hormones, the most powerful of which is testosterone; large amounts secreted by testes, small amounts by ovaries and by adrenal glands of both sexes.

Androsperm   Mature sperm that possess a Y chromosome.

Anilingus   Oral-anal stimulation.

Antibody   A substance produced by the body that attaches to a foreign substance (antigen) and renders it harmless.

Antigen A foreign organism or substance that invades one's body, causing the production of antibodies.

APGAR rating evaluation Scoring system performed to obtain a tentative and rapid assessment of newborn infants' vital signs.

Aphrodisiac Any food, drug, or beverage that when ingested increases one's sexual motivation.

Areola Dark, pigmented area around the nipple of each breast.

Arousability The rate at which an individual changes arousal levels; how fast orgasm is reached.

Arousal A person's level of sexual excitement at any one moment.

Artificial insemination Artificially transferring sperm to a female's genital tract.

Atresia Normal degeneration of follicles in the ovary.

Atrophy Degeneration of an organ or tissue.

Attitude Posture of the fetus; relationship of one fetal body part to another.

Autonomic nervous system Part of nervous system regulating smooth muscle contraction and gland secretion; it controls involuntary activities.

Axillary hair Hair located in the armpits.

Barr body A tiny clump of material at the edge of the nucleus in a cell of a human female—actually represents one X chromosome; the number of Barr bodies is one less than the number of X chromosomes in a cell.

Bartholin's glands A pair of glands located under the labia minora, each communicating with the outside by a short duct, opening directly on each side of the hymen; function unknown.

Bilateral Being present on both sides of the body.

Bisexual An adult who seeks out sexual contact with individuals of either sex.

Breasts Mammary glands.

Breech presentation Fetus' buttocks or legs are born first.

Capacitation The process of stimulating the final maturation of sperm so that fertilization can occur; takes place in the vagina and uterus.

Carpopedal spasms Muscle contractions of hands and feet occurring during peaks of sexual tension.

Castration Usually surgical removal of the gonads.

Celibacy (1) Refraining from sexual contact; (2) in religious orders refers specifically to the state of remaining unmarried.

Cervix Neck of the uterus.

Cesarean operation Fetus is delivered through an incision in the abdominal and uterine walls.

Chancre A tiny, painless sore that often is the first sign of syphilis.

Cholesterol The chemical basis of androgens, estrogens, and progesterone.

Chromosomes Structures within a cell that contain the genes responsible for a person's characteristics.

Circumcision Surgical removal of the foreskin of the penis.

Clitoris Organ located in the upper vulva between the labia minora; receptor and transformer of erotic stimuli; clitoridectomy is surgical removal of the clitoris.

Cohabitation Living together with a sexual relationship.

Coital induction Induction of ovulation by coitus (rabbits, ferrets) as contrasted with spontaneous ovulation (humans, rats).

Coitus Penetration of penis into vagina.

Coitus withdrawal Withdrawal of the penis from the vagina before ejaculation—a contraceptive technique.

Colostrum   A watery, alkaline secretion of the breast usually present the last few weeks of pregnancy and for 3 to 4 days after delivery; lower in fat and carbohydrate content but higher in protein and vitamin A than mother's milk.

Conception   Fertilization of an egg by a sperm.

Condom   A latex or "intestinal" sheath placed over the erect penis during coitus; acts as a contraceptive device; also helps prevent transfer of genital-tract infection.

Congenital   Existing at birth.

Contraception   Chemical or mechanical techniques that prevent fertilization from taking place and are relatively easy to reverse.

Coprophilia   Sexual pleasure derived by viewing someone defecating.

Copulation   Sexual intercourse.

Cornification   Hardening of cells (examples: vaginal mucosa, skin) due to normal formation within these cells of certain proteins such as keratin.

Corpora cavernosa   Paired columns of erectile tissue in the penis and clitoris.

Corpus albicans   Nonfunctional remnant of a corpus luteum.

Corpus luteum   Endocrine gland developed from the remaining tissue of a Graafian follicle after an ovulation; secretes progesterone and estrogens.

Corpus spongiosum   A column of erectile tissue in the penis surrounding the urethra; at tip of penis it expands to form substance of glans penis, and in area over scrotum it expands to form bulb of penis.

Courtship   Act of paying attention to someone in order to derive something in return—love, marriage, financial security, coitus, companionship, and so on.

Cowper's glands   Paired glands which provide water, mucus, and buffers for the seminal plasma.

"Crabs" (*Phthirius pubis*)   Lice that congregate in and around pubic and anal hair causing a severe itch; the disease is called pediculosis pubis.

Cremaster muscle   A voluntary (striated) muscle located in the scrotum; contracts in response to sexual excitement, fear, and anxiety, increasing the flow of blood from the testes back into the body.

Cryptorchidism   A condition where one or both testes fail to descend from an embryonic location in the abdomen to the scrotal sacs.

Cunnilingus   Oral contact with the vulva and vagina.

Detumescence   Return of an erect penis to the flaccid state.

Diaphragm   A thin latex dome designed to fit over the cervical opening of the uterus; a contraceptive device usually used with spermicidal jelly or cream.

Diastolic blood pressure   Blood pressure in the arteries during the time the heart fills with blood.

Dildo   Artificial penis.

Dimorphism   A characteristic difference between the sexes.

Diploid   Number of chromosomes found in almost all cells except the gametes.

Döderlein's bacilli   Normal bacteria inhabiting the vagina which continually convert sugar to lactic acid.

Douche   Washing the contents of the vagina.

Ectopic pregnancy   A pregnancy located somewhere in the body other than in the uterus.

Ejaculate   The semen; specifically the amount of semen released at a given ejaculation.

Ejaculation   Propulsion of semen from the penis.

Embryo   In humans, the unborn young beginning with the first week following fertilization to the end of the second month.

Endometrium   Mucus membrane forming inner layer of uterine wall; site of implantation of a fertilized egg; portion of this lining sloughed off during the menstrual flow.

Enzyme   A protein catalyst serving to increase the rate of chemical reactions.

Epididymis   Highly coiled duct interposed between tubules of the testis and vas deferens; location of sperm maturation, accumulation, and selection.

Episiotomy   An incision made in the vulvar skin to expedite delivery and prevent tearing of tissue.

Erection   Widening, lengthening, and hardening of penis as it becomes congested with blood.

Erogenous zones   Any part of the skin containing numerous receptors that when stroked cause sexual arousal.

Erotic   Any factor that causes an increase in sexual motivation.

Estradiole   Most powerful estrogen.

Estrogens   Female hormones responsible for characteristics of female; secreted by ovaries and adrenal glands.

Estrone   One of the estrogens.

Estrus cycle   The sex hormone cycle of many nonhuman female mammals; the female is sexually receptive (in heat) during only one phase of the cycle; menstrual flow generally lacking. In some species light spotting may occur during heat.

Excitement phase   First phase of human sexual response; gradual rise in sexual arousal.

Exhibitionist   One who preferentially and habitually gets sexual gratification from exhibiting his genitals to unwilling observers.

Fallopian tubes (oviducts)   Paired tubes extending between the ovaries and the uterus; function as conduits for the transport and maintenance of sperm, oocytes, and zygotes.

Fellatio   Oral contact with the penis.

Fertilization   Union of sperm and egg.

Fetish   Sexual gratification derived from an inanimate object.

Fetus   In humans, the unborn young beginning with the third month following fertilization to birth.

Fixed action patterns   Inherited patterns of behavior.

Follicle-stimulating hormone (FSH)   Hormone secreted by the anterior pituitary; stimulates follicle development in the ovaries and spermatogenesis in the testes.

Forcible rape   An act of penile-vaginal contact that is forced upon a woman without her consent.

Foreplay   Physical contact which purposely increases sexual motivation prior to coitus; serves to heighten and synchronize the arousal levels of the partners.

Fornication   Voluntary coitus between an adult male and female who are unmarried.

Frenulum   Thin fold of skin that attaches the foreskin to the glans penis.

Frigidity   Refers to a woman with a low or nonexistent sex drive.

Frottage   Obtaining sexual pleasure by rubbing one's genitals (usually when fully clothed) against the body of a female in a crowded place.

Gametes   Sperm and eggs.

Gender identity   Private feeling of one's own maleness or femaleness (see sexual identity).

Gender orientation   Orientation toward a particular sex for purposes of sexual contact (heterosexual, homosexual, bisexual).

Gene   A segment of the genetic material inside a chromosome that is the mold for a specific protein. Genes are inherited but may become altered (mutated).

Genital folds   The embryonic structure that develops into the labia minora in a genetic female and into the shaft of the penis in a genetic male.

Genitalia   Sex organs located in or near the reproductive tract and excluding the gonads.

Genital swelling   The embryonic structure that develops into the labia majora in a genetic female and into the scrotum in a genetic male.

Genital tubercle   The embryonic structure that develops into the clitoris in a genetic female and into the glans penis in a genetic male.

Gerontophilia   Deriving sexual pleasure and gratification by sexually assaulting elderly persons.

Gestation   Period of pregnancy.

Glycogen   A carbohydrate.

Gonads   Ovaries and testes.

Gonorrhea   A venereal disease of the mucous membranes caused by a coffee-bean-shaped bacterium—*Neisseria gonorrhaeae.*

Graafian follicle   A secondary ooctye surrounded by fluid and several layers of granulosa cells: a mature follicle ready for ovulation.

Granulosa cells   Cells of the ovary that surround an oocyte.

Gynecomastia   A condition in which the male breast enlarges.

Gynosperm   Mature sperm that possess an X chromosome.

Haploid   The chromosome number found in gametes—usually half that of other body cells.

Hermaphrodite (true)   A human who has both ovarian and testicular tissue.

Heterosexual   An adult who seeks out and prefers members of the opposite sex for purposes of sexual contact.

Hirsutism   State of being excessively hairy.

Homologous organs   Organs that have a similar embryological history.

Homosexual   A gay person; an adult who seeks out and prefers members of the same sex for sexual contact.

Human chorionic gonadotropin (HCG)   Hormone produced by the placenta that helps maintain the corpus luteum and thus the pregnancy.

Hymen   Tissue partially enclosing the vaginal opening; no known biological function.

Hypothalamic-releasing factors   Hormones secreted by the hypothalamus which regulate pituitary functions.

Hypothalamus   Part of the brain known to regulate the pituitary and many bodily functions (sexual, metabolism, salt and water balance, growth, etc.).

Hysterectomy   Removal of the uterus.

Hysterotomy   A minor Cesarean section performed as an abortion technique sometime between the sixteenth and twentieth week of gestation.

Implantation   The burrowing of the fertilized egg into the endometrium lining of the uterus.

Impotence   The inability to achieve or maintain an erection sufficient for coitus to take place.

Incest   The crime of performing coitus or getting married to a biologically close relative; the degree of relationship is determined by law in each state.

Inguinal canals   A pair of canals in a male connecting the abdomen with the scrotal sacs; each testis usually descends through a canal before birth; canals generally close off at birth.

Inguinal hernia   Part of intestine protrudes into the scrotal sacs through the open inguinal canals.

Intercourse (sexual)   Generally refers to coitus; other types of sexual contact are indicated by other modifiers, e.g., anal intercourse.

Intersex   An individual with characteristics of both male and female; a person with ambiguous genitalia.

Interstitial cell-stimulating hormone (ICSH)   Identical to luteinizing hormone in the female; secreted by anterior pituitary in the male; stimulates testosterone production by Leydig cells in the testes.

Intrauterine device (IUD)   A device placed in the uterus which prevents implantation; usually plastic.

Intromission   Penis penetration into the vagina.

Labia majora   Outer, thick folds of skin that protect the vaginal opening, labia minora, and the urinary opening.

Labia minora   Thin folds of skin lying between the labia majora that guard and protect the vaginal opening.

Labor   A group of processes responsible for the expulsion from the uterus of the fetus, placenta, and membranes of pregnancy.

Lactation   Milk secretion from a female breast.

Lesbian   A gay female.

Leydig cells   Cells located between seminiferous tubules in the testes; they manufacture and secrete testosterone and possibly estrogen.

Libido   Sexual motivation, urge or desire for sexual activity.

Linea nigra   Dark, pigmented line extending from the pubic hair to the umbilicus of some pregnant women.

Longitudinal presentation   The long axis of the fetus is parallel to the long axis of the mother.

Luteinizing hormone (LH)   Hormone secreted by the anterior pituitary—in females, causes ovulation and corpus luteum formation; in males, it stimulates testosterone secretion from the testes and is called ICSH (Interstitial-cell–stimulating hormone).

Masochism   Obtaining sexual pleasure and gratification by experiencing physical or mental pain and humiliation.

Masturbation   Self-stimulation of the genitalia and/or other parts of the body in order to derive erotic pleasure.

Meiosis   Two cell divisions which result in the formation of haploid sperm and eggs.

Menarche   The first menstrual cycle in a woman's life.

Menopause   The cessation of menstrual cycles in a woman's life.

Menses   The menstrual flow consisting of blood, endometrial tissue, some vaginal cells, mucus, and various chemicals.

Menstruation   Same as the menses.

Miscarriage   Spontaneous abortion; pregnancy that terminates on its own for any reason.

Mitosis   A type of cell division resulting in two daughter cells each containing the diploid number of chromosomes and thus genetic material that is identical to the parent cell.

Mons veneris   Pressure-sensitive fatty tissue beneath the pubic hair.

Mosaic chromosome constitution   A person with cells containing differing chromosomal numbers, arrangements and types.

Mucosa   Mucus membrane lining a cavity—e.g., vagina, uterus.

Müllerian ducts   A pair of embryonic ducts or tubes that develop into the fallopian tubes, uterus, and upper third of the vagina in a genetic female.

Müllerian inhibitor   A substance produced by the fetal testes that inhibits Müllerian duct development and its differentiation into female internal genitalia.

Mutation   A change in the genetic material (DNA); usually occurs spontaneously but may be caused by some environmental factor—temperature, radiation, chemical, etc.

Myotonia   Increased muscular tension.

Naegele's rule   Method of calculating a pregnant woman's date of delivery.

Necrophilia   Deriving sexual pleasure by sexually assaulting a corpse.

Neonate   Newborn young.

Nondisjunction   Failure of members of a chromosome pair to separate during meiosis so that one germ cell receives both members and the other receives neither.

Oocyte   Egg from time of replication of genetic material (before female's birth) until fertilization.

Oogenesis   The process of meiotic divisions that transforms an oogonium into the mature oocyte component of a zygote.

Oral contraceptive   A drug that prevents conception, taken orally.

Orgasm   An extremely pleasurable response involving the feeling of physiological and psychological release from maximum levels of sexual excitement.

Orgasmic dysfunction   A woman who is nonorgasmic in coitus and/or masturbation.

Orgasmic platform   Vasocongestion in the outer third of the vagina during sexual excitement.

Orifice   A body opening.

Os clitoris   Small bone present in the clitoris of rodents, bats, carnivores, whales, and many primates excluding humans.

Os penis   A bone present in the penis of rodents, bats, carnivores, whales, and many primates excluding humans.

Ovaries   Paired primary sex organs in the female which produce eggs and secrete estrogens, progesterone, and androgens.

Oviducts   Fallopian tubes.

Ovulation   The periodic discharge of an egg from the Graafian follicle in the ovary.

Oxytocin   A hormone secreted by the posterior pituitary which causes uterine contractions during breast stimulation; involved also in milk let down from the breast.

Parasympathetic nervous system   Part of autonomic nervous system that activates the body's restorative functions such as digestion.

Parturition   Childbirth.

Pathogenic   Disease-producing.

Pedophiliac   A person who obtains pleasure by sexually molesting a child.

Penicillin   The primary antibiotic used to fight many types of bacterial infections, including venereal diseases.

Penis   A male organ of copulation.

pH   Hydrogen ion concentration; provides information on the degree of acidity of a solution or substance; neutral = 7, acid = less than 7, alkaline = more than 7.

Pheromones   Any chemical substance produced by one individual that changes the behavior of another.

Phimosis   An unusually long, tight, and unretractable foreskin.

Pituitary gland   A small gland located beneath the hypothalamus; secretes several hormones regulating many bodily functions.

Placebo   A pill composed of an inactive substance.

Placenta   Organ of fetal and maternal exchange of oxygen, carbon dioxide, nutritive materials, and waste products.

Plateau phase   A period when sexual excitement is intensified penultimate to orgasm.

Postnatal   After birth.

Potency   The ability of a male to sustain an erection for sexual intercourse.

Premarital intercourse   Coitus occurring between puberty and the first marriage.

Premature ejaculation   The process of ejaculating sooner than a man desires.

Prenatal   Prior to birth.

Prepuce   Foreskin covering glans of the penis and clitoris.

Presentation   Relationship of the long axis (from head to foot) of the fetus to the long axis of the mother.

Primary follicle   A primary oocyte and a single layer of granulosa cells immediately surrounding it.

Procreation   Production of offspring; reproduction.

Progesterone   A hormone secreted by the corpus luteum involved in regulating the menstrual cycle.

Prolactin   Hormone secreted by the anterior pituitary; known to stimulate milk secretion.

Prostaglandins   Substance produced by the body that causes contractions of uterus and fallopian tubes; found in semen.

Prostate gland   Gland in the male that provides up to 33 percent of the seminal plasma.

Prostitution   Indiscriminate sexual relations for hire, usually without affection.

Puberty   Physical maturation leading to the ability to reproduce.

Quickening   Fetal movements in the uterus.

Rape   See forcible rape.

Refractory period   A temporary lack of receptor and nervous response to sexual stimuli occurring during the resolution phase of human male sexual response.

Regeneration   Regrowth; replacement of removed parts or substances by new growth.

Resolution phase   The period after orgasm during which a physiological return to prearousal states occurs.

Rhythm method   Abstaining from coitus during the fertile period of the menstrual cycle.

Sadism   Receiving sexual pleasure and gratification by physically or mentally hurting someone.

Scoptophilia   Sexual pleasure derived from viewing other people's genitalia.

Scrotum (scrotal sacs)   An outpouching of the abdominal wall in the groin which houses the testes.

Sebaceous glands   Oil-producing glands in the skin.

Secondary sex characteristics   Sexual differences in anatomy that are not directly concerned with reproduction, e.g., hair distribution, breast development, quality of voice, and certain characteristics of bones and musculature.

Seduction   Legal term meaning voluntary sexual intercourse where a man gives his unconditional promise of marriage to an unmarried woman.

Semen   Sperm and seminal plasma making up the ejaculate material.

Seminal plasma   Fluid medium that both transports and energizes sperm.

Seminal vesicles   Pair of glands in the male that produce up to 80 percent of the seminal plasma, including fructose sugar and mucus.

Seminiferous tubules   Highly coiled tubules in the testes where sperm are manufactured.

Sensate focus exercises   Physical exercises that help identify each partner's erogenous zones.

Sertoli cells   Certain cells in the seminiferous tubules which regulate spermatogenesis.

Sex chromosomes   The XX and XY chromosome pairs in humans.

Sex flush   A skin rash developing during sexual excitement due to vasocongestion of blood vessels in the skin.

Sex-role assignment   Assignment of a person into a particular sex at birth; decision made by physician on the basis of external genitalia.

Sex-role identity   All the things a person does or says to indicate to others the degree that one is either male or female (see sexual identity).

Sex skin   Color changes of the labia minora which occur during sexual excitement and are due to vasocongestion.

Sexual identity   A person's feelings of and about his or her own maleness or femaleness and the ways in which he or she expresses these feelings. Includes both gender identity and sex-role identity.

Sexual motivation   The urge for sexual activity, libido, sex drive, sexual desire.

Smegma   Oil gland secretions and dead cells that accumulate under the foreskin.

Sodomy   Multiple legal meanings: coitus with animals; penis-anus intercourse; any sex act other than face-to-face coitus between a man and a woman.

Sperm (spermatozoon)   Mature gamete in a male.

Spermatogenesis   Sperm production.

Spermicidal cream or jelly   A substance used as a contraceptive which kills or incapacitates sperm in the vagina.

Spirochaete   Corkscrew-shaped bacteria.

Sterilization   Surgical techniques which remove or block a portion of the reproductive tract, thereby preventing conception.

Steroid   The basic chemical structure of several sex hormones.

Stressors   Severe or unusual stress that activates the adrenal glands.

Subcutaneous   Beneath the skin.

Superfemale   A person with three X chromosomes in each body cell.

Supermale   Generally refers to a person with XYY genotype.

Sympathetic nervous system   Increases activity when an organism faces a situation that may be taxing to the functions of the body. Portion of autonomic nervous system that becomes highly activated in the presence of a stressor or of high sexual arousal.

Syphilis   A venereal disease of the blood caused by the spiral-shaped bacterium, *Treponema pallidum.*

Systolic blood pressure   Pressure in the arteries when the heart contracts.

Testes   The primary sex organs of males; manufacture sperm and secrete androgens and estrogen.

Testicular feminization   A person with XY sex chromosomes who shows female anatomy, psyche, and rearing.

Testosterone   The most powerful androgen; secreted by the Leydig cells of the testes.

Transsexual   A person who psychologically is one sex but physically is the opposite sex.

Transverse presentation   The long axis of the fetus lies at an angle or cross-wise with respect to the long axis of the mother.

Transvestite   A person who derives pleasure and/or increased sexual arousal from wearing clothing of the opposite sex.

Trichomoniasis   An infection of the vagina caused by a single celled organism, *Trichomonas vaginalis;* symptoms include a frothy, greenish yellow discharge and inflammation of the vulva and vagina.

Tubal ligation Tying off and excising part of the fallopian tubes or fusing them shut with an electric current.

Tunica dartos A smooth muscle whose contraction causes the scrotum to move closer to the body in response to low surrounding temperatures.

Umbilicus Navel; "belly button"; site of cord attachment joining fetus to placenta in the uterus.

Universal flexion The various parts of the fetus' body are flexed so that the arms are folded across the chest, the thighs are folded on the abdomen, the legs are bent on the thighs, and the chin touches the chest.

Unlawful intercourse (statutory rape) Act of coitus with a female under the age of consent.

Urethra The canal through which urine passes from the bladder; in the male, semen also passes through this canal.

Urogenital system The genital and urinary systems.

Urophilia Obtaining sexual gratification by being urinated on or by viewing others urinating.

Uterus Pear-shaped organ connecting the vagina with the fallopian tubes; normal site of implantation of a fertilized egg.

Vagina Internal organ that connects the vulva to the uterus; encircles penis during intercourse, part of the birth canal.

Vaginal mucosa Lining of the vagina.

Vaginal thrush (Candidiosis, Monilia, fungus) A vaginal infection caused by a fungus, *Candida albicans;* symptoms include a cheesy-white discharge and inflammation of vagina and vulva.

Vaginismus Irregular and involuntary contractions of the muscles surrounding the outer third of the vagina whenever coitus is attempted.

Vas deferens The sperm duct; acts as a conduit for sperm between the epididymis and the ejaculatory duct; cut during a vasectomy.

Vasectomy The blocking or cutting of each sperm duct preventing the passage of sperm during an ejaculation.

Vasocongestion Accumulation or pooling of blood in various parts of the body.

Venereal disease An infection transmitted primarily by sexual intercourse.

Vertex presentation The back of the fetus' head is born first.

Voyeurism Being sexually aroused by viewing someone in the nude or persons having sexual intercourse.

Vulva Female external genitalia consisting of clitoris, labia minora, labia majora, hymen, vaginal and urethral openings, and vestibule.

Wolffian ducts A pair of embryonic ducts that develop into the sperm ducts, seminal vesicles, and epididymis in a genetic male.

Zygote The fertilized egg.

INDEX

3 1862 005 223 256

University of Windsor Libraries

DATE DUE

DATE DUE

RETURNED

RETURNED

MAR 2 3 1993

RETURNED

RETURNED